International Handbook of Public Health

INTERNATIONAL HANDBOOK OF PUBLIC HEALTH

EDITED BY
Klaus Hurrelmann and Ulrich Laaser

GREENWOOD PRESS
Westport, Connecticut • London

Library of Congress Cataloging-in-Publication Data

International handbook of public health / edited by Klaus Hurrelmann and Ulrich Laaser.
p. cm.
Includes bibliographical references and index.
ISBN 0-313-29500-X (alk. paper)
1. Public health. 2. World health. I. Hurrelmann, Klaus. II. Laaser, Ulrich, 1941- .
RA427.I54 1996
362.1—dc20 95-46131

British Library Cataloguing in Publication Data is available.

Library of Congress Catalog Card Number: 95-46131
ISBN: 0-313-29500-X

First published in 1996

Greenwood Press, 88 Post Road West, Westport, CT 06881
An imprint of Greenwood Publishing Group, Inc.

Printed in the United States of America

The paper used in this book complies with the Permanent Paper Standard issued by the National Information Standards Organization (Z39.48-1984).

10 9 8 7 6 5 4 3 2 1

CONTENTS

Part III Addresses of Public Health Organizations

TABLES AND FIGURES

THEORY AND TRAINING IN PUBLIC HEALTH

BASIC AND APPLIED RESEARCH

BRAZIL

GERMANY

ISRAEL

ITALY

JAPAN

KOREA

MALAYSIA

PHILIPPINES

POLAND

RUSSIA

SOUTH AFRICA

TANZANIA

THAILAND

UNITED STATES

PREFACE

The concept of public health—the health of the public—since the early times of Hippocrates has been seen in an ecological context, including environmental and social "conditions of living" as well as the individual and collective "ways of living." As such, it must not be perceived as an exclusively analytical scientific approach; it has always been linked to a basic interventive intention aiming at population-wide improvement of health.

The following definition by the World Health Organization (WHO) seems to be widely accepted: "Public Health is the science and art of preventing disease, prolonging life and promoting health through the organized efforts of society." It might be illuminating to compare this definition to a description of public health that stems from a political process, namely, the negotiations between the member states of the European Union leading in 1993 to the Treaty of Maastricht on European Union. Its Article 129.1 on public health reads: "The Community shall contribute towards ensuring a high level of human health protection. Community action shall be directed towards the prevention of diseases, in particular the major health scourges, including drug dependence, by promoting research into their causes and their transmission, as well as health information and education. Health protection requirements shall form a constituent part of the Community's other policies."

There are certain characteristics that are common to both wordings. First, and most important, both definitions refer to the society and its organization as a state, not to the individual per se. Although health is a personal good, it is not only an individual responsibility but a collective responsibility as well. Whereas monitoring and restoration of individual health mainly constitute a task of the curative sector in medicine, the health of the entire population is subject to the society and the state. It goes far beyond the present reality but opens a wide and important field when reference is made by the European Union to "other policies" such as agriculture, traffic, and education.

Second, both citations refer to science and research, respectively. It should be underlined that the improvement of the population's health requires a scientific base. Public health cannot be built on either uncritical administrative execution, top down, or likewise uncritical action movement, bottom up, without careful evaluative analysis and monitoring.

Third, both wordings stress prevention: The first one accentuates health promotion; the second, health protection. There is a narrow interpretation of prevention as preventive medicine; obviously, that is not appropriate here. Rather, a wide understanding is meant relating to the three dimensions of maintaining good health, preventing impaired health from worsening, and enabling people to live with reduced health. In this sense, for example, setting up a motivational and organizational framework for nursing of the elderly or for assisting the dying is an important issue of public health promotion.

Fourth, a striking omission is common to both paragraphs: Medicine is not mentioned. What, then, is the relationship between public health and medicine and the medically determined health care system? One aspect is obvious—the medical sciences relate to the public health sciences; medical subdisciplines such as social medicine, medical sociology, medical psychology, behavioral medicine, and environmental medicine get a common focus only around the issue of the public health. To describe the relationship between medicine and public health from the public health point of view, a modified quote of Thomas Aquinas (originally on the role of theology) might serve: "Like the architect thinks out a plan and directs the construction according to it, so the public health professional designs a system for the delivery of medical care." Medical care is subject to public health reasoning, and public health should no longer be considered an appendix of clinical medicine.

The system of delivery of curative care, which consumes about 90 percent of all financial resources invested in the health sector—that is, between 5 and 10 percent of the gross national product—is legitimately a subject to be considered with regard to its impact on the public health, for example, in the context of benefit-to-cost analyses. Although the problem would be misunderstood if an economic calculus were applied to the patient-physician relationship directly, the society as a whole must not hesitate to set explicit priorities for resource allocation wherever possible.

Four cornerstones of public health can be derived from the two definitions cited: the societal dimension, the scientific foundation, the preventive orientation, and the independence of clinical care. As both editors of this book have been involved with the renaissance of a new public health in Germany since 1989, let us refer to the German history of public health in order to illustrate another inherent principle that likely should not be exclusively a European perception alone: Look back to the year 1883 when Bismarck presented his legislation on sickness funds—the *Krankenversicherungsgesetz*—to the Reichstag in

Berlin. He based it on four principles: obligatory membership for almost everyone, variety of competing funds, partition of cost between employers and workers, and salary compensation during temporary disablement. What we consider to be an inherent principle of public health is the attempt of Bismarck—who by no means can be called a socialist—to balance solidarity and free choice in such a way that the highest possible degree of equity and social security is achieved.

At the end of the twentieth century, many of the major health problems facing the world populations stem from social disruption, environmental destruction, and inhibitional imbalances. The scope of public health in the last part of the twentieth century has greatly expanded. Not only have the number of recognized health hazards to the public increased, but the strategies available to resolve them have grown commensurably. Holland, Detels, and Knox have already pointed out in their 1984 *Oxford Textbook of Public Health* that public health has borrowed and adapted knowledge from the medical, biological, physical, social, behavioral, ecological, and mathematical sciences and has been quick to recognize the potential of new fields.

The *International Handbook of Public Health* is an important work to facilitate worldwide orientation for public health professionals. Public health professionals must act as linchpins between theory and practice, between politics and people, and between research and practice. They will have to be able to communicate with a wide variety of other professionals in academia, administration, and field organizations. Thus, all public health training must have a strong foundation in biostatistics and epidemiology, policy studies, human biology, and social sciences like sociology and social psychology. Interdisciplinarity is a keyword, not just in the sense that various disciplines have their specific course offerings in public training but in the sense that throughout the educational curriculum the learning process is driven by the recognition of the multilayered and multidisciplinary nature of public health problems. The *Handbook* delivers information about different solutions to these problems worldwide.

Throughout the world, training in public health and "health sciences" has acquired more attention than ever before, at the undergraduate, graduate, and postgraduate levels. Most facilities are presently found at the latter level; they offer training to professionals such as medical doctors, lawyers, economists, managers, and so on, who would like to increase their knowledge base and bring their skills up to the requirements of modern-day public health. However, most of these institutions outside the United States are firmly based in schools of medicine and therefore run the danger of overrepresentation of the medical model for health. Recently, new facilities that are based outside medical schools establish strong links with other academic units and institutions for public health training. The *Handbook* gives an overview of this development.

Presently, curricula in public health are offered through college-style institutes, through separate Schools of Health Sciences or Public Health (with capacities ranging between 10 and 3,000 students), postgraduate institutes linked to medical schools, and separate course offerings aimed at specifics in the public health realm. Obviously, much valuable expertise is being built up. But this is happening without clear standards and definitions regarding exit competences. The *Handbook* documents this development.

The *International Handbook of Public Health* provides a synopsis of the state of the development of public health in different countries. Individual countries vary considerably in national policies for organizing health services. The *Handbook* is a forum for systematic surveys of the situation of public health in different countries, allowing for comparative analysis.

The *Handbook* has three parts. Part I gives an overview of the state of scientific developments in public health. Part II surveys public health in different countries: industrial countries on different continents with democratic and pluralistic cultural and political systems and with market economies; industrial countries with the tradition of centrally planned cultural, political, and economic systems that are in the process of becoming pluralistic market systems; and developing and/or newly industrialized countries with a wide range of cultural, political, and economic systems.

The diversity of countries surveyed, both in terms of the type of sociocultural and economic systems and in terms of regional differences across the continents, provides rich national experiences and allows for a comparison of the development of public health institutions worldwide and the political activities directed toward public health in each of the countries included.

Each chapter is devoted to a particular country and appears in alphabetical order. The chapters are designed so that they will be uniform in structure and comprehensive in coverage. Each chapter presents specific categories of information about the selected countries that represent dimensions along which cross-national comparisons may be made. To make comparisons readily applicable, each chapter employs the same basic headings, with minor exceptions.

1. Major health problems facing the country
2. Provision, utilization, and impact of health services
3. The infrastructure of training and research in public health
4. Major challenges for the health services

And finally, Part III documents addresses for public health organizations worldwide.

PART I

Public Health—Theory, Training, and Research

THEORY AND TRAINING IN PUBLIC HEALTH

Klaus Hurrelmann, Ulrich Laaser, and Jacques Bury

THEORETICAL BASE OF PUBLIC HEALTH

Chronic diseases, above all, heart and circulatory diseases, malignant growths (cancers) and diseases of the respiratory and alimentary organs, infections, and diseases of the muscular and skeletal systems, are the great "killers and incapacitators" of today. They are created by long-term excess strain on the physical, emotional, and social adaptation and/or control capacities. Except for infections, they cannot be ascribed to a single or a decisive cause. There is, rather, a whole bundle of personal, social, ecological, and somatic initiatory conditions to be identified whose individual factors stand in a complex relationship to one another (Holland, Detels, and Knox 1984).

Even in the industrial countries, where infectious diseases have been repelled to a great extent, the state of health of the population is far from being satisfactory. Many people suffer from diseases that could be avoided and are affected to a considerable extent by premature death. In spite of the starting position, which is considerably better than that of nonindustrialized countries—better medical system, countrywide health insurance system, wide-ranging inoculation programs and medical examinations in schools, efficient hygiene measures, sufficient food, and so on—completely new types of health risks and problems are occurring that represent great challenges to researchers working in medical services supply systems.

The new spectrum of diseases that dominates in present-day societies, and new types of syndromes such as, for example, immunodeficiencies, cannot be solely or decisively explained by means of a biomedical model and also cannot be effectively dealt with by a curative medical system based on this. Medical professionals and medical apparatus have both specialized in the search for causal mechanisms in the body and in repelling corresponding biochemical and physiological errors. Chronic diseases, however, come into existence through a combination of genetic information, infections, way of life, and environmental conditions, and for this reason, they cannot be controlled solely with the methods of basic biological and medical research. The methods and findings of research with a background of epidemiology, sociology, and behavioral science have to be added. What diagnosis and treatment require is a multiperspective ''holistic'' way of looking at things (Hurrelmann and Laaser 1993).

The Need for an Interdisciplinary Approach

With regard to the structures of medical services, it will be increasingly important to create conditions that will encourage multiprofessional cooperation and enable an interlacing of outpatient and inpatient treatment. It is obvious that in the future a new division of labor between medical and nursing services will be necessary in these fields. The subordination of nursing with respect to medical services is increasingly proving to be obsolete and dysfunctional. The lack of nursing staff is becoming more and more critical and will presumably intensify pressure to reorganize occupational activities in this sector of the health services, leading to an independent position of nursing.

Also, the preventive sector of the health services is still not receiving enough attention. It is a characteristic feature of all chronic diseases that they start at an early stage in a person's life and development. Smoking, drinking alcohol, using drugs, incorrect diets and overfeeding, not enough exercise, insufficient hygiene, and other behavior detrimental to health induce in part the early stages of heart and circulatory diseases or cancer. Dangerous driving, autoaggressive behavior, and unprotected sexual acts are decisive causes for morbidity and mortality rates that are still high and are, above all, early and premature with regard to life histories. These are ''risk factors'' that are largely behavioral—in other words, potentially under the control of the individual. However, the risk factors are based on behavioral patterns that are fully integrated in the habitual patterns of a sociocultural lifestyle and that are formed by the life situation in each case.

For this reason, all preventive approaches must have behavioral and situational components (Hurrelmann and Lösel 1990). Chronic diseases, for example, are very seldom fully curable once they have manifested themselves, but they are—at least in principle—preventable. For this reason, it would be logical if a larger share of the total expense for health would be spent for preventive services. Such investment should alter the starting conditions that contribute to the development of chronic degenerative diseases. Appropriate strategies will have to combine means of behavior-oriented prevention (health education, behavioral modifications, etc.) and situation-oriented prevention (promotion of health in the fields of work, housing, recreation, education, and medical services).

In the future, not only at the level of etiological research but also at the level of the supply of medical services, greater account should be taken of the multidimensional interlacement of the causes of impairments to health so that each phase of the triple step ''Health Promotion/Prevention—Treatment/Cure—Care/Rehabilitation'' should receive sufficient attention. The undue emphasis placed on the middle step of treatment and cure with expensive diagnosis and therapy that characterizes our present health services should be rapidly reduced, and for this, the cooperation of different disciplines will be necessary (Omenn, Fielding, and Lave 1991).

The structural problems referred to above can only be mastered by means of interdisciplinary cooperation. This also applies to the infrastructural and organizational problems facing the health services. Organizational structures and services in the fields of clinical and ambulatory services are constantly changing. The increasing claims made on the medical system in the face of increasingly scarce public funds mean that it is essential that flexible and efficient organizational structures are provided. As knowledge of the operations of the health service is still in its infancy, there is a great deal of catching up to be done in the field of research. This is a further field in which it is imperative that there is cooperation between the scientific traditions of biomedicine and social and organizational research, above all in areas that have been neglected up to now, such as health economics, health systems research, administration, organizational research, and evaluations research.

Interdisciplinary Enrichment Strategies

Up to now, interdisciplinary approaches to research have been effective in which biomedical scientists and hospital doctors have cooperated with psychiatrists, psychologists, sociologists, and ecologists. This collaboration has resulted in initial findings with regard to psychological, social, and physiological influences on the origins and course of sickness and health. Several areas for research have already been established that are characterized by intensive interdisciplinary cooperation. Examples are research into stresses at work and critical life events, research into the effects of social support resources on health, and research into the effects of the ecological environment on the health of population groups.

In these research fields, a systematic examination is made of how psychological and social factors, and ecological factors as well, influence the origins and course of chronic degenerative diseases. Many studies have been able to find connections between stressful and critical events in private and working lives (the death of a close relative, loss of a job, forced early retirement, etc.) and heart disease, cancer, and gastrointestinal diseases. The literature on the subject also provides evidence for the connection between personal characteristics—in particular, certain styles of coping with stress and the controller's own lifestyle—and the diseases that have been mentioned. Personal and social factors were identified not only for the origin but also for the course of diseases, which are responsible for the way in which the individual copes with an illness and also for the course of treatment and rehabilitation.

The subject matter of environmental medicine includes health hazards that result from situations and events in the physical environment, in particular, as well as the explanation of active mechanisms and quantifying and assessing risks. Environmentally related measures for health promotion and protection are also analyzed in this branch, including prevention of risk, risk management and communication, and their respective evaluation. Up to now, research has been faced with tremendous challenges because of the immense dynamics of the various cross-linked material and energy flows. For this reason, an exact evaluation of individual environmental factors that are potentially relevant to health has only been possible within narrow limits. One of the most important steps in the development of this sector has been environmentally related health reporting as an instrument for the empirical foundation of health planning and health policies oriented toward prevention. Environmentally related health reporting proves to be useful where it extends above and beyond the requirement of medical and environmental statistics and takes up systematically developed and scientifically based reports with interpretations of the data and including elements of prognosis.

If we analyze working methods in the various interdisciplinary research fields referred to, strictly speaking there is no deviation from the traditional biomedical model to be seen but, rather, an enrichment of this model by means of factors from research into psychology, social sciences, and environmental sciences. In other words, there has been no fundamental paradigmatic change, no complete change of basic theoretical assumptions, but rather an extension in that mental, social, and ecological factors have been absorbed into the model as additional marginal conditions along with genetic, endocrinological, neurological, and physiological factors. This research mainly uses the risk factor concept as its orientating epistemological model, whereby the risks of the origins, development, and course of a disease and not those of health are the focal point of the research (Hurrelmann and Laaser 1993).

It is difficult to assess whether a model for explaining illness aggravated by mental, social, and ecological dimensions can overcome the problems referred to above of the fundamental biomedical model. An extended risk factor model of the origin and development of a disease or illness quite naturally takes into consideration the anchoring of various diseases in the context of daily life to a narrow extent only. The model assumes that diseases are isolated states that are treated as such, without sufficient attention being paid to case histories and their interweaving with biographies and personal development and with a society that is in part pathogenically structured. It tends toward a mechanico-technicalized orientation that lives from the ideal of eliminating or minimizing identified risk factors; in this, too little attention is still paid to the subjective embedment of risk factors in behavioral patterns, lifestyles, ambiences, and societal structures.

Even if these delimitations can perhaps be overcome by further development of the theory model, it is still unsatisfactory that all theoretical efforts are directed at diagnosing diseases and not at clarification of preconditions for health. If further research follows this development, it will move in the direction of interdisciplinary cooperation that in the end would still remain under the guidance and leadership of medicine as an ''illness science.'' Psychology, social sciences, environmental sciences, and other disciplines would to a certain extent be ''complementary subjects'' to medicine, which would retain under its direction the overall coordination of gathering and applying the results of research.

Perspectives for a Comprehensive Health Science Orientation

If health research is to be in the foreground, instead of research into diseases, it will be necessary to construct an interdisciplinary, organizationally independent field of ''health sciences'' in cooperation on an equal footing between medicine, biology, psychology, sociology, economics, and possibly other fundamental sciences. In order to be able to constitute this new field in this area of science, a fundamental theoretical orientation point is required that is suitable for, and acceptable to, all participating disciplines. This orientation point could be a ''bioecopsychosocial'' model of the development of health and disease that contains biomedical, ecological, sociostructural, and psychosocial components as equally valid constitutive elements (Hurrelmann 1989; Hurrelmann and Laaser 1993). This approach can be considered to be the focus of ''public health.''

It should be the central goal of public health, understood as applied and interdisciplinary health sciences, to direct itself toward the somatic, mental, social, and ecological conditions for the retention of health and the prevention of illness, in separation from, and as a counterbalance to, biomedical and clinical research, which focus on the origin of diseases and their cure. The central questions for public health are the conditions under which people remain healthy, how the frequency of disease can be reduced, and which opportunities can be seized in order to create these conditions for as many people as possible. In contrast, the leading questions for scientific medicine and fundamental biomedical research are the ways in which diseases of a single individual person can be recognized and the measures that have to be taken to halt or reverse the process of the disease. In the field of public health, interest is directed to a greater extent toward whole population groups and the living conditions relevant to their health, including medical services structures.

Public health is composed of various branches of research and science. It is extremely important for their efficiency that they receive impulses not only from biomedical paradigms but also from behavioral and social science paradigms and that they carry on from as many existing tried and tested branches of the relevant disciplines as possible. Among established branches in the field of medicine, industrial, social, environmental, behavioral, and preventive medicine provide access to health sciences. These branches are concerned with conditions for keeping people healthy, for preventing and guarding against illnesses insofar as these are caused by environmental and behavioral conditions, and they concentrate on caring aspects such as the promotion of psychological and physical welfare. Together with epidemiology, they form one of the supports of modern health sciences.

The second support is provided by the field of behavioral, social, and organization sciences. As we have already mentioned, there are quite distinctive branches of research, above all in psychology and sociology, such as stress, assimilation, and behavioral research, that look into the health situation of whole population groups and attempt to lead this back to social, political, cultural, economic, and ecological environmental factors. In addition, there are economics, management, and organization-related branches and ecological working areas.

It can therefore be seen that there is coexistence based on a division of labor between biomedical and clinical research in the framework of "illness sciences," on the one hand, and sociomedical, behavioral, social, environmental, and organization research in the framework of public health as "health sciences" on the other (Hurrelmann and Laaser 1993).

Illness sciences are concentrated in the first place on the clarification of biological phenomena: Basic biological and medical research is concerned with knowledge of cellular and molecular-biological processes in humans, with the aim of compiling fundamental rules of physical functions and malfunctions and of finding out the regulatory mechanisms for biological phenomena and their functioning. This fundamental area consists above all of the branches of cell and molecular biology, immunology, virology, parasitology, biochemistry, biophysics, genetics, microbiology, botany, and zoology. In the field of human medicine, the theoretical directions of anatomy, physiology, pathophysiology, pharmacology, toxicology, human genetics, and medical biometrics work in addition; and finally, clinical-medical research is concentrated on areas of application such as orthopedics, dermatology, neurology, pediatrics, and psychiatry.

The strand of public health is composed of fields whose focal points are sociomedically oriented, such as socioepidemiology; industrial, behavioral, environmental, and preventive medicine; nursing and rehabilitation research; of basic behavioral and social science research (assimilation, stress, social support, resources and inequality research, socialization and personality research); and, in addition, of system and medical services supply research with the fields of health economics, planning, administration, and management.

It is important to remember that from the point of view of their working methods the two research strands contrasted here on the basis of a division of labor are organized for interdisciplinary work. Obviously, there are many difficulties in cooperation emerging in recent years in the illness sciences, which result, among other things, from the tension existing between foundation and application references. Naturally, the tension between the branches of the health sciences (public health) is even greater, as here disciplines meet that have extremely different epistemological and methodological bases. In the public health, paradigm and system borders within the disciplines are transcended: Because they start from different interests with regard to knowledge, doctors specializing in industrial, social, and preventive medicine, on the one hand, and medical psychologists and sociologists, clinical psychologists, social psychiatrists, behavioral researchers, sociopedagogues, environmental researchers, systems analysts, management, and administration researchers, on the other, speak different languages.

Health Supply Systems

A focal point of public health lies in research into systems and supplies—in other words, investigations of whether the structures of the supply and health systems are tailored to suit the needs of the market, effective, and efficient. This involves a broad spectrum of branches that are on the whole concerned with an analysis of medical supply systems and the supplementary and adjacent service systems in the fields of psychology, psychiatry, nursing, teaching, and rehabilitation. The relevant branches from the spectrum of behavioral and social science disciplines are organizational sociology, health economics, planning and administration in the health service, management research, health policies, health law, and research into quality assurance and evaluation, nursing, health systems, rehabilitation, and supply. From the narrow field of social medicine, the subject of applied epidemiology plays an important role, as do mixed subjects such as nutritional research, industrial medicine, medical sociology, and behavioral and environmental medicine (Holland, Detels, and Knox 1984; Schwartz and Badura 1991).

One main task area in this respect is research at the interface between environment and health to analyze the connection between environmental toxins, causes, and progress of diseases and to delineate consequences for the corresponding organizational fields in the health system. Another area is health systems research, which analyzes the tailoring of supplies to requirements and the cost-effectiveness of administration and services throughout the health system. Evaluation research belongs here as well, and health economics, with the help of which the performances of insurers and health insurance services and other public welfare health institutes are examined with regard to their efficiency.

As research up to now quite clearly shows, social, psychological, and physical health disorders arise with environmentally related and/or societal conditions in the background that bring excessive stress and adjustment requirements for individuals and groups who do not have the resources necessary for coping. Inequalities in society result in unequal risks, depending on social situations and class, cultural integration, gender, age, and so on. Many of these stresses originate in the personal environment of those affected, and in the long run, the resources are also anchored in this personal environment (Hurrelmann 1989).

For this reason, when medical care systems are developed, the decisive objective is to strengthen resources found in personal environments and not to weaken them further by inappropriate interventions. The individual's capabilities for self-help and those of his social environment must therefore logically be included in the analysis of starting conditions and courses of health and disease developments. Precipitate interference from professionals brings the risk of social isolation and "hospitalization."

The aim must be to utilize and promote existing self-help capabilities, instead of dismantling and trimming them by means of highly perfected intervention and medical care supplies that are foreign and inimical to the personal environment. Here it is important that the persons affected participate in the analysis of the problem and even that alternative solutions are run through with them—in other words, that participation is aimed for at all levels. The medical care structures that would take account of this type of approach have to involve many professions.

DIFFERENT TRAINING POLICIES IN PUBLIC HEALTH

As Frenk (1993) has written, it is essential to place the bases of production (research), reproduction (teaching), and use of knowledge (practice) within their conceptual context, which involves rigorously defining what constitutes public health. We think that these three elements are to be seen as components of a system with interlinks and feedbacks. Moreover, we strongly argue against the apparent separation of production and reproduction (where research is equated with production and teaching with reproduction). We consider it especially critical to clarify these interlinks now, when the prominent role of learning over teaching has been established. Concepts such as teaching as a learning experience (i.e., learning through teaching) and learning as a research experience (i.e., the similarities in the cognitive processes involved) are emerging alongside the well-established view of research as a learning process.

Even if there have been numerous initiatives in training programs in public health in many countries over the last 15 years, nevertheless, these innovations remain too often isolated and have not brought forward the radical revision of existing programs that is needed. The persistence (or renewal) of the split between the traditional hygiene role of public health and the roles of administration of services and especially hospital services is the most problematic feature of the current situation. Most of the renewed interest by the field of management in the health sector remained narrowly centered on management and by the focus of hospitals on a biomedical model of disease. The real challenge is to develop competences in management for health, which implies the broad conception of public health described above. The challenge is to develop an approach to public health training in which public health managers require a combination of specialist clinical skills and general management skills. Combining these skills in a group of individuals will be vital in the future in meeting the challenges posed by health care systems and by policy-makers (Laaser, de Leeuw, and Stock 1995).

Today, most postgraduate training programs are generally discipline based and often monoprofessional. When it is not at the admission of students—for example, programs accessible only to medical doctors—then it is at the outcome level: There are as many public health training programs as public health professional careers.

Where new programs, such as health economics, health education, and health promotion, have been added, this has been done most of the time in parallel to the existing ones. While their creation is to be welcomed, they still reflect a continuation of the trend toward hyperspecialization: The overall result of existing training policies and methods has been an overemphasis on producing specialists with very specific skills and competences, rather than generalists with broad vision who are capable of integrating their own work with that of others, both within and outside the health sector (WHO/EURO 1991).

Teaching careers in public health are based on hyperspecialization and publications in international scientific journals. Credit is not awarded by academic peers for contributions to health policy developments at national, regional, or local levels; for popular books contributing to an increase in population awareness and information; or for other ''nonscientific'' activity.

Establishing an Interdisciplinary Training Culture

The general public health knowledge base, where it exists, is limited and traditional. This is a major constraint to building the interdisciplinary policy and planning inherent in the approach targeted to health gains. There is an urgent need for a critical mass of professionals within the health system with a broad understanding of public health, including the management of health issues, in order to support the reform process as well as lend support and critical contributions to the implementation and evaluation of health care system reforms.

What is needed is a common core curriculum or track for all public health students, which should provide a common understanding of public health and a focus on the health of populations and on a global and social model of health and of health gain. This would provide a common language, methodologies, and tools for all students, including those coming from the social sciences. This could take the form of a common partial track, which is possibly the real role for a master's of public health that is accepted worldwide.

Table 1 lists the subjects that most frequently constitute the core program of compulsory subjects in the curriculum of the basic general public health course. Groups (1), (2), and (3) represent a decreasing frequency of inclusion as compulsory subjects. Many institutions also offer courses in the public health aspects of a specialized discipline, such as occupational health, nutrition, or tropical medicine. The curriculum for these courses consists of different compulsory subjects according to the discipline being studied.

A student in a basic general public health course is ordinarily expected to

Table 1
Compulsory Subjects in Public Health Education

Most common title of the subject:

1. *Basic sciences*

   Biostatistics/biometry/statistics
   Epidemiology
   Microbiology

   Applied disciplines

   Environmental health and sanitation
   Environmental sanitation
   Health education
   History and philosophy of public health
   Introduction to public health
   Organization of health services

2. *Basic sciences*

   Behavioral sciences
   Demography
   Medical sociology
   Social aspects of public health
   Social sciences and health

   Applied disciplines

   Food and nutrition
   Health administration and management
   Health care management
   Health planning
   Maternal and child health services
   Occupational health

3. *Basic sciences*

   Health care evaluation
   Health economics
   Health services research

   Applied disciplines

   Community organization
   Family planning and population
   Mental health services
   Population problems
   Primary health care

Table 2
Elective Subjects in Public Health Education

1. Chronic disease epidemiology
   Health law and legislation
   Hospital administration
   International and comparative health
   Records and information systems
   School health
   Social security and social policy
   Tropical medicine
2. Accident prevention
   Computers and data processing
   Genetics and public health
   Gerontology
   Health manpower development
   Human relations and management
   Public health nursing
   Rehabilitation of the disabled
3. Air and water pollution
   Dental health
   Educational methods
   Food hygiene
   Hygiene of housing
   Malaria control
   Screening programs
   Tuberculosis control
   Venereal disease control
   Veterinary public health

take a minimal number of elective subjects. Any of the subjects listed in Table 1 that are not compulsory at a particular institution may be available as an elective subject. Such advanced subjects are sometimes taught in another department of the university.

Table 2 lists the additional subjects that are most frequently available as elective subjects. Groups (1), (2), and (3) represent a decreasing frequency of availability.

Teaching and Learning Methodology

In the basic general public health course, much use is made of methods outside the classroom. In addition to lectures, the following three teaching/learning methods are used at numerous institutions:

1. The *general open-topic seminar*, during which diverse subjects are discussed, often with the participation of faculty members from various departments.
2. The *dissertation*, *thesis*, or *essay*, prepared by a student on an assigned subject or one he has chosen himself. This is not a major dissertation, such as that for a doctoral degree, but a task that may reasonably be completed within a one-year period of study.
3. *Field practice*, for which a student is assigned to a community or an organization for a certain period of time—often one or two months. There, he or she works under the supervision of an experienced public health specialist, sometimes examining a special problem and preparing a report on his or her findings. Some institutions have permanent administrative relationships with communities or organizations where student field assignments can be carried out.

There are still many challenges to cope with in public health training. One key factor is the need to get away from professional protectionism and the rigidity expressed by some groups of providers, where training programs are considered primarily as a means to guarantee the professionalization of a special group. There is no single public health role, and the traditional roles are breaking down; inherent in public health are more loosely defined and overlapping roles. Therefore, there can be no one totally standard public health training; in an environment in which people come to a profession with multiple backgrounds and pursue multiple careers after graduation, the only possible way forward is diversity (Badgley 1992; Colomer 1994).

Shaping Adequate Learning Environments

Intersectorality for health policy development is essential. Public health must be capable of engaging in a dialogue with actors beyond the health sector. This will require leadership and negotiation skills. Other important aspects of the learning process are related to the World Health Organization (WHO) Health for All policy (Bury 1989) such as multiprofessional training—in other words, "learning together to work together" (WHO/Geneva 1988)—and involvement in intersectoral activities. This refers also to the whole concept of an adequate learning environment (Barnard and Köhler 1994).

The great challenge facing the Schools of Public Health is to learn to incorporate the new complexity of health conditions and response systems. In order to do so, the schools should become more familiar with their changing reality so as to become leading agents of change in health (Frenk 1993). In other words, this means that while the traditional concept of excellence is still of prime importance, the relevance of the training has to be considered as well (Fineberg et al. 1994; Köhler 1991).

Various means can contribute to foster this relevance. Among the factors in the learning environment, the teachers are crucial: Besides their academic quality, their past and present experience and activities in the health sector are important. This also contributes to facilitating the learning process with regard to the relations with, and the involvement of, the community, as well as promoting links to the policymakers.

For instance, a reasonable percentage of the teachers should be part-time teachers coming from the health services, and a substantial percentage of the learning activities should take place in the community, especially as concrete projects implementation. A few full-time chairs can be created in Schools of Public Health, funded by the Ministry of Health or the Ministry of Science, offering three- to five-year fixed-term contracts on a rotation basis for different top-level administrators of health services, selected by the school. Other feedback mechanisms from the health services should be sought regularly, such as periodic consultations, questionnaires, surveys, and workshops on the perceived training needs, satisfaction with graduates, and so on (Normand 1994).

At the level of postgraduate training, whether complementary training or continuing education program, "learning by doing" means less by the classical problem-solving approach than learning by actually solving real professional problems—and by doing it while integrating a research component, as in action research. In other words, it is training by research rather than training for research (WHO/Geneva 1988). There is a great deal of consensus that research can be used to increase the relevance of training, especially in relation to policymaking and service delivery. This is especially evident in the example of evaluative research.

The competencies needed as a program manager and policy adviser include the ability to critically review and use research results and to evaluate research (including a good knowledge of evaluative research and meta-analysis) for policy-making, planning, and assessing projects. This is expressed as possessing critical thinking and writing skills, analysis, and synthesis; being able to review an issue, including commissioning relevant further applied research when needed; knowing how and when to use experts; and being able to summarize the key points for different audiences. There is definitely a need to train public health generalists to deal with the researchers and the experts of particular fields in public health in order to be able to negotiate with them and make a relevant contribution to problem solving in a spirit of partnership. For this, training programs must introduce students to the methodologies of research; its potential; and its limits, indications, costs, and time frames. Research workers themselves, in institutions and universities, must participate in the creation of a climate of understanding of research and encourage the collaboration of managers and caregivers in research activities (Davies 1991).

It is obvious that the key partners in the process must be universities, since by definition they are multidisciplinary and integrate training and research. The idea is not new (WHO/Geneva 1984), but the partner does not seem to have met the expectations. The link between training and research is often more present within the person of the professors than in their training programs, and the multidisciplinarity is more a coexistence within an institution than a joint practice in training or research activities, which is really what interdisciplinarity is about. The interlinks with health policy and programs in countries are usually weak, notably as professors are not often involved in health policy development or services management.

The independence of universities is good inasmuch as it is the guarantee for academic freedom that has permitted universities to be the place for innovations and resistance to authoritarianism all over the world. But, obviously, this independence that gives the possibility to change gives at the same time the possibility not to change, and this has been a contributing factor to the so-called ivory tower syndrome. Of course, universities have to be understood as such and not as medical faculties; indeed, their major potential for contributing to health development comes from outside the medical faculty—for example, from sociology, demography, anthropology, economics, political sciences, psychology, education, law, or ethics (Bury 1989).

A recent promising trend may be found in the concept of an interfaculty and interinstitution School of Public Health, cofunded and coadministered by the university with representatives from the different faculties and by the government with representatives from the different ministries involved in the health field, in research, and in higher education. This could start and remain at a more modest level but with the same spirit, such as by contractual service agreements where a university is linked with some health services for practical courses for students or with research teams or by getting teachers for research modules with ministries, for exchanging staff or joint involvement in policy-making (Laaser 1994).

The other major existing model is the National School of Public Health under the authority of the Ministry of Health. In principle, the links with health services are embedded in the mission of the school; however, it is less obvious in practice. Moreover, one of the pitfalls in this construction may be a too-pronounced lack of independence from political power. The involvement in relevant research activities is usually limited. The overall level of quality is frequently questioned. The other dangers with a School of Public Health under the Ministry of Health are political appointments, lability in funding linked to changes in government, and less of a contribution to research.

The two models of Public Health Schools mentioned above might be somewhat restrictive, especially for the countries-in-transition. There may possibly be other solutions coming from the experiences and traditions of countries themselves, or the development of fully fledged schools could be undertaken in stages. Another possibility is consortium arrangements. A scheme for combined universities and public health institutes may be very difficult to devise but is often considered necessary.

The setting in which training takes place will obviously reflect the priorities within the country's health development (Laaser 1994). In other words, it has to be multidisciplinary, it has to encourage community participation, and it has to be health promoting and linked with research. Taking for granted the fact that the problems are different for the different countries and that they should be addressed in each specific situation, some suggested approaches or strategies for typical situations should be identified to assist countries in formulating their responses. The culture and traditions of a country and the past and existing organizations and systems in the field of health, education, research, and science are extremely important in determining the range of possibilities for future models of public health.

REFERENCES

Badgley, R. F. (1992). Public health: Trends and challenges. In: Pan American Health Organization: *The Crisis of Public Health: Reflections for the Debate*. Scientific Publication no. 540. Rio de Janeiro. 53–67.

Barnard, K. & Köhler, L. (1994). Creating a learning environment in a school of public health. *European Series on Training and Research in Public Health*, 2, 20–28.

Bury, J. A. (1989). *Approaches to Integrate the Basic Themes of Health for All in the Education of the Health Personnel.* Copenhagen: WHO/EURO. (unpublished)

Bury, J. A. (1993). *WHO Health for All Research Policy and the New Challenges in Countries of Central and Eastern Europe*. Working paper for the WHO/EMRC Workshop. Prague. 75–89.

Colomer, C. (1994). *Context for MPH Programmes*. Discussion paper for First NMPH Conference. Granada. (unpublished)

Davies, A. M. (1991). *The Evolving Science of Health Systems Research*. Geneva: WHO.

Fineberg, H. V., Green, G. M., Ware, J. H. & Anderson, B. L. (1994). Changing public health training needs: Professional education and the paradigm of public health. *Annual Review of Public Health*, 15, 237–257.

Frenk, J. (1993). The new public health. *Annual Review of Public Health*, 14, 469–490.

Holland, W. W., Detels, R. & Knox, G. (Eds.). (1984). *Oxford Textbook of Public Health.* Oxford: Oxford University Press.

Hurrelmann, K. (1989). *Human Development and Health*. New York: Springer Verlag.

Hurrelmann, K. & Laaser, U. (Eds.). (1993). *Gesundheitswissenschaften. Handbuch für Lehre, Forschung und Praxis.* Weinheim: Beltz.

Hurrelmann, K. and Lösel, F. (Eds.). (1990). *Health Hazards in Adolescence*. Berlin: De Gruyter.

Köhler, L. (1991). Public health renaissance and the role of Schools of Public Health. *European Journal of Public Health*, 1, 2–9.

Laaser, U. (1994). The contribution of the Schools of Public Health to public health in Europe. *German Journal of Public Health*, 2, 109–118.

Laaser, U., de Leeuw, E. & Stock, C. (Eds.). (1995). *Scientific Foundations of a Public Health Policy in Europe*. Weinheim: Juventa.

Maynard, A. (1993). *The Future of Health Services Research*. Centre for Health Economics Newsletter. York: University of York Press.

Normand, C. (1994). *Structure and Organisation of Masters in Public Health Programmes.* Discussion paper for First NMPH Conference. Granada. (unpublished)

Omenn, G. S., Fielding, J. E. & Lave, L. B. (Eds.). (1991). *Annual Review of Public Health.* Vol. 14. Palo Alto: Annual Reviews.

Pan American Health Organization (PAHO). (1992). *The Crisis of Public Health: Reflections for the Debate.* Scientific Publication no. 540. Rio de Janeiro.

Schwartz, F. W. & Badura, B. (Eds.). (1991). *Public Health.* Berlin: Springer Verlag.

WHO/EURO. (1985). *Targets for Health for All. Targets in Support of the European Regional Strategy for Health for All.* Copenhagen.

WHO/EURO. (1991). *Targets for Health for All. The Health Policy for Europe.* Summary of the updated edition. Copenhagen.

WHO/EURO. (1993). *Research Administration in the Countries of Central and Eastern Europe.* Report from a joint WHO/EMRC Workshop. Prague.

WHO/EURO. (1994). *Training and Research in Public Health.* Copenhagen.

WHO/Geneva. (1984). *The Role of Universities in the Strategies for Health for All. A Contribution to Human Development and Social Justice.* Geneva.

WHO/Geneva. (1988). *Learning Together to Work Together for Health. Report of a WHO Study Group on Multiprofessional Education of Health Personnel.* Technical Report Series no. 769. Geneva.

World Bank. (1993). *Investing in Health. World Development Report.* Washington, D.C.: World Bank.

ORGANIZATIONAL STATUS OF BASIC AND APPLIED RESEARCH IN PUBLIC HEALTH

Roger Detels, Walter W. Holland, and Heizo Tanaka

In this chapter, we present the organizational status of basic and applied research in public health as it is conducted in three of the leading research countries of the world: the United States, the United Kingdom, and Japan.

THE UNITED STATES

Organization of Public Health Research

In the United States, there is no single federal agency, private organization, or professional association that has the responsibility of setting the national research agenda for public health. On the other hand, there are many organizations that influence the type of research being conducted.

In 1979 the Department of Health, Education and Welfare published *Healthy People: Surgeon General's Report on Health Promotion and Disease Prevention*, which for the first time established a series of measurable and achievable public health goals for reduction of disease and health promotion in the United States. This publication was followed in 1980 by *Promoting Health/Preventing Disease: Objectives for the Nation*, which established 15 priority areas and 226 specific and measurable goals for the nation to achieve by 1990. These goals were published by the Department of Health and Human Services (DHHS) (the Department of Health, Education and Welfare was renamed early in 1980). Based on the experience of working toward these goals, DHHS published *Healthy People 2000 National Health Promotion and Disease Prevention Objectives* in 1990, which reset goals for the nation to achieve by the year 2000. For the year 2000 the number of priority areas was increased from 15 to 22, and more emphasis was placed on the groups that had not achieved nor progressed in the 1990 goals. These included children, adolescents, older adults, minority groups, people with disabilities, and the poor.

DHHS does not have jurisdiction over the state and local health agencies or the other public and private organizations committed to improving the health of the public. They, therefore, have attempted to recruit these various agencies in the process of achieving these goals by holding a series of hearings on establishing the goals that they published in 1980 and 1990 and have encouraged many of the federal and local agencies to participate in the process of developing these goals. Further, they encouraged and assisted the American Public Health Association to publish *Model Standards: A Guide for Community Preventive Health Services* in 1985, which presented a template to be used by local health agencies in setting targets and implementing programs for improvement in health in their communities. By 1987, 87 percent of the states and territories had established health objectives for 1990, and now most have also established health objectives for the year 2000. In 1991 the American Public Health Association published a sequel to the earlier publication entitled *Guide to Implementing Model Standards*. The process of building a consensus and motivating agencies to adopt these goals is described in a chapter entitled ''Objectives-Based Strategies for Disease Prevention'' in the third edition of the *Oxford Textbook of Public Health* (McGinnis et al. 1996).

The Congress of the United States can establish priority areas for research by allocating funds to federal institutions to be used for specific purposes. Alternatively, both the federal and legislative branches of the government can establish commissions to review specific issues and provide recommendations to them. The legislative and the executive branches may also establish ''offices'' to set agendas and monitor research in specific areas in federal agencies, as they recently have done with the establishment of the Office of AIDS Research within the National Institutes of Health (NIH). Often, they take these actions in response to lobbying efforts by professional associations (such as the American Public Health Association [APHA]), disease-oriented societies (such as the American Cancer Society), and groups of concerned citizens (such as the various ''gay'' organizations, which have lobbied for more research in the area of HIV/AIDS [human innumodeficiency virus/acquired immunodeficiency syndrome]).

The individual federal agencies also establish priorities for research reflecting either the concerns of the agency leadership or the concerns of their advisory councils. They stimulate research in these priority areas using a variety of administrative techniques, which are discussed below.

Finally, individual investigators also play a role in setting research priorities by deciding the areas in which they will develop research proposals for consideration of funding by the various federal, state, local, and private organizations. The basic philosophy of research in the United States is to allow scientists to determine their own research agenda, and thus a high proportion of the research funded in the United States is investigator initiated. This basic philosophy to support the individual creativity of the scientist may have played a key role in establishing the United States as a leader in the field of health research.

Research in public health issues in the United States is conducted in a variety of settings. These include schools of public health, schools of medicine, research institutions, federal agencies, and state and local departments of health services. With the exception of the last two, however, specific research on public health issues is, for the most part, not the exclusive agenda of any one of these institutions. Thus, schools of medicine will conduct research relevant to public health, primarily through departments for preventive and community health or their equivalents, and schools of public health may conduct research that has more clinical than public health relevance. Research in public health issues is also conducted by research institutions such as the RAND Corporation in Santa Monica, California. Research relevant to public health may also be conducted in departments of anthropology, social sciences, and the physical sciences and schools of business, social work, policy, and law.

Organization of Funding for Public Health Research

The founding concept of the United States—the union of separate, autonomous, self-governing units, the states—has tended to suppress coordination and planning of all aspects of social organization at the federal level as compared with Europe and other areas of the world. The organization and funding of public health research reflect this philosophy of autonomy and freedom to choose.

Further reflecting this philosophy, funding for public health research comes from a variety of sources including public and private funds. With the exception of research funds from state and local departments of health services, these funds are usually not specifically designated for research in public health. Further, there is no national agency with the responsibility of coordinating funding of research, let alone public health research. Although there is a national professional organization for public health professionals, the APHA, this association does not set broad agendas for public health research, although it does provide a forum for research at its annual meetings. The APHA does, however, vigorously lobby the U.S. Congress on public health issues, which may in turn generate funds for research in specific public health issues. From time to time, the Congress does pass initiatives for research on special topics, as it has in the past for cancer, multiple sclerosis, toxic wastes, and more recently, AIDS.

In the United States, public health research falls under the broad rubric of biomedical research. The United States spends more money than any other country in the world on biomedical research, but the proportion of that funding that is specifically spent on public health issues is difficult to determine, although it is probably not a large proportion of the total. Funding for public health research comes from both public and private funds, although the larger proportion of the total funds is from public sources.

Public Sources of Public Health Research Funding

Of the public sources of research funding, the major funding agencies are in the federal government and include the NIH, the U.S. Centers for Disease Control and Prevention (CDC), the Environmental Protection Agency (EPA), the Agency for Health Care Policy Research (AHCPR), the Healthcare Financing Corporation (HFC), the National Center for Health Statistics (NCHS), and the Food and Drug Administration (FDA), as well as other federal agencies that provide lesser funds. The major funder of health research is NIH.

The National Institutes of Health. NIH is a collection of 21 agencies, the majority of which are oriented to specific diseases (for instance, the National Cancer Institute and the National Heart, Lung Institute). Exceptions include the National Institute of General Medical Sciences, which supports research in areas not covered by the other institutes; the Fogarty International Center, which supports international research and training; the National Institute of Environmental Health Sciences, which supports research on environmental hazards affecting health; the National Institute on Drug Abuse, which supports research on problems related to illicit use of addicting drugs; and the National Center for Nursing Research, which supports research to improve the quality of nursing. Figure 1 gives the administrative structure of NIH, including a listing of the various institutes. There is no institute committed to public health research. The larger institutes support both intramural and extramural research, but the emphasis in all the agencies is on support of extramural research.

Extramural support is distributed using a variety of mechanisms. The majority of research funds from NIH are for projects that are generated by individual investigators, groups of investigators, or research institutions. Each of the institutes of NIH has a council, which is made up of leaders from the research community, the concerned constituency, and the general public. One of the tasks of these councils is to set priorities for the institute. Individual institutes may promote research in specific areas recommended and/or approved by its council by contracting for research in that area with academic institutions and research agencies. Usually, bidders are solicited through mechanisms such as requests for proposals (RFPs), which invite institutions to bid for research on a specific topic. Under the contract mechanism, the institute is able to maintain reasonably tight intellectual and fiscal control of the direction of the research supported by the contracts. Institutes desiring to promote research in specific areas of interest may also issue requests for applications (RFAs), which alert researchers that funds may have been set aside for research in these areas and that proposals in these areas may receive priority funding. These proposals are funded as grants, rather than contracts, so that the intellectual control of the research remains with the investigator. The setting of priorities for research may also come from the office of the director of NIH and from congressional mandates implemented though special provision of funds for NIH that are designated for specific areas of research.

Figure 1
The Administrative Structure of NIH

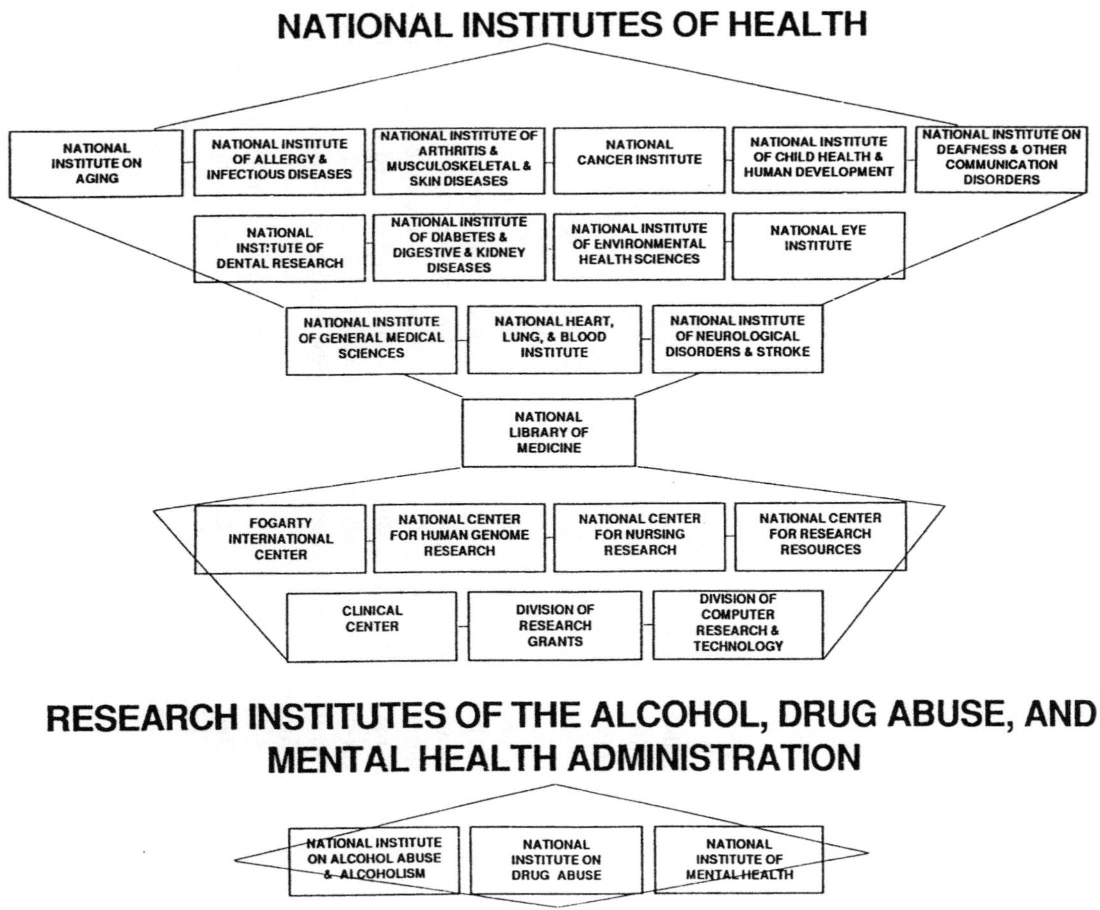

The NIH has established a rigorous peer review system for establishing the priority for funding. Proposals are submitted to the Division of Research Grants, which subjects them to review by a committee of scientific peers. This committee ranks the proposals on scientific merit. The Division of Research Grants assigns the grant to a specific institute or institutes. The councils of the individual institutes then subject the proposals to a second review, which also considers the research priorities of the institute. The proposals are then funded by the institute according to the ranking established by both the peer review committee and the council.

The Centers for Disease Control and Prevention. The CDC is the federal agency that is responsible for disease control in the United States. Although its primary role is in surveillance of disease and control of disease outbreaks, in recent years it has increasingly taken on the task of research in public health issues of importance to the country. Much of this research is conducted by research staff of the CDC. Although the CDC does not provide funding for investigator-generated research, it does provide funding for research in specific areas that it designates usually through the contract mechanism. In addition, the CDC has also established an arrangement with the Association of Schools of Public Health to offer limited funding in designated areas of public health research to interested investigators in the schools of public health.

Environmental Protection Agency. The EPA has the responsibility for protecting the U.S. public from environmental health hazards. In accordance with this responsibility, the agency conducts both intramural and extramural research. Extramural research is funded through both the contract mechanism and the grant mechanism. Contracts are usually given for specific tasks in support of the intramural program, but for which an outside institution may be better qualified. The mechanism for funding grants is similar to that used by the NIH. Investigator-generated proposals in environmental health sciences are submitted to the EPA, which subjects them to peer review and agency review to set priorities for funding.

Agency for Health Care Policy Research and the Healthcare Financing Corporation. The AHCPR and HFC are the major federal agencies that fund health services research in the United States. Although they also conduct research intramurally, the majority of their funds are spent on extramural research.

The Other Federal Funding Agencies. A wide variety of federal agencies, some mentioned above, provide some funds for research on public health issues. They use a variety of mechanisms for allocating funds, although most attempt some level of peer review in the process.

Funding at the State Level. The resources of the states vary widely. Most states do not have sufficient funds to provide funding for public health research. However, the most populous states, such as California and New York, do allocate limited funds for public health research, usually through their departments of health services or related agencies. For example, the state of California has an agency, the California Air Resources Board (ARB), that supports both intramural and extramural research in support of clean air. The extramural program uses a mechanism of peer review similar to that of the NIH in allocating research funds. They support both investigator-initiated research and ARB-initiated research. In addition, the legislature of the state of California has designated research funds for specific agendas, often through the public and private universities of the state. These have included initiatives on smoking prevention research, toxic hazards, and AIDS research.

Funding at the Local Level. Most U.S. counties and cities do not have sufficient funds to support public health research, but again, the larger cities and counties such as New York and Los Angeles do provide limited funds, primarily for applied research. For example, in Los Angeles, the Southern California Air Quality Management District occasionally supports research projects on specific issues of interest to it. The Los Angeles County Department of Health Services supports both intramural research and extramural research, usually on a contract basis. Counties and cities that include a school of public health will often contract with them to carry out joint research on public health issues. There have been numerous examples of this between the departments of health in the San Francisco Bay area, Los Angeles, and San Diego and their respective schools of public health.

Private Sources of Funding for Public Health Research

Nonpublic funds for public health research are offered by a variety of organizations. These range from the large private foundations (such as the Rockefeller Foundation, the Robert Wood Johnson Foundation, the Milbank Foundation, the Commonwealth Foundation, the Ford Foundation, the Kaiser Family Foundation, and the Carnegie Foundation), which fund research in many different areas, to smaller foundations (such as the Thatcher Foundation), which fund specific areas of research. Private foundations, especially the Robert Wood Johnson, Kaiser Family, and Commonwealth Foundations, are the largest source of funding for health services research. Disease-specific voluntary associations (such as the American Heart Association, the American Cancer Society, the Lung Association of America, and the American Foundation for AIDS Research [AmFAR]) fund research in their own areas. Although these foundations and associations provide a relatively small proportion of the total U.S. research funds, they are often able to fund "high-risk" research, which the NIH system is unlikely to fund. An example of the important types of public health research that the disease-specific societies provide is the early support of research on the adverse effects of tobacco use on heart disease and cancer, supported by the American Cancer Society and the Lung Association of America. Similar research on the adverse effects of high levels of cholesterol was supported by the American Heart Association.

The mechanisms that these foundations and societies use to identify priority areas of research for funding vary. Some of the foundations set specific areas of priority with their advisory boards and directly approach research organizations that they feel are likely to provide outstanding research in those areas, rather than to solicit proposals from the research community at large. Other organizations, particularly the disease-oriented voluntary associations such as the American Heart Association, solicit research proposals and prioritize them using a system similar to the NIH peer review system.

The disease-oriented societies also play a very important additional role in promoting research funds in specific areas through their lobbying efforts aimed at state and federal legislatures. These lobbying efforts have sometimes stimulated the formation of commissions to evaluate the need for research in specific areas such as AIDS. Inevitably, these commissions themselves become advocates of increased funding for these areas of research and have a direct impact on stimulating legislature to appropriate funds to areas based on their recommendations.

Funding Levels for Research in the United States

Figure 2 gives the change in funding for health research between 1983 and 1992 in total dollars, as a percentage of total research and development, and as a percentage of the total health costs. Health research as a percentage of total research and development grew by 17.9 percent but remained at approximately the same level when considered as a percentage of total health care costs. The national support for health research and development by source of funds and performer is given in Table 1. The government support of research has more than doubled between 1983 and 1993 ($6,117 million to $14,017 million). During this same interval industry support of research and development has grown more than threefold, from $4,205 million to $15,562 million. A similar increase was observed in the research supported by national private nonprofit foundations ($456 million to $1,248 million). Funds for NIH have grown from $3,789 million in 1983 to $9,763 million in 1993.

Problems with the Organization of Research in the United States

The United States is the leading country in the world in the field of public health research, but the system that supports that research machine appears to be a ''hodgepodge'' system, which is disorganized and lacks a unifying planning approach. Its success despite the lack of a tightly planned approach may be due, in part, to the magnitude of funding that is provided to the research community through public and private sources of funds. This democratic approach to research funding may actually promote entrepreneurship by researchers desiring to work in meaningful areas, which will have the maximum impact on science and the health of the community. Rigorous peer review may ensure that only the best research is funded. On the other hand, peer review tends to select

Figure 2
National Expenditures for Total Health Costs, Total R&D, and Health R&D, 1983–1992

Health R&D as a Percentage of Total R&D, and of Total Health Costs, 1983 and 1992

(Dollars in Billions)

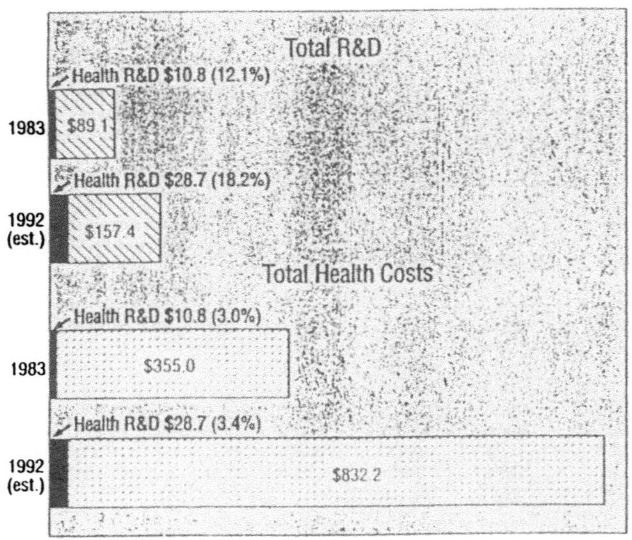

Percentage Change Since 1983 in Total Health Costs, Total R&D, and Health R&D, 1984–1992

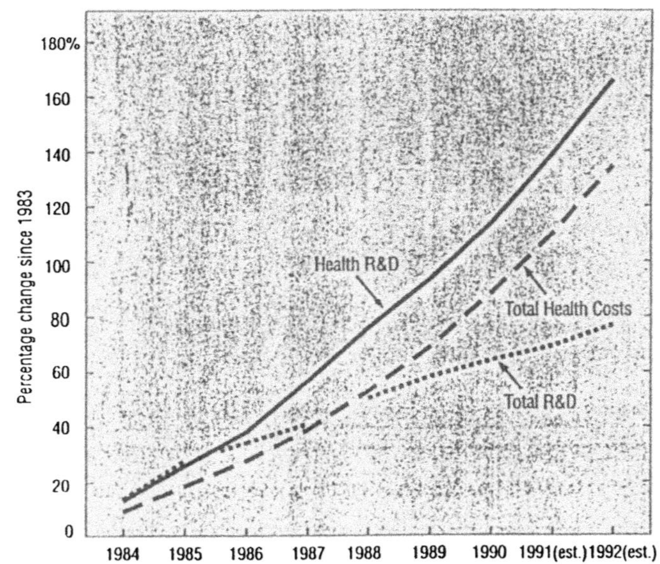

Source: Letsch, Lazenby, Levit, and Cowan 1992.

Table 1
National Support for Health R&D by Source or Performer, 1983–1993[a]

(Millions of Dollars)

Sector	1983	1984	1985	1986	1987	1988	1989	1990	1991 (est.)	1992 (est.)	1993 (proj.)
Total of A or B	$10,778	$12,154	$13,558	$14,894	$16,931	$18,996	$20,914	$23,094	$25,753	$28,717	$30,828
A. BY SOURCE OF FUNDS											
Government	6,117	6,883	7,669	7,924	9,028	9,725	10,628	11,418	12,429	13,626	14,017
Federal	5,399	6,087	6,791	6,895	7,847	8,431	9,163	9,791	10,602	11,727	11,978
NIH	(3,789)	(4,257)	(4,828)	(5,005)	(5,852)	(6,292)	(6,778)	(7,136)	(7,696)	(8,407)	(9,769)
State & local	718	796	878	1,028	1,182	1,294	1,465	1,628	1,828	1,900	2,040
Industry	4,205	4,765	5,352	6,188	7,104	8,433	9,405	10,717	12,234	13,870	15,562
Private nonprofit	456	506	538	782	799	838	881	959	1,091	1,221	1,248
Foundations	89	111	122	129	161	155	129	155	178	236	211
Voluntary health agencies	206	205	233	260	285	323	354	363	393	420	447
Howard Hughes Medical Institute[b]	54	79	51[c]	247	183	179	197	215	250	273	268
Other	107	112	133	146	170	181	201	226	270	293	322
B. BY PERFORMER											
Government	1,813	1,997	2,139	2,155	2,388	2,590	2,576	2,862	2,991	3,382	3,479
Federal[d]	1,577	1,741	1,869	1,848	2,042	2,214	2,162	2,403	2,480	2,837	2,898
State & local	236	256	270	307	346	376	415	460	511	544	581
Industry[e]	3,668	4,216	4,660	5,293	6,003	6,929	7,901	8,877	10,101	11,370	12,620
Private nonprofit	4,665	5,245	5,954	6,471	7,400	8,035	8,977	9,575	10,729	11,760	12,254
Higher education[e]	3,779	4,269	4,839	5,314	6,048	6,573	7,201	7,699	8,684	9,279	9,668
Other[e]	887	976	1,115	1,157	1,352	1,462	1,777	1,877	2,044	2,481	2,586
Foreign	631	697	805	975	1,140	1,443	1,459	1,779	1,932	2,205	2,475

[a] *Revised.*
[b] *These figures report support for the direct conduct of biomedical research. In addition, HHMI's Office of Grants and Special Programs provides support for scientific career development, which is not included here.*
[c] *Total includes only eight months of operations due to change in fiscal year.*
[d] *In addition to in-house research, includes program management and direct operations attributable to health R&D.*
[e] *Includes Federally Funded R&D Centers.*

Source: Letsch, Lazenby, Levit, and Cowan 1992.

"safe" research with little risk of failure. Unfortunately, cutting-edge advances rarely result from safe research.

The argument could be raised that federal funding for public health research should be provided through a separate funding mechanism or through special allocations from the Congress. Although this might bring a higher profile to public health research, it is probably unlikely to result in an increase in research dollars for public health issues. Public health has traditionally been very unsuccessful in recruiting support except when the country is confronted with a very clear health threat. Therefore, given this past history, separating funding for public health research from biomedical research (traditionally, a popular area) might actually reduce the funds spent for research on public health issues.

The Future of Health Research in the United States

The U.S. approach to funding of research and its success may be severally challenged in the near future. The ascendancy of conservatives in the government and the need to balance the budget may severally reduce the public research funds in coming years. Such an outcome will test whether this system for research support is the result only of the vast amount of money spent or the creativity and entrepreneurship of the research community when it is allowed to establish its own priorities.

THE UNITED KINGDOM

The support of public health research is as much of a problem in the United Kingdom as in other countries. Although public health has been, and is, firmly embedded in the national health service, its academic base is less secure. The duties and responsibilities of the subject have been outlined in the Acheson Report, published by the Department of Health in 1988 (Acheson Report 1988). Each Health Authority (of which there are about 120 in England) has a director of public health and two to six additional consultant positions as well as trainees and support staff. There also are academic departments of public health or their equivalent in each of the medical schools in the United Kingdom. Finally, one school, the London School of Hygiene and Tropical Medicine, undertakes postgraduate education exclusively. Each of these departments and institutions conducts public health research.

Public health research at universities is supported by a series of funding agencies, the most important of which is the central government through its Department of Health. The Medical and Social Science Research Councils also provide some support. Private foundations, particularly the King Edward Fund and the Nuffield Provincial Hospitals Trust, provide grants as do other charitable foundations, industry, and the National Health Service (NHS) itself. The major sources of funding and amounts have been summarized in three recent reports

(House of Lords Select Committee on Science and Technology 1988; Peckham 1991; Braun 1994).

Public health research in the United Kingdom is defined as "a wide ranging field, covering strategic and applied research into the health needs of the population as a whole and the provision of services to meet those needs." (House of Lords Select Committee 1988). Obviously, in order to meet the needs that are identified, public health research must necessarily encompass health education and promotion, epidemiology, economics, statistics, and behavioral sciences.

As part of the reforms of the NHS in 1991, a new Research and Development Directorate was created within the service (Department of Health 1991). The purpose of the National Directorate is to establish a coordinated strategy and framework of health research that is designed to strengthen the scientific basis for health care. Management responsibilities have been devoted to eight regions, each of which has its own director. Each region undertakes both national and locally determined research.

The first initiatives stemming from this directorate have included the start of the Cochrane Centre at Oxford, designed to aid understanding through the use of meta-analysis studies and research on mental illness, the first nationally determined priority area (Anonymous 1992; NHS Management Executive 1992). Other research initiatives on cancer, cardiovascular disease and stroke, among others, have also been identified and started.

One of the main problems in public health research has been the paucity of staff available to fill vacancies in academic departments (Clarke and Kurinczuk 1992). The shortage of public health physicians is compounded by insufficient research staff from other professional disciplines. Good public health research frequently involves close collaboration with clinicians and is usually the product of work by groups of researchers, drawn from public health physicians, statisticians, demographers, nurses, social scientists, economists, medical physicists, engineers, geographers, and psychologists. In the absence of clear, reasonably secure, and adequately remunerated career structures for people from these disciplines, it has been difficult to recruit and retain sufficient research staff of the right quality.

There are few, if any, formal arrangements for the training of researchers. Some of the eight regions of the NHS have a small number of research positions, but these places are usually taken by clinicians in training. Most medical practitioners involved in higher specialist training are expected to spend time in research, although few make a career in the field. Public health physicians in training have opportunities to rotate into academic departments, but a minority avail themselves of these opportunities, and frequently, they do not have a clear view of their future role. Further, sparse consultant/senior lecturer staffing means that the formal training in research methods that is being provided is often of poor quality. Formal training for people from other professional disciplines is equally hit-or-miss.

Views of Public Health Research

There are beliefs and images that need to be broken down before improvements in the quality of public health research can be made. These barriers can be summarized briefly:

1. Politicians always know the "right" way to run health services, based on their "experience." They will not accept that their experience might be unrepresentative. They do not like pilot studies, trials, or comparisons, which might confound their beliefs.
2. Managers like to foster "good practice," defining it from "common sense." They "do not wish to wait for doctors to define the ultimate proof."
3. Some public health practitioners subscribe to similar views, backing instinct rather than scientific inquiry. Most, however, are too busy to marshal the evidence necessary to confirm or confound the beliefs of others.
4. A persistent complaint of public health research workers is that they are neglected by comparison with those undertaking nonapplied or "pure" research. It is certainly true that universities can be unsympathetic in supporting health service research that does not fulfill the requirement of being original and is seen as service rather than research. Conversely, health authorities have expectations that academic departments should be undertaking this work.
5. NHS managers perceive academic public health as pursuing its own interests in its own time and only secondarily concerned with contributing to the needs of the NHS.

Although anecdotal evidence can be adduced to underpin some of these derogatory views, none are wholly true. More important, effort needs to be put into breaking down the barriers these attitudes create, which are inimical to the commissioning, support, and conduct of public health research.

Places. Research implies new ideas and their testing, development, and application to the solution of problems. To promote such research requires that appropriate structures be in place. Where they have existed, they are now threatened. Paradoxically, although introducing research and development to the NHS formally for the first time, the reforms of 1991 and associated proposals to reduce the number of medical schools in London threaten some of the existing research structures and institutions (Tomlinson 1992). Similarly, a recent report to the director of Research and Development questioned the utility of existing research units and suggested the establishment of fewer, much larger, multidisciplinary centers designed to answer specific questions (Williams 1992).

Although one applauds the multidisciplinary approach, a fear exists that restricting the number of centers might be inhibitory to public health research. A careful balance is needed between the laudable objective of assembling a "critical mass" in a context of many institutions with few researchers and the stimulus provided by competition in a context of multiple research centers. Research in specific directions clearly has a place but should not inhibit spontaneous interests, creativity, and initiative, which are the heart of good research. Economies of scale, which can lead to the "big is beautiful" approach, need to be balanced against the loss of personal identity and initiative that ensues.

Information. Despite the huge expenditure on information systems in the NHS, the information available to researchers remains poor. In part, this is because the basic data are themselves poor (Holland 1995).

Public health research needs, just as does clinical research, data about people, their lives, ailments, treatments, and ultimate fate. The difference is that public health can often manage with aggregated and anonymous data. Both clinicians and public health researchers rely on data derived from the patient interview, and they need the data to be accurate. Unfortunately, much of what is processed on a large scale in the NHS is designed for the needs of management for information about the processes without any capacity to relate them to demand or outcome. The imposition of targets arising from the NHS reforms has increased pressure on management to show changes in health over time (HMSO 1992). This pressure is likely to change the manner in which data are recorded. The resulting increased emphasis on disease instead of process will facilitate the use of the information for public health research, as will the ability to relate different episodes of disease and treatments in different places. Despite the existence over many years of the Oxford Record Linkage Study, it is impossible in most places to trace people who move from one location to another over time. Current developments in medical and clinical audit will accommodate accurate linkage of data. Of course, the ability to so trace people, a factor of importance in public health research, has ethical connotations, which need to be faced.

Health of the Nation. The publication of a strategy for health incorporating key areas and targets, *Health of the Nation*, provides a focus for present and future public health research (HMSO 1992). Clearly, one of the major challenges for public health for the year 2000 is to tackle the biggest public health problem currently facing the Western world—ischemic heart disease. The attack will be made on two fronts: first, the development of methods to identify those most at risk of developing this condition, through the use of appropriate biochemical and genetic tests; and second, the use of large-scale clinical trials to determine the effectiveness of these tests and the modification of lifestyles or introduction of preventive treatment to reduce disease incidence.

Research into ischemic heart disease and the other key areas identified in *Health of the Nation* underscores the need for health technology assessment, about which the Department of Health has published a report (Drummond, Crump, and Little 1992). New diagnostic tests and treatments developed from the advances in molecular and genetic biology will need careful evaluation through randomized control trials and other methods. Similarly, developments in imaging and minimally invasive surgery will continue to need critical evaluation.

Within the more traditional health care sector, public health research must continue to work toward the development of the most appropriate models of provision for prevention via primary care, such as identification of the most efficacious and economical methods of treatment so that the maximum benefit for health can be achieved within the resources available. Sometimes this will mean giving up established practices of dubious worth. Enormous strides have been made. For example, there is increasing acceptance of the view that screening, viewed as a panacea by many, is not always appropriate and that inappropriate screening is not only expensive but can also carry with it risks of producing iatrogenic effects in some of those screened.

Problems with the Organization of Public Health Research in the United Kingdom

The Select Committee inquiring on medical research stated that public health research was particularly badly supported (House of Lords Select Committee on Science and Technology 1988). The committee suggested that public health research needed its own distinct institutional identity, as far removed as possible from competition with biomedical and clinical research and the self-interests of the Department of Health. The committee suggested that a National Health Research Authority should be developed with the Medical Research Council (MRC), which should be funded by the NHS. This never happened, and the Research and Development Directorate was created instead (Department of Health 1991). The major problem for public health research is that it often requires follow-up of populations or groups over a long time period and, thus, requires a stable, secure base and career structure. This has never been achieved. Braun has described the consequences in detail (Braun 1994). As he has noted, although there is a broad academic base, the public health disciplines—with the exception of epidemiology and health economics—have a relatively weak position in the universities and in research. A problem for almost all academic public health departments is that they are much too small to carry political weight compared to the clinical and basic science departments.

Although cores of public health research exist in universities, the institutionalization in the university and the simultaneous dependence on Department of Health grants put the public health researcher in a double bind. This has had two effects: There has been little success in the establishment of a solid academic presence within the universities, which consider the subject to be too applied and thus "not respectable." Second, the Department of Health is often more interested in a rapid solution than in a long, academic discourse. This has had the consequence that Department of Health funding has become less easily available. As Braun has noted, "Politics and the still rather weak public health disciplines appear to be increasingly less 'united by a common fate' as utilitarian government policy runs its course. The government is increasingly inclined to employ commercial research institutes that are able to provide the appropriately exploitable research" (Braun 1994).

The MRC has also not yet proven itself to be the proper authority for effectively establishing a scientific community in public health, even though it has created the organizational foundations for such a community within the MRC itself. It remains unclear whether the especially tenuous position of public health research will be given due attention in the allocation of grants. As long as basic biomedical research provides the evaluative criteria for awarding this funding, it remains doubtful whether it will actually be possible to establish a critical mass of university-based researchers. Moreover, the MRC continues to insist on developing public health research in accordance with a biomedical approach. This might limit success to those few subfields of public health that are thematically connected to clinical practice.

England does have opportunity structures for establishing a public health function and public health science that are not available in other countries. The key here is the nationalized health service, which gives the government much greater leeway in defining the activities and functions of the health care system. Such an opportunity structure alone is not enough. The question is whether the new DH (Department of Health) director of Science and Development will be in the position to make a significant contribution to a reform of the function of public health (within the NHS). Given the short-term and multiple interests at the Department of Health, there is a great probability that fragmented and decentralized research funding will continue (Department of Health 1991)

Public health research is also clearly underfunded in England. The funds that went into this field, already meager by comparison to those going to medical research, actually shrank in real terms in the 1980s. It is becoming increasingly more difficult for the departments to maintain their research function and to keep their autonomy by means of a high percentage of grants.

The situation of the research centers and research units outside of the medical schools has also been changed by the shift in strategy of the DH. In 1991, the attempt was made to integrate public health into the university as a scientific discipline by means of the government department funding of its own research units and centers. The Department of Health was, thus, not content to take the usual course and make a call in the scientific system for research specifically required and then receive it in directly usable form within a short period of time. It was recognized from the outset that this could never serve as the basis for establishing qualified and ultimately valuable policy consultation.

Nevertheless, politics still did not succeed in establishing a scientific community in public health with its funding. The study emphasized two reasons for this. On the one hand, an element of tension developed in all the research units that were affiliated with the university between their integration into science and their usefulness for politics. As public health became a recognized scientific discipline and part of the academic canon, at some point in its theoretical development it produced a paradigm in which it distinguished itself from all nonscientific influences. Thereafter, it was no longer reasonable for the Department of Health to fund these institutions, since it could not remove itself from the short-term character of the political time frame. The Department of Health sought to have public health research become part of the academic canon without exhibiting the patience necessary for such a task.

There were also political developments that induced the Department of Health to curtail funding for these research units. Primary responsibility here falls to the austerity policy of the government. Given the scarce resources, it became increasingly difficult to provide research units with long-term funding. It had simply become too expensive.

The research institutions that were financed on the basis of basic-facility funding also impeded the required flexibility of political action, which became more urgent in the 1980s in the face of new challenges such as AIDS and government demands for greater cost-effectiveness and productivity. The Department of Health found itself compelled to be in a position to present the useful results of its own activities in an ever more rapid fashion. In this context, it no longer seemed to make sense to draw upon academically oriented public health research, with its long-term development time frame. For this reason, grants were given to commercial facilities (and not to university-based research units), since the former were able to deliver useful results more rapidly. Thus, in this field, too, government policy and the system of contracting funding led to transformed conditions of action and to difficulties in the implementation of the research function.

Despite the institutional arrangements made to ensure the autonomy of funding agencies and scientific organizations in England, the policies of the Thatcher administration had lasting effects on the conditions of action and, thus, on the strategy formation of the organizations and actors involved in the funding and scientific systems. Both the Select Committee and the Advisory Board of Research Councils (ABRC) warned the government of the consequences of these policies on the research productivity of the English scientific system. In terms of its austerity program, the government remained unswayed; in terms of its neoliberal policy, several small changes were made in the Department of Health, and the NHS aimed at reviving the research function. It is doubtful whether these corrections can alter the despondent atmosphere of the scientific system. As promising as certain new approaches to funding policy might be (e.g., in clinical research), without the confidence and trust of researchers in the future of their activities, such efforts will hardly be able to renew enthusiasm in health research (Department of Health 1991).

Recommendations for the Future of Health Research in the United Kingdom

If public health research is to flourish in the United Kingdom in the presence of these problems, a number of conditions will need to be met:

1. The development of a proper, valid, reliable information system (Braun 1994).
2. The organization of research in centers with an appropriate, critical mass of researchers.

3. The willingness of researchers to tackle areas of deficiency, ignorance, and weakness in our knowledge base.
4. A sustained program of recruitment and commitment to researchers in all the disciplines of the field.

As changes in the health service and society in the United Kingdom are beginning to reveal the need for public health, knowledge is increasing, and thus it is possible that the change in status that has been observed on the "service" side of public health will also spread to the academic side.

JAPAN

Recent Advances in Public Health Research

From a socioeconomic point of view, as shown in Figure 3, Japan's twentieth century can be divided into four periods: privation (–1950), reconstruction (1950–1960), high economic growth (1960–1975), and low economic growth (1975–) (Tanaka 1992). Japanese public health issues including research were influenced by the social and economic state (Tanaka 1995).

In the seventeenth century, Japanese rulers decided that Japan's existing relations with Europeans should be discontinued and inaugurated the policy of a "closed country," which lasted until the middle of the nineteenth century when the United States forced the Japanese to give American ships access to their ports. As soon as the country was opened, communicable diseases, for example, cholera, black plague, and small pox, became epidemic. In around 1900 when Japan fought its giant neighbors, China in 1894–1895 and Russia in 1904–1905, the industrialization and movement of population led to the serious worsening of environmental conditions in urban areas.

As industrialization advanced more before and after World War I, many laborers suffered under the burden of long working hours and low wages, and the gap between the rich and the poor was widened. Social services to relieve the poor and the disabled were implemented.

Japan before and during World War II was a nation committed to a large standing army. There were dangerous future implications for the military in the low population increment resulting from a falling birthrate and high maternal and infant mortality rates. Furthermore, tuberculosis was a great threat to adults aged 20 to 30 years who were to be soldiers. The government encouraged the Japanese to have more babies and to build up their physical strength under the propaganda slogan, "Enrich the country, strengthen the military."

Defeat in World War II brought a great and sudden food crisis to Japan. The Japanese were poorly housed and poorly clothed and lacking the essentials of sanitation. Communicable diseases and malnutrition were common among them. They were also exposed to helminthic diseases, for example, ascariasis and ancylostomiasis.

Figure 3
Socioeconomic State and Public Health in the Twentieth Century, Japan

Public Health Research	Period	Year	Socioeconomic State
Communicable disease Environmental health in urban areas Social services for the laborers, the poor, and the disabled	Privation	1900	Japan-China War Japan-Russia War World War I
		1940	Japan-China War Pacific War
Tuberculosis Maternal and child health Physical strength Tuberculosis, communicable disease Helminthic disease Malnutrition		1945	Defeat
Water supply, sewerage Health insurance	Reconstruction	1950	Independence of the USA
Stroke and hypertension Cancer Air pollution Occupational disease in laborers and farmers Mental health Environmental pollution So-called intractable disease Health and welfare for the elderly	High Economic Growth	1960	Program for doubling general income Oil crisis
Cancer, stroke Health and welfare for the elderly and the disabled So-called intractable disease Mental health Health promotion Global environment Quality of life	Low Economic Growth (Stable Period)	1975	
		1990	Bubble economy

In the early period of reconstruction after Japan became independent of the United States, the policy shifted to prevention of tuberculosis, maternal and child health, and urban garbage and industrial waste treatment. The water supply and sewerage system started to be modernized. With the increasing importance of chronic noncommunicable disease, epidemiological studies and preventive measures for hypertension, stroke, and gastric and cervical cancers were initiated. It was noteworthy that the health insurance system that covered all the nationals was enforced.

Health problems were characterized by stroke, mental disorders, environmental pollution, so-called intractable diseases (connective tissue diseases, neuromuscular diseases, etc.), and occupational diseases among laborers in industrial factories and among farmers in depopulated districts during the period of high economic growth. With the aging of the population, health and welfare for the elderly were also highlighted. Currently, during the low economic growth period, health promotion, active or total health, quality of life, and global environmental problems are being emphasized.

Public health research reflects the changing picture of health. For example, Figure 4 shows the trends in the presentations at the Annual Scientific Meetings of Japanese Society of Public Health from 1970 through 1988 (Nekota and Anzai 1989). In the 1970s, 20.1 percent of all the presentations were occupied by environmental health, being followed by chronic noncommunicable disease (16.3 percent), community health (14.2 percent), maternal and child health (9.7 percent), and infectious disease (8.7 percent). In the 1980s, reports on chronic noncommunicable disease took the first rank, and those on health and welfare for the elderly and health promotion/education increased. Hypertension and stroke accounted for more than 50 percent of chronic noncommunicable disease presentations, while hypercholesterolemia and coronary heart disease were not studied so much. The proportion of cancer to the chronic diseases was 25 percent. Reports about infectious disease remained at the upper level, about 10 percent of all the presentations. Epidemiological methodology, biostatistics, food and nutrition, and mental health were relatively frequently presented, 3 to 7 percent, respectively.

The number of presentations at the Annual Scientific Meetings of Japanese Society for Hygiene in 1975–1984 and in 1985–1994 are shown in Table 2 (Shima 1995). The annual number of presentations increased from 3,436 in 1975–1984 to 4,555 in 1985–1994. Reports of environmental health and toxicology of chemicals and heavy metals decreased year by year, although increasing trends were observed in the number of reports on epidemiology and prevention of cancer, cardiovascular diseases (particularly hypertension and stroke), so-called intractable diseases, and other chronic noncommunicable diseases (particularly diabetes mellitus and osteoporosis), as well as health and welfare for the elderly, nutritional problems, disease control, and health promotion and education.

Figure 4
Main Fields of Public Health Presented at the Annual Scientific Meetings of Japanese Society of Public Health, 1970–1988

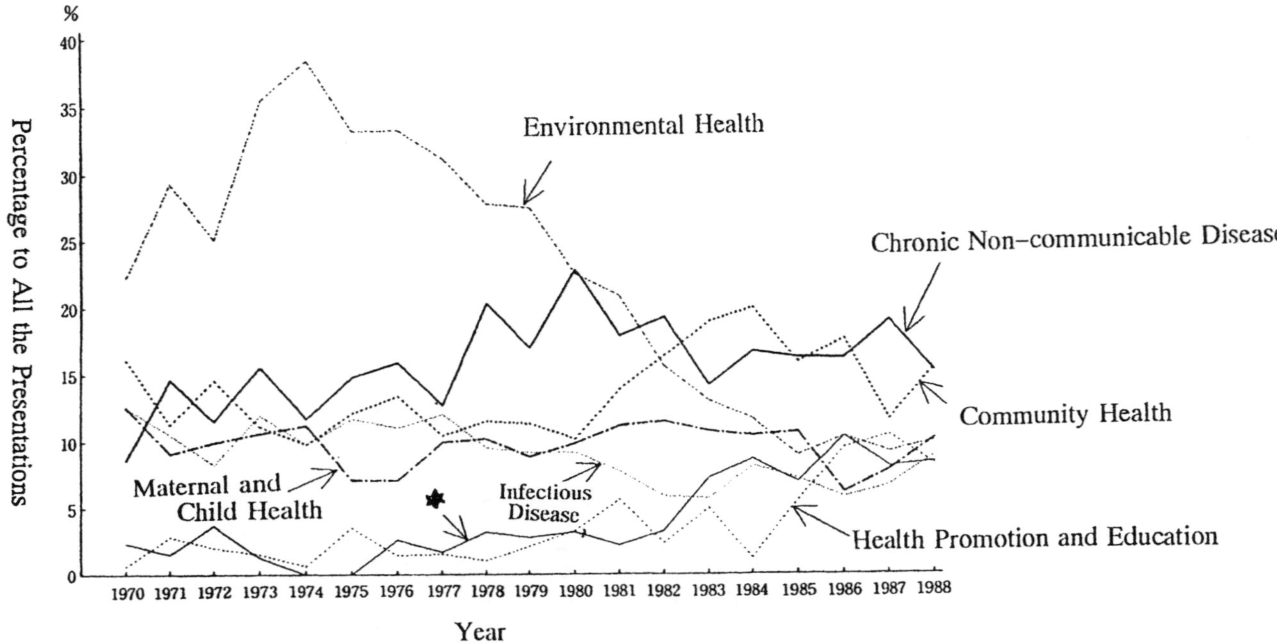

★ Health and Welfare for the Elderly

Source: Nekota and Anzai 1989.

Table 2
Number of Presentations at the Annual Scientific Meetings of Japanese Society for Hygiene, 1975–1984 and 1985–1994

Field	1975-1984(%)	1985-1994(%)
Air pollution	195(5.7)	183(4.0)
Water pollution	74(2.2)	60(1.3)
Housing, Clothing	54(1.6)	48(1.1)
Environmental health, environmental physiology	384(11.2)	302(6.6)
Infectious disease	94(2.7)	112(2.5)
Mercury	165(4.8)	141(3.1)
Cadmium	282(8.2)	266(5.8)
Zinc	50(1.5)	61(1.3)
Silicon, asbestos	0(–)	32(0.7)
Lead	149(4.3)	98(2.2)
Inorganic deleterious substances, other metals	274(8.0)	353(7.7)
Pesticides	46(1.3)	82(1.8)
Organic solvents	90(2.6)	78(1.7)
Other deleterious substances	195(5.7)	128(2.8)
Biological monitoring, measurement methods	7(0.2)	52(1.1)
Dietary survey	109(3.2)	161(3.5)
Nutritional physiology	6(0.2)	196(4.3)
Food hygiene	80(2.3)	60(1.3)
Maternal and child health	92(2.7)	123(2.7)
School health	78(2.3)	158(3.5)
Cancer	145(4.2)	314(6.9)
Cardiovascular disease	158(4.6)	244(5.4)
Other chronic non-communicable disease	67(1.9)	151(3.3)
Health and welfare for the elderly	49(1.4)	189(4.1)
So called intractable diseases	65(1.9)	103(2.3)
Mental health, stress	0(–)	58(1.3)
Health control	125(3.6)	239(5.2)
Health promotion	16(0.5)	86(1.9)
Immunology	0(–)	51(1.1)
Community health, Medical service	127(3.7)	163(3.6)
Health education	0(–)	29(0.6)
Biostatistics, population, disaster, accident	176(5.1)	199(4.4)
Others	84(2.4)	35(0.8)
Total	3,436(100%)	4,555(100%)

Source: Shima 1995.

Academic Societies

There are several academic societies related to preventive medicine and public health in Japan. Among them, the Japanese Society of Public Health covers almost all of the fields in public health and has more than 10,000 members who consist of not only researchers in medical schools and research institutes but also physicians, public health nurses, dietitians, dentists, and pharmacists in local health centers in prefectures and cities.

In 1991, the Japan Epidemiological Association was founded, and its journal is the only English-language one published in Japan in the field of public health. The Japanese Society for Hygiene, one of the oldest societies, makes environmental health and toxicology its main field of study, with the experimental laboratory as its primary site, while the Japanese Association of Industrial Health uses the workplace as its research site.

Organizations of Public Health Research

Basic or applied research in public health is centered within medical schools and national or local government research institutes. On the other hand, reports of public health activities are presented at academic societies by health personnel in local health centers (848 centers as of 1994).

There are 43 national medical schools under the administration of the Ministry of Education, Science and Culture, 8 schools under the local governments (prefectures or major cities), and 29 private schools, each of which has one to three, mostly two, departments of public health, hygiene, environmental health, or community health (Health and Welfare Statistics Association 1994). Each department or chair (*koza*) is made up of a professor, an assistant professor, and one or a few lecturers and assistants, that is, four to five members in total. According to the *Asahi Shimbun*, one of the leading newspapers with a daily circulation of 8.2 million, the medical schools in Tohoku, Tokyo, Tokyo Medical and Dental, Keio, Kanazawa, Nagoya, Kyoto, Osaka, Kyushu, and Kumamoto Universities (the order is from the north to the south) rank among the best ten in terms of published papers in the journals with the high-impact factor on the basis of MEDLINE (The Asahi Shimbun 1995).

There are seven affiliated national laboratories of the Ministry of Health and Welfare. They are financed by the general account and conduct innovative and pioneering research activities that respond to the respective administrative requirements (Table 3) (Health Sciences Division 1994). Five national research centers are financed by the special account: the National Cancer Center, the National Cardiovascular Center, the National Center of Neurology and Psychiatry, the Medical Center Hospital, and the Children's Medical Research Center, some of which have a department of epidemiology with three to five researchers. Moreover, studies are carried out on the welfare of the disabled at the National Rehabilitation Center for the Disabled. In addition, 73 institutes of public health

Table 3
Research Institutes of the Ministry of Health and Welfare, Japan

Institute	Research	Number of Researchers
Institute of Population Problems	Survey of population, demography	25
Institute of Public Health	Training public health personnel	111
National Institute of Health and Nutrition	Health promotion, nutrition, food science	34
National Institute of Health	Infectious disease, food hygiene, pharmaceuticals, laboratory animals	310
National Institute of Leprosy Research	Leprosy	18
National Institute of Health Services Management	Medical care issues medical institutions and facilities, hospital administration	9
National Institute of Health Sciences	Pharmaceuticals food science, food additives, chemical reagents	200

Source: Health Sciences Division 1994.

Figure 5
Number of Researchers in Five Selected Countries

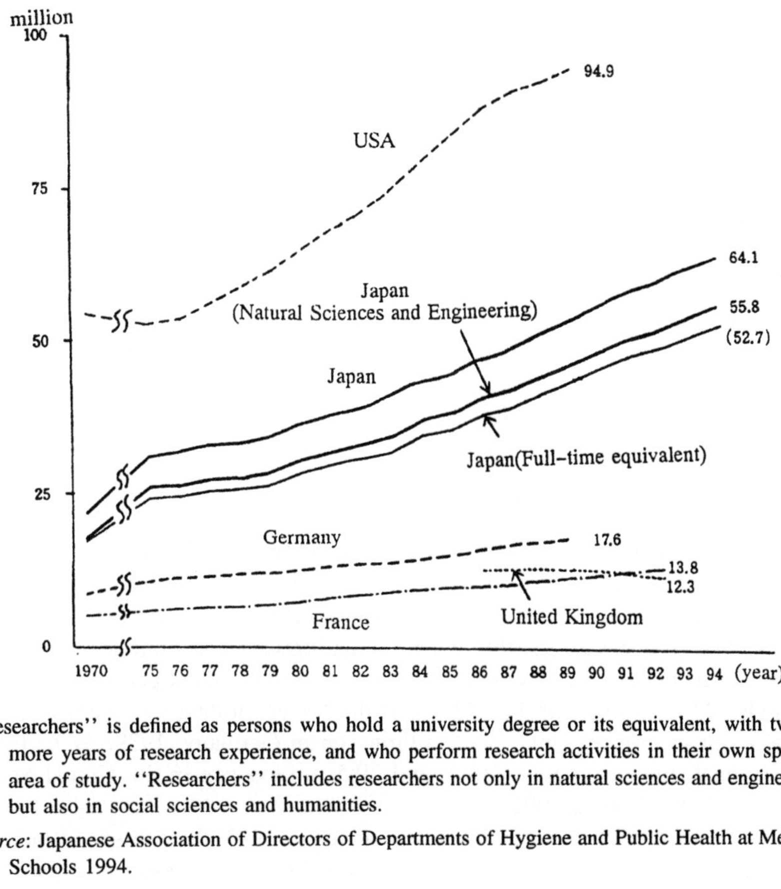

"Researchers" is defined as persons who hold a university degree or its equivalent, with two or more years of research experience, and who perform research activities in their own specific area of study. "Researchers" includes researchers not only in natural sciences and engineering but also in social sciences and humanities.

Source: Japanese Association of Directors of Departments of Hygiene and Public Health at Medical Schools 1994.

or environmental health and several cancer or cardiovascular centers are under the control of local governments, that is, prefectures and major cities (Health and Welfare Statistics Association 1994).

Research Personnel

In the number of researchers, the United States stands out above other countries (Figure 5). The number has increased more markedly in Japan as well as in the United States than in Germany, France, and the United Kingdom. In terms of the number of researchers per 10,000 population, however, Japan takes first position (50 per 10,000), while the rate is 38 in the United States, 28 in Germany, 24 in France, and 21 in the United Kingdom (Science and Technology Policy Bureau, 1995; Statistics Bureau 1995)

The sector of researchers is classified into industry, research institutes, and universities/colleges. The number of researchers in industry has increased most markedly among the three sectors in Japan. In 1994, the number was 367,000 in industry, 151,000 in universities, and 40,000 in research institutes (Science and Technology Policy Bureau 1995; Statistics Bureau 1995).

The professional field is divided into science, engineering, agriculture, and "health," which includes medical science, dentistry, pharmacy, and others. In 1994, the percentage of all researchers in the field of health was 10.0 percent (3,961/39,581) in research institutes and 57.0 percent (86,390/151,448) in universities, although the data were not available in industry (Statistics Bureau 1995). The number of public health researchers in universities was 855 (855/86,390 = 1.0 percent) (Japanese Association of Directors of Departments of Hygiene and Public Health 1994). Although there were 707 health researchers in the national research institutes, public health researchers, in the strict sense of the word, were the minority.

Research and Development Expenditures

The research and development (R&D) expenditures in five selected countries during the period from 1975 to 1993 are shown in Figure 6. R&D expenditures in Japan ranked second after the United States and tended to increase from 1975 to 1992 and to decrease in 1993 when the nationwide economic abnormality—the so-called bubble economy—arose. However, the amount per researcher, for example, 23.2 million yen in 1993, was the lowest among the countries: 35.5 million yen in France, 1992; 34.2 million yen in Germany, 1989; 31.1 million yen in the United Kingdom, 1992; and 29.5 million yen in the United States, 1989 (Statistics Bureau 1995).

In terms of the R&D expenditures by sector in 1993, the amount in industry accounted for 72.3 percent of 12,528,354 million yen for natural science and technology: 14.3 percent for research institutes and 13.5 percent for universities. According to the R&D expenditures by science field in 1993, health received 108,901 million yen in research institutes and 674,882 million yen in universities (Statistics Bureau 1995).

Funding for health research in research institutes and universities comes from a variety of sources including public and private funds but mainly from the Ministry of Education and the Ministry of Health and Welfare. The Ministry of Education provides 3 to 5 million yen annually, with one department of public health in national medical schools. In addition, the Grants-in-Aid for Science Research are available for any researcher. About 35 percent of the applicants for the Grants-in-Aid are funded, and 75 percent of the requested budget is provided for each study. In 1994, as shown in Table 4, the researchers in the field of public health succeeded in obtaining 481 million yen of the Grants-in-

Figure 6
Research and Development Expenditures in Five Selected Countries, 1975–1993

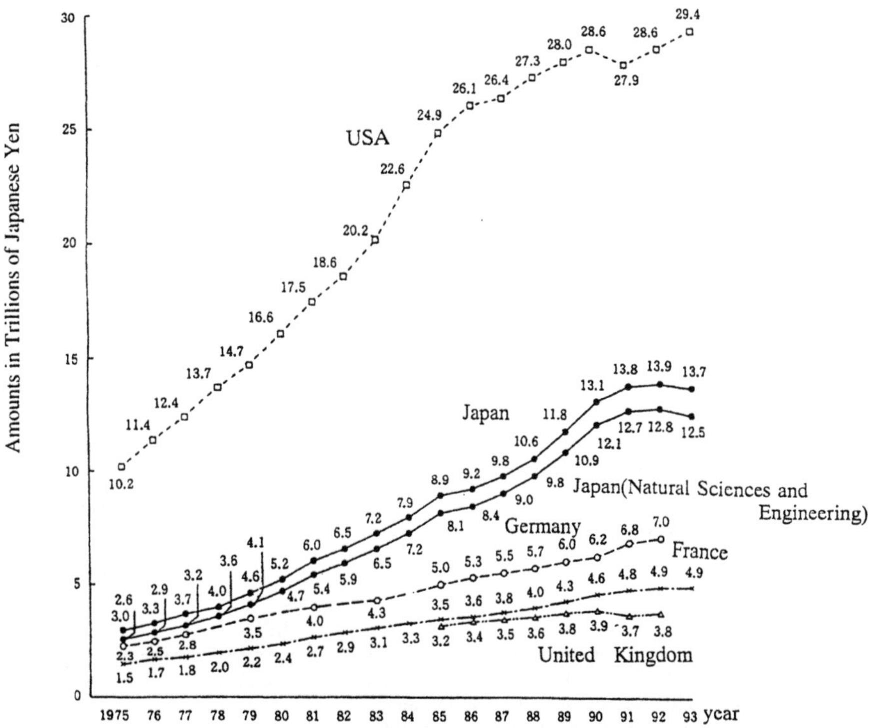

R&D expenditures in four countries plus Japan are converted according to Organization for Economic Cooperation and Development (OECD) purchasing power parity in each year. For example, purchasing power parities to Japanese yen in 1994 are as follows: 185 yen/U.S. dollar; 84.9 yen/Deutsche mark; 28.4 yen/French franc; and 289 yen/UK pound.

Source: Statistics Bureau 1995.

Aid, less than 17 percent of the total (Association of Grant-in-Aid for Scientific Research 1994).

The Health Science Research Grants have been appropriated since 1951 by the Ministry of Health and Welfare in order to support researchers for expenses required for conducting research activities on topics recognized as necessary for securing the scientific promotion of administrative measures and improving the technical levels of national health and welfare.

Some basic studies in public health are also supported by the Science and Technology Agency, and environmental health studies are supported by the Environment Agency. Most prefectures and major cities also provide funds to support public health research that is conducted by health centers, local institutes of public health, and others, as mentioned earlier.

Table 4
Grant-in-Aid for Scientific Research, Ministry of Education, Science and Culture, Japan, 1994 (millions of Japanese yen)

Grant-in-Aid for	*"Health"*[1]	*Public Health*[2]	*All Fields of Sciences*[3]
Specially promoted research (50–300)[5]	—	—	2,560.0
Scientific research on priority areas	—	—	20,800.0
Cooperative research	(839.2)[4]	29.4	2,740.0
General scientific research			
A (10–50)[5]	(2,349.0)[4]	61.8	5,720.0
B (3–10)[5]	(4,565.1)[4]	135.0	9,720.0
C (3)[5]	4,727.0	147.0	12,560.0
Encouragement of young scientists (1.2)[5]	2,319.3	57.3	5,820.0
Developmental scientific research (30)[5]	—	50.2	7,520.0
Others	—	—	6,860.0
Total	—	480.7	74,300.0

[1]Medical sciences (including public health), dentistry, pharmacy, and others.
[2]Hygiene, public health, medical sociology, and others.
[3]Natural sciences, engineering, social sciences, and humanities.
[4]Biological sciences—all fields of sciences excluding social sciences, humanities, physics and chemistry.
[5]The budget that an applicant can request, amounts in millions of Japanese yen.

Source: Association of Grant-in-Aid for Scientific Research 1994.

The Foundation Library Center of Japan estimated that there were 497 private foundations as of July 1991 and conducted a survey to investigate the actual state (Foundation Library Center of Japan 1991). Out of 497 foundations, 290 responded to the questionnaire in 1991. They had 802 programs and subsidized 24,950 million yen annually, of which 35.5 percent was shared by the field of "health." Although the data specific to public health research were not available, the percentage was estimated to be less than 5 percent of the amount for health. There are also some funds, mainly from life insurance companies, that support studies of public health alone.

Perspectives of Public Health Research

Japan has succeeded in reducing not only infectious diseases and malnutrition but also cardiovascular disease and cancer and now boasts the longest life expectancy of any country in the world. Public health research has contributed to this success, although the funds allocated for public health research have been substantially less than those allocated for biomedical and clinical research.

We have to continue to eliminate the threats of infectious disease, cancer, and cardiovascular disease to promote health, to prolong life expectancy, to improve the quality of people's lives, and to challenge global environmental problems. Only public health research can respond to these various needs, rather than biomedical research, because public health research focuses on human groups, individuals, and ecosystems, elucidating relationships to disease and health between and among many other levels, while biomedicine pursues studies on a microlevel.

Clearly, we must continue to expand funding for public health research.

REFERENCES

Acheson Report. (1988). *Public Health in England: The Report of the Committee of Enquiry into the Future of the Public Health Function.* London: HMSO.

American Public Health Association. (1985). *Model Standards: A Guide for Community Preventive Health Services.* Washington, D.C.: APHA.

American Public Health Association. (1991). *Guide to Implementing Model Standards.* Washington, D.C.: APHA.

Anonymous. (1992). Cochrane's legacy. *Lancet*, 340, 1131–1132.

The Asahi Shimbun. (1995). *The University Ranking for 1996, Asahi Original.* Tokyo: The Asahi Shimbun. 64–67. (in Japanese)

Association of Grant-in-Aid for Scientific Research. (1994). *Grant-in-Aid for Scientific Research, Ministry of Health, Science and Culture in 1994 (ISBN 4–324–04195–4).* Tokyo: Gyosei. (in Japanese)

Braun, D. (1994). *Health Research and Its Funding.* Country Reports, Vol. II, France and England. Sponsored by the Federal Ministry for Research and Technology. Bonn: Bock.

Clarke, M. & Kurincz, J. J. (1992). Health services research: A case of need or special pleading? *British Medical Journal*, 304, 1675–1676.

Department of Health. (1991). *Research for Health: A Research and Development Strategy for the NHS.* London.

Drummond, M. F., Crump, B. J., & Little, V. A. (1992). Funding research and development in the NHS. *Lancet*, 339, 230–231.

Foundation Library Center of Japan. (1991). *1992 Directory of Grant-Making Foundations. Guide to Private Grant Sources (ISBN 4–474–00169–9C2000 P4500E).* Tokyo: Foundation Library Center of Japan. (in Japanese)

Health and Welfare Statistics Association. (1994). Health services in Japan (Kokumin eisei no doko). *Indices of Health and Welfare (Kosei no shihyo)*, 14(9)(Supp.), 7–21, 189–198. (in Japanese)

Health Sciences Division, Ministry of Health and Welfare. (1994). *Health Sciences Annual Report in 1994 (ISBN 4–905690–11–0).* Tokyo: Institute of Health Sciences Co. Ltd. 21–37. (in Japanese with English summary)

HMSO. (1992). *The Health of the Nation: A Strategy for Health in England.* London: Royal Commission on Medical Education.

Holland, W. W. (1995). An ethical health service: Its information needs [Queen Elizabeth, Queen Mother Lecture]. *Journal of Public Health Medicine*, 17 (2), 41–52.

House of Lords Select Committee on Science and Technology. (1988). *Priorities in Medical Research.* Vol. 1, Report HL 54–1. Session 1987–1988. London: HMSO.

Japanese Association of Directors of Departments of Hygiene and Public Health at Medical Schools. (1994). *List of Names of Faculty Members in Departments of Hygiene and Public Health in 1994.* Okayama: Japanese Association of Directors of Departments of Hygiene and Public Health at Medical Schools. (in Japanese)

Letsch, S. W., Lazenby, H. C., Levit, K. R. & Cowan, C. A. (1992). National health expenditures. *Health Care Financing Review.* 14 (2), 1–30.

McGinnis, J. M., Harell, J. A., Artz, L., Files, A. A. & Maiese, D. R. (1996). Objectives-based strategies for disease prevention. In *Oxford Textbook of Public Health* (eds. R. Detels, W. W. Holland, J. McEwen, & G. Omenn). 3rd ed. Oxford: Oxford University Press.

Nekota, Y. & Anzai, S. (1989). Trends in public health research according to the presentations at the Annual Scientific Meetings of Japanese Society of Public Health, 1970-1988. *Japanese Journal of Public Health,* 36, 324–331. (in Japanese).

NHS Management Executive. (1992). NHS R&D call for outline proposals in mental health. *British Medical Journal* [classified advertisement, 20 June].

Peckham, M. (1991). Research and development for the National Health Service. *Lancet,* 338, 367–371.

Science and Technology Policy Bureau, Science and Technology Agency. (1995). *Indicators of Science and Technology (ISBN 4–17–152270–6).* Tokyo: Printing Bureau, Ministry of Finance. (in Japanese with English titles)

Shima, S. (1995). *A List of the Presentations at the Annual Scientific Meetings of Japanese Society for Hygiene.* Aichi: Department of Public Health, School of Medicine, Fujita Health University. (in Japanese)

Statistics Bureau, Management and Coordination Agency. (1995). *Report on the Survey of Research and Development in 1994 (ISSN 0447–5089).* Tokyo: Japanese Association of Statistics. (in Japanese with English titles)

Tanaka, H. (1992). Nutrition and cardiovascular disease, A brief review of epidemiological studies in Japan. *Nutrition and Health*, 8, 107–123.

Tanaka, H. (1995). A brief history of public health in Japan. In *Health Control* (ed. H. Tanaka), Tokyo: Japanese Association of Nursing Press. 13–19. (in Japanese)

Tomlinson, B. (1992). *Report of the Inquiry into London's Health Service, Medical Education and Research.* Presented to the Secretaries of State for Health and Education. London: HMSO.

U.S. Department of Health and Human Services. (1980). *Promoting Health/Preventing Disease: Objectives for the Nation.* Washington, D.C.

U.S. Department of Health and Human Services. (1990). *Healthy People 2000. National Health Promotion and Disease Prevention Objectives.* Publication no. PHS 91–50212. Washington, D.C.

U.S. Department of Health, Education and Welfare. (1979). *Healthy People: Surgeon General's Report on Health Promotion and Disease Prevention.* Publication no. PHS 79–55071. Washington, D.C.

Williams, P. O. (1992). *Review of the Role of DH-Funded Research Units.* Report to the Director of Research and Development of a review team chaired by Dr. P. O. Williams. London: Department of Health.

PART II

Country Reports

AUSTRALIA

G. Dennis Calvert

MAJOR HEALTH PROBLEMS IN AUSTRALIA

In general, the major health problems are those found worldwide in relatively affluent, technologically advanced countries. Australia contains some pockets of poverty, particularly in some rural areas where Aboriginal communities may bear the brunt of unemployment and social disadvantage, in some inner-city areas where a number of homeless or unemployed people may be found, and in city suburbs where unemployment or the breakdown of family structures may be a problem.

Measures of Ill Health

There are many deficiencies in statistics on the health of Australians for a number of reasons. A national body, the Australian Institute of Health and Welfare, has been established to remedy this, and much of the data in this chapter on health status have been obtained from the institute.

There is no national register of Australian residents (citizens and noncitizens) that can be used to report health status. National or state registers (e.g., of those entitled to vote in national or state elections, or registers used for assessing income tax) are, generally speaking, used for one specific purpose and cannot be linked with health data. Some surveys recruit subjects from the electoral rolls on which particular groups of people (e.g., younger people, those without citizenship) are underrepresented or not represented.

There are no national data on the incidence of mental disorders or on the welfare of mentally ill people in the community. Data on use of mental health services are sparse and are confined mainly to data on the use of hospitals and other institutions. In the absence of a linked medical record system (in which admission of a single patient to more than one institution can be distinguished from admission of a different patient to each of these institutions), we cannot produce reliable data on the *incidence* of psychiatric (or other) conditions requiring hospital admission from the statistics on hospital admissions.

Increasingly, the actuality or likelihood of case-mix-based funding is driving hospitals to produce more accurate statistics on conditions requiring hospital admission. There are few data on the incidence of the many disorders in Australia that are nonlethal or that do not require hospital admission.

A number of indicators of ill health are available. Some indicators that give a national picture are discussed below.

Mortality

The most readily available indicators of the impact of ill health are mortality statistics. Life expectancy in Australia has been rising over this century; in 1920–1922, life expectancy at birth was 59.2 years for boys and 63.3 years for girls (d'Espaignet et al. 1991), while in 1992 the figures, respectively, were 74.5 years and 80.4 years. The major causes of death are circulatory disorders, with neoplasms the second major cause of death. (The mortality figures are taken from the Australian Institute of Health and Welfare [AIHW] publication *Australia's Health 1994*. The AIHW houses the National Death Index, which will contain records of all deaths in Australia since 1980.)

There are considerable differences in death rates between different states in Australia. The Northern Territory had a higher age-standardized death rate in 1992 (1,217 per 100,000 population for men, 924 per 100,000 population for women) than the total Australian population (855 per 100,000 and 520 per 100,000, respectively), reflecting increased mortality in the Aboriginal people (31 percent of the population in the Northern Territory). Other differences in death rates between states are not so large, and the explanation is unclear.

Following a steady rise in mortality from cardiovascular disease from 1920, a phase of decline began in about 1968 and has continued. In 1968 age-standardized cardiovascular disease death rates per 1,000 population were at their highest, 8.1 deaths per 1,000 for males and 5.3 deaths per 1,000 for females. In 1992 the death rates had fallen to less than half at 3.6 per 1,000 for males and 2.4 per 1,000 for females. Coronary heart disease (CHD) has been, and is, the main cause of cardiovascular death. CHD mortality is declining at an annual rate of 4.0 percent in men and 2.7 percent in women. Stroke mortality is declining at about 4.5 percent per year in men and women. The decline in death rate, occurring in all age groups affected by cardiovascular disease, has been attributed to both primary prevention (declining incidence of CHD, probably the main effect, associated with improvements in risk factors in the population) and improved medical care and treatment (ensuring that those who have a heart attack now have a better chance of survival).

In spite of this dramatic fall, cardiovascular disease is still the major cause of death for both men and women, accounting for 44.4 percent of deaths from all causes among Australians in 1992. The death rate for CHD and cardiovascular disease in Australia is still higher than in many other industrialized countries. The death rate from CHD in men is more than twice that in France and Spain, 60 percent more than in Italy, and almost five times that in Japan. Differences for women are of similar magnitude.

By contrast with cardiovascular disease, the death rate from cancers has remained relatively steady over the last 70 years. In 1965, death rates for males and females were, respectively, 2.0 and 1.3 per 1,000, while in 1992 this had risen slightly to 2.3 and 1.4 per 1,000, respectively. Cancer accounts for 27 percent of male deaths and 24 percent of female deaths, second only to circulatory disease deaths. Cancer registration is mandatory in each state and the Northern Territory.

Lung cancer in men and breast cancer in women account for 15.8 percent and 24.8 percent, respectively, of all cancers (excluding nonmelanocytic skin cancers), and each is the leading cause of death from cancer in that sex. Since about 1980 the death rate from lung cancer in men has been declining (probably the result of a fall in the number of men smoking). The death rate from lung cancer in women has been rising since 1970, and this may be the result of increased cigarette smoking by women.

Transport-related injury, particularly road accidents, is an important health problem, both because young people are disproportionately affected and because transport injuries use a substantial number of health services. Deaths per 100,000 population have been falling since 1970 when they were about 46 per 100,000 (in men) to 1992 when they fell below 20 per 100,000. This improvement has been ascribed to compulsory seat belt legislation, compulsory helmets for motor cyclists, better roads and cars, and better retrieval services.

Disability

Another index of the impact of chronic diseases is obtained by surveys of disability. Surveys from 1981 have used a definition of disability related to the World Health Organization's (WHO's) International Classification of Impairments, Disabilities, and Handicaps (ICIDH) conceptual framework (World Health Organization 1980), that disease or disorder or loss may lead to impairment, which may in turn lead to disability, which may in turn lead to handicap.

The 1993 Australian Bureau of Statistics survey of disability of aging and carers (Australian Bureau of Statistics 1993b) estimated that 18 percent of Australians were disabled in some way. The proportion of people reporting one or more disabilities rose with age, from 7 percent at 0 to 14 years to 67 percent of people aged 75 years or more. The most frequently reported primary disabling conditions were those of the musculoskeletal system and connective tissue, with 4.9 percent of Australians being disabled by these conditions. The next most frequently reported primary disabling conditions were hearing loss (2.6 percent) and mental disorders (2.0 percent). There must be some reservations about these percentages: For various reasons, hearing loss and mental disorders may be underreported in a national survey of disability. Continuity of care, for instance, for people with chronic mental illness, is a major problem, the dimensions of which are not completely clear (National Health Strategy 1993a). The true impact of dementia in older people is unknown. Alzheimer's disease, especially, is common and may not come to medical attention for some years if caregivers manage effectively.

All in all, the available data do not indicate that the overall health expectancy—that is, years of disability-free life, as distinct from life expectancy—is improving, at least not in the last few years (Mathers 1991).

Notifiable Communicable Diseases

A further index of disease impact is provided by notifiable communicable diseases. There is a statutory obligation on medical practitioners to notify these to health authorities. Although efforts are made to ensure accurate figures, it is accepted that the apparent incidence is less than the true incidence for all notifiable diseases, in part because of incomplete reporting.

Measles. Currently, the major immunization-preventable disease causing concern is measles. The impact of measles on morbidity and mortality has been reduced by an immunization program and antibiotic availability, but the disease is by no means controlled. Between 1921 and 1925 the mortality from measles was 5.7 per 100,000 per year for children up to 14 years. This fell steadily to 0.6 per 100,000 per year between 1961 and 1965, and to 0.1 per 100,000 per year between 1981 and 1985. By the early 1980s, there were an equal number of deaths from subacute sclerosing panencephalitis, a late complication of measles. Since 1991, measles has been a notifiable disease in all states and territories of Australia (figures from Australian Institute of Health and Welfare 1994, see also Communicable Diseases Network—Australia 1993).

The 1989–1990 National Health Survey found that approximately 90 percent of children aged one to six years were reported to be fully immunized against measles. However, serology surveys are generally lacking; there are few data on the prevalence of measles antibody in children in whom immunization has been reported. Causer et al. (1994) found that about 90 percent of children who had documented proof of immunization were antibody positive, and 80 percent of children who reported immunization but did not have documentation were antibody positive.

Since 1990, there has been a pattern of sporadic outbreaks of measles in the various states of Australia. In 1988, there were 45 cases of measles reported and in 1989, 69 cases. In 1990 this jumped to 221 cases, and the annual number of cases has remained above 200 ever since.

HIV Infection and AIDS. The AIDS (acquired immunodeficiency syndrome) epidemic in Australia is made up of several subepidemics, all of which appear to have peaked. After notifications rose from 127 in 1985 to 763 in 1991, they declined slightly to 692 in 1992. Those notified with AIDS are overwhelmingly males (since 1986, over 95 percent are males), and the mean age for males and females with AIDS is about 38 to 40 years. Over 50 percent of those notified are in New South Wales, 20 to 30 percent in Victoria, about 10 percent or less in Western Australia. The largest category is homosexual or bisexual men (about 80 percent or more of notified cases). Heterosexual contact accounts for about 6 percent of cases. People with hemophilia, and those receiving blood transfusion, had a peak incidence in 1989 and 1985, respectively, and currently about 2 percent of cases fall in this category. Injecting drug users are an important subgroup; heterosexual drug users account for about 1 to 3 percent of those with AIDS and homosexual or bisexual men who use drugs about 2 to 6 percent (figures from Australian Institute of Health and Welfare 1994).

Australia has had, by comparison with a number of countries, a very successful strategy to control and lessen the spread of AIDS. The goals are to eliminate transmission of the human immunodeficiency virus (HIV) and to minimize the personal and social impact of HIV infection (National HIV/AIDS Strategy 1993), and methods have included various means of health promotion, education, research, and the establishment of specialized services.

Sexually Transmitted Diseases. Perhaps the two most important notifiable sexually transmitted diseases, apart from AIDS, are gonococcal infection and syphilis. In 1992, there were almost 3,000 cases of gonococcal infection notified and almost 2,700 cases of syphilis. Major differences between states are apparent; in the Northern Territory the notification rate for gonococcal infection is 441 per 100,000 population, whereas in Tasmania and the Australian Capital Territory it is 3 per 100,000. Similarly for syphilis, the notification rate varies from 276 per 100,000 population in the Northern Territory to 2 in Victoria, the Australian Capital Territory, and Tasmania. Although there is scope for improvement in statistical collections, there is also an indication of high prevalence of sexually transmitted diseases in certain population groups (figures from Australian Institute of Health and Welfare 1994).

Population Subgroups

Low Socioeconomic Status. People with the most limited economic and educational resources experience poorer health as measured by standardized death rates and measures of illness (National Health Strategy 1992; Australian Institute of Health and Welfare 1994). Overall, those of low socioeconomic status are:

- More likely to suffer disability (men and women on low incomes are 138 percent and 38 percent, respectively, more likely to suffer disability than men and women on high incomes);
- More likely to have serious chronic illnesses (men and women on low incomes report

58 percent and 32 percent, respectively, more serious chronic illnesses than men and women on high incomes);

- More likely to have suffered recent illnesses (low-income men and women report about 25 percent more recent illnesses than men and women on high incomes); and
- Most likely to report being in fair/poor health as opposed to good/excellent health (low-income men and women are 167 percent and 148 percent, respectively, more likely than high-income men and women to view their health in this way) (all figures from Australian Institute of Health and Welfare 1994).

A number of health-related variables are disproportionately associated with low socioeconomic status. For instance, low-income men are 40 percent more likely to smoke than high-income men. Women who have received low levels of education are 68 percent more likely to be overweight than women who have received high levels of education. Men in the most socioeconomically disadvantaged areas are 26 percent more likely to be inactive than those in the least socioeconomically disadvantaged areas (National Health Strategy 1992).

Compared with people of high socioeconomic status, those of low socioeconomic status make greater use of hospitals, outpatient clinics, and doctors. For instance, low-income men are 71 percent more likely to have a hospital episode, 36 percent more likely to visit the doctor, and 138 percent more likely to use an outpatient clinic than high-income men. Low-income women are 19 percent more likely to visit a doctor and 152 percent more likely to visit an out-patient clinic than high-income women (National Health Strategy 1992).

Australians Living in Nonmetropolitan Areas. The provision of equity in health, including redressing those imbalances and improving health care provision and outcomes, is seen by many as a major health problem. About 36 percent of Australians live outside capital cities, half in major regional centers and the remainder in rural and remote areas. Among men and women aged 25 to 64 years, nonmetropolitan residents experience higher mortality than metropolitan residents; 15 percent higher for men and 9 percent higher for women during 1985–1987. Nonmetropolitan residents have higher mortality rates for a number of causes of death including coronary heart disease, cerebrovascular disease, diabetes (in women only), traffic accidents, and pneumonia/influenza (Australian Institute of Health and Welfare 1994). Differences between metropolitan and nonmetropolitan areas in terms of morbidity are not easy to interpret, and the picture is confounded by the difficulty of access of health care in some rural locations.

Older People. The proportion of older people in the Australian population is rising. In 1989, 11 percent of the Australian population were age 65 or more, but by the year 2031, the proportion will have risen to over 20 percent (Australian Bureau of Statistics, 1990). The cost of health care rises with age, with increased use of major surgical procedures (e.g., coronary artery bypass grafts), implants and prostheses, treatments for cataract, and insertions of cardiac pacemakers in the aged. Techniques including laparoscopic surgery, catheter-based techniques, and noninvasive techniques such as extracorporeal shock wave lithotripsy allow effective surgery to be carried out at an older age than previously. The use of drugs increases with age. It is expected, therefore, that if the current rates and types of treatment persist, the total cost of health care will rise with an expansion of the need for health care for the elderly.

Aboriginal and Torres Strait Islander People. Aboriginal people, although in better health now than some 20 years ago, still carry a greater burden of ill health as manifested by increased rates of hospitalization, maternal mortality, mortality in adults, and disability than non-Aboriginal Australians. They are more likely to be unemployed and in poor housing than other Australians, and there is no doubt that these factors contribute to poor health. A great deal has been written on Aboriginal health (see Thomson and Merrifield 1988) without very great advances being made in health status, at least for Aborigines living in rural/remote areas.

Death rates of Aboriginal people greatly exceed the corresponding total Australian rates at all ages, with the ratio of age-standardized mortality rates being 2.8 for males and 3.3 for females (Australian Institute of Health and Welfare 1994). This excess mortality is not evenly spread; Aboriginal people in rural/remote areas and those living on the fringes of country towns take the brunt of excess mortality; those living in urban areas appear, on the whole, to have an excess mortality little different from that of non-Aboriginal people in similar socioeconomic circumstances. (In the Northern Territory the difference between Aboriginal and non-Aboriginal mortality rates is considerable. The Aboriginal death rate in the 30–34 age group was seven times greater than that of non-Aborigines for males and 13 times greater for females in 1979–1983 (Northern Territory Department of Health 1986), and the overall picture for adults in rural and remote areas appears to have changed little since then (Australian Institute of Health and Welfare 1994).

The major improvements that have been wrought in Aboriginal life expectancy over the past 20 years have been achieved mainly through reduction in infant mortality. However, the expectation of life at birth still remains lower for Aboriginals than the total Australian population. The proportion of newborn boys that can expect to live to age 65 is 45 percent for Aboriginals but 81 percent for non-Aboriginals; and for girls 54 percent of newborn Aboriginal girls can expect to live to 65, compared to 89 percent of newborn non-Aboriginal girls. The major cause of death in Aboriginal men and women is cardiovascular disease, in many cases, secondary to the insulin resistance syndrome (which includes abdominal obesity). Other contributing causes of cardiovascular disease include alcoholism or excess alcohol intake (which may also be a cause of injury, the major component of the second highest cause of premature death in Aboriginal men) and cigarette smoking. There is, however, increased mortality in Aboriginal adults (c.f. non-Aboriginals) for almost all causes of mortality, and ischemic heart disease, cerebrovascular disease, cancers, injury, and poisoning account for most deaths.

Immigrants and Refugees. The 1991 Australian census noted that 22.3 percent of Australians were born outside Australia, and 12.9 percent were born in countries where English was not the main language. In general, recent migrants enjoy better health in terms of mortality and morbidity than people born in Australia, and there appear to be no substantial short-term health disadvantages associated with immigrant status. Refugees are a heterogeneous group, and there are some among them who have suffered physical or psychological trauma and even torture, and who will bear scars. As the period of residence increases, overall health may decline, and this may be associated with deficient skills in English language or socioeconomic dislocation and loss of status in Australia (Donovan et al. 1992).

PROVISION, UTILIZATION, AND IMPACT OF HEALTH SERVICES

Organization of Health Services

The health care system in Australia is complex and involves each of the three levels of government—Commonwealth and state and local governments—as well as public and private providers.

The government of the Commonwealth of Australia includes a Department of Health, which bears various other responsibilities as reflected in the departmental name (currently, the Department of Human Services and Health). A good description of its structure and functions may be found in Commonwealth Department of Human Services and Health (1994b). The Commonwealth Department of Health administers major benefit schemes that include medical, pharmaceutical, hospital, and nursing home services. It manages a number of other health programs, many of which involve specific funding. The Commonwealth out of its taxation income provides specific-purpose grants to states for the health care system.

Other Commonwealth government agencies are variably responsible for aspects of health. The health of Aboriginal and Torres Strait Islander people has been of Commonwealth concern, and an office for Aboriginal and Torres Strait Islander Health Services has been established within the Department of Human Services and Health in 1995.

State and Territory Health administrations are responsible for hospital services; mental health programs; systems of extended care; child, adolescent, and family health services; dental health services; women's health programs; health promotion; rehabilitation systems; and regulatory functions. In addition, State Health Departments have systems in place for monitoring items such as expenditure and standards of performance.

Local government authorities (e.g., city or county councils) employ health surveyors to survey environmental hygiene and sanitation practices, including food practices. Other state government or semiautonomous authorities are responsible for air quality monitoring and regulation, the quality of piped water, and sewage disposal and drainage (e.g., Environmental Protection Agency, Water Boards).

Provision of Hospital and Medical Care

In 1991–1992, while most hospitals were in the public system, just over a quarter of acute hospital beds were in private hospitals, run either by religious or charitable organizations or proprietors operating for profit (Australian Institute of Health and Welfare 1994). In 1995, these figures are substantially unchanged.

Medical care outside hospitals is based on general practitioners, mostly in private practice, who can refer people to hospitals. Medical specialists are employed by hospitals or health organizations but can also work in a private practice as specialist consultants, in many cases earning income from hospital work.

The Commonwealth Department of Veterans' Affairs arranges medical care for ex-service personnel and beneficiaries, in most cases through the general medical system.

Public and Private Health Insurance

Medicare is a universal system of health insurance that has been in operation since 1984. An outline is given in *Australia's Health 1994* (Australian Institute of Health 1994). Medicare is administered by a Commonwealth statutory authority, the Health Insurance Commission, which also administers the Pharmaceutical Benefits Scheme, and is funded from taxation revenue. All people normally resident in Australia except foreign diplomats and their dependents are eligible for Medicare benefits. A schedule for fees has been established, and benefits for medical services in the community relate to that schedule. Doctors are not obliged to adhere to the scheduled fees, but if they direct bill the Health Insurance Commission for any service, the amount payable is the Medicare benefit and the patient is not required to pay any additional amount. Doctors may charge the patient directly, and the patient may be, in part or wholly, reimbursed by Medicare. Benefits are also paid for services provided by optometrists and for oral surgery by dental surgeons.

Agreements between the Commonwealth and state and territory governments provide for all Medicare beneficiaries to obtain inpatient and noninpatient care at public hospitals without charge. Medical care is provided for such "public" patients at no cost to them by doctors appointed by the hospitals.

Private health insurance can be purchased to cover charges in private hospitals and for private status in public hospitals. Private health insurance may also be purchased to cover other costs, for example optometry, physiotherapy, and ambulance fees.

The Pharmaceutical Benefits Scheme subsidizes the cost of a wide range of drugs and medicinal preparations. There is a set price for every item covered by the scheme. Concessional beneficiaries pay $2.60 for each item, and others pay the first $16 for each item, and in some cases where a specific brand costs more than the basic level for the drug, they pay an additional amount.

Health Care Financing

In 1992–1993, health expenditure by Australian governments and individuals was $34.338 billion, an average of $1,944 per person (Australian Institute of Health and Welfare 1994). Health expenditure represented 8.5 percent of gross domestic product (GDP), an increase of 0.8 percent from recent years. Of the total amount expended on health, governments provided $23.2 billion, the Commonwealth government providing $15.1 billion and state and local governments $8.1 billion, and the private sector $11.1 billion. When expressed in absolute terms, health expenditure has been rising steadily, about 2.7 times between 1971 and 1993. As a percentage of GDP, expenditure has risen from about 5.3 percent in 1970 to about 8.5 percent in 1993. The excess health care inflation rate is low, at 0.1 percent, and it appears that a major contributor to control of growth and ratio of health expenditure to GDP is the control of price increases in the health sector.

THE INFRASTRUCTURE OF TRAINING AND RESEARCH IN PUBLIC HEALTH

Training in Public Health

The Public Health Education and Research Program provides funds to nine universities to strengthen postgraduate education and research in public and tropical health (Commonwealth Department of Human Services and Health 1994b). The Master of Public Health (MPH) degree is taught in these, and other, universities. Those taking MPH degrees include medical and nursing personnel and some with backgrounds in other fields. In those universities supported by the Public Health Education and Research Program, public health was until recently (generally) taught in a Department of Public Health or Community Medicine within a Faculty of Medicine. In other universities, public health is generally taught by a Department of Public Health in a Faculty of Health Sciences (or similar name), which may include disciplines such as nursing and psychology.

Current Public Health Education and Research Program funding rules encourage public health consortiums, with two or more universities collaborating in teaching public health in a city or state, and there are several such consortiums.

State governments are individually responsible for public health within the state. Each state has a public health system, which allows medical and nonmedical personnel to train "on the job" in public health. For instance, the most populous state, New South Wales, has a network of public health units, and public health trainees have an opportunity to gain experience in several units during a two-year training program.

A professional body involved in accrediting rather than training public health practitioners, the Australasian Faculty of Public Health Medicine is affiliated with the Royal Australasian College of Physicians. It accredits individual training programs for medical graduates and examines candidates in public health medicine for membership to the faculty. A Commonwealth program for accrediting public health training programs in universities has been recommended and will be implemented in 1996.

Research in Public Health

Research in public health is largely financed by Commonwealth and state government agencies, though some nongovernment agencies (e.g., National Heart Foundation, Diabetes Australia, Cancer Councils) may direct some funds to research in public health.

Health research is funded by the Commonwealth in several ways (Commonwealth Department of Human Services and Health 1994b). The National Health and Medical Research Council (NHMRC) recommends funding by two mechanisms: the Medical Research Endowment Fund, administered by the Medical Research Committee (MRC) (which funds research and training in health and medical research), and the Public Health Research and Development Council (PHRDC), which funds research into social and public health. Although some funding provided by the MRC is for public health initiatives, most is not. In 1994 the PHRDC funded 51 project grants, 6 larger program grants, and 23 small grants; the success rate for project grant funding was 18 percent.

The Commonwealth government through the Research and Development Grants Advisory Committee also funds social and behavioral research in areas of direct relevance to the department's policy and program responsibilities. In recent years, these areas have included rural women's health, rural and remote service provision, child poverty and adversity, child health, aging and well-being, and postnatal depression. These projects are generally investigator driven.

Both Commonwealth and state governments may tender for public health research to be carried out in areas relevant to government policy.

MAJOR CHALLENGES FOR THE HEALTH SERVICES

Equity of Access

Equity of access to health services has not been fully achieved. Rural areas, particularly those remote from major population centers, containing some 3 million Australians, are not as well served as urban areas. This is of particular concern when the population in some rural or remote communities is substantially Aboriginal. A combination of unemployment, poverty of resources, and poor education can lead to the demoralization of Aboriginal communities and poor health outcomes, and this may be compounded by lack of access to health services.

Those mentally ill people whose illness incapacitates but does not bring them to effective contact with the health services may also be said to lack equitable access to health services. Many support services for such people are in the hands of religious groups or other nongovernmental organizations, and access to services is unevenly distributed through Australia.

Equity of Outcomes

Good health is not equally accessed by all groups of society, and a great many factors contribute to this apart from lack of access to health services. Aboriginal people, poor people, and unemployed people in general suffer worse health than those not in these categories. The solutions to achieving equity in health involve other sectors in society as well as the health services. Achievement of effective targeted intersectoral collaboration for good health is a difficult task, not least because it is difficult to define such interventions in ways that can be politically implemented and give measurable health outcomes.

Even in areas of health promotion that are the responsibility of the health system, there are difficulties in reaching and influencing all who might benefit. Programs are usually more likely to benefit middle-class educated people than poorer people or people with a non-English-speaking background.

The Overall Structure and Financing of the Health Services

The Commonwealth government distributes funds for health services through a variety of arrangements to each state (including, especially, hospital funding grants). It also makes payments to local government (for aged and disabled persons' homes and hostels, children's services, etc.). Other services are directly paid for by the Commonwealth, including the system of universal health insurance, Medicare, which will pay for some or all of a consultation with a general practitioner. The Commonwealth also directly funds a pharmaceutical benefit scheme.

This system of divided responsibilities does not always lead to the most effective use of health service resources. State-supported hospitals may prefer to conserve their budgets and promote the use of private practice medical care (paid by the Commonwealth) where possible, although hospital-based delivery of care may be preferable on other grounds (e.g., a hospital may best be able to provide specialist multidisciplinary outpatient clinics or highly specialized treatment). If a patient is discharged early to the care of a general practitioner, and asked to collect drugs from a pharmacy outside the hospital, the Commonwealth will fund much of the cost. Such cost-shifting between state and Commonwealth has been recognized as a problem, but the solution would require a major health service restructuring that does not appear likely in the near future.

Many aspects of the structure and financing of the Australian health services were canvased in a series of background and issues papers known as the National Health Strategy (Division of Health, Housing and Community Services, 1990–1993, e.g., National Health Strategy 1993b). These have stimulated a debate on reform of the Australian health system. The debate has been formed also by the many changes that have been taking place internationally as countries attempt to contain health care costs and at the same time ensure a tolerable degree of equity in the health care system.

Health Goals and Targets

At the national level, goals, targets, and strategies are being developed as an initial step toward improving health outcomes. Definition of goals and targets should advance efforts to restructure the health system, improve data collection, and rationalize roles, responsibilities, and resource allocation.

The initial focus on cardiovascular disease, cancer, mental health, and injury is set within the broader framework of the National Health Policy, which specifies national goals in the areas of social justice, access and participation, intersectoral action, and healthy lifestyles. The goal in the area of social justice is to reduce the level of health inequalities in Australia, with emphasis particularly on Aboriginal and Torres Strait Islander peoples, people of non-English-speaking backgrounds, and socioeconomically disadvantaged Australians. Goals in the area of healthy lifestyles relate to the prevalence of smoking; to premature death, illness, and injury associated with alcohol use; to increasing participation in regular physical activity; and to reducing the consequences of diet-related cardiovascular disease (with a focus on blood cholesterol, obesity, and high blood pressure).

Goals in cardiovascular health include a number of specific goals relating to risk factors and to treatment and continuing care. Three major strategies relate to the development of specific strategies for priority groups, the development of best practice guidelines for a number of areas, and better data monitoring systems.

Goals for cancer control relate to lung cancer (with emphasis on smoking control), skin cancer (both melanotic and nonmelanotic), cancer of the cervix, breast cancer, colorectal cancer, and prostate cancer.

Prevention of injuries includes strategies aimed at suicide, transport-related injury, work-related injury, fall injury, sport injury, interpersonal violence, consumer product–related injury, burns and scalds, poisoning, drowning, postinjury management, and rehabilitation.

Mental health strategies are directed primarily at depression, schizophrenia, and suicide.

Health Outcomes, Marginal Benefit Analysis, and Resource Allocation

Together with definition of targets, there is an emphasis throughout Australia on the measurement of health outcomes. The concept of health outcome measurement is simple: What is the effect of a health service intervention? The practice is rather less simple. The outcome of a diagnostic procedure or a specific treatment may be easy to estimate, although planners tend to lose sight of the fact that to measure outcomes in terms of duration of life or quality of life or long-term morbidity may be an extremely expensive and difficult exercise—witness the many millions of dollars that have had to be spent to show that lowering blood cholesterol decreases the risk of subsequent heart attack, or prolongs life, or that the intensive treatment of insulin-dependent diabetes delays the onset of neural or renal or visual complications. The outcome of a recommendation designed to prevent disease, say one recommending dietary change or more exercise, may in the real world be impossible to measure.

Similarly, the analysis of marginal benefits (''If I take away $\$\times000$ from this health service program, what will be the disbenefit, and if I allocate it to any of these other programs, what will be the benefits? By making a number of judgments of this kind, can I improve the allocation of resources in the health service?'') promises much, but there is a considerable amount of work to be done before this can be counted a useful tool in health service resource allocation.

The rational allocation of health resources will continue to preoccupy much of the time of those who develop health service policy, and for the foreseeable future policymakers will steer a difficult course between the rocks of politics and public opinion and the whirlpools of economic theory and rationalism.

REFERENCES

Australian Bureau of Statistics. (1990). *Estimated Resident Population by Sex and Age. States and Territories of Australia.* Catalogue no. 3201.0. Canberra.

Australian Bureau of Statistics. (1993a). *Deaths Australia.* Catalogue no. 3302.0. Canberra.

Australian Bureau of Statistics. (1993b). *Disability, Ageing and Carers: Summary of Findings.* Australia 1993. Catalogue no. 4430.0. Canberra.

Australian Institute of Health and Welfare. (1994). *Australia's Health 1994.* The Fourth Biennial Health Report of the Australian Institute of Health and Welfare. Canberra: Australian Government Publishing Service.

Causer, J., Karr, M., Fett, M., & Mira, M. (1994). *The Prevalence of Serological Evidence of Immunity to Measles, Mumps and Rubella in Preschool Children.* Paper presented at the Thirteenth Scientific Meeting of International Epidemiological Association, Sydney, 26–29 September 1993.

Commonwealth Department of Human Services and Health. (1994a). *Better Health Outcomes for Australians. National Goals, Targets and Strategies for Better Health*

Outcomes into the Next Century. Canberra: Australian Government Publishing Service.

Commonwealth Department of Human Services and Health. (1994b). *Department of Human Services and Health. Annual Report 1993–94*. Canberra: Australian Government Publishing Service.

Communicable Diseases Network—Australia. (1993). *Annual Report of the National Notifiable Diseases Surveillance System 1991*. Communicable Diseases Intelligence 16. Canberra: Australian Institute of Health and Welfare.

Crowley, S., Antioch, K., Carter, R., Waters, A.-M., Conway, L. & Mathers, C. (1992). *The Cost of Diet-Related Disease in Australia*. Australian Institute of Health and Welfare. Canberra:

d'Espaignet, E. T., van Ommeren, M., Taylor, F., Briscoe, N. & Pentony, P. (1991). *Trends in Australian Mortality 1921–1988*. Australian Institute of Health Mortality Series no. 1. Canberra: Australian Government Publishing Service.

Donovan, J., d'Espaignet, E., Merton, C. & van Ommeren, M. (Eds.). (1992). *Immigrants in Australia: A Health Profile*. Australian Institute of Health and Welfare: Ethnic Health Series no 1. Canberra: Australian Government Publishing Service.

Mathers, C. (1991). *Health Expectancies in Australia 1981 and 1988*. Australian Institute of Health. Canberra: Australian Government Publishing Service.

National Health Strategy. (1992). *Enough to Make You Sick. How Income and Environment Affect Health*. National Health Strategy Research Paper no 1. Canberra: Department of Health, Housing and Community Services.

National Health Strategy. (1993a). *Help Where Help Is Needed. Continuity of Care for People With Chronic Mental Illness*. National Health Strategy Issues Paper no. 5. Canberra: Department of Health, Housing and Community Services.

National Health Strategy. (1993b). *Pathways to Better Health*. National Health Strategy Issues Paper no. 7. Canberra: Department of Health, Housing and Community Services.

National HIV/AIDS Strategy. (1993). *National HIV/AIDS Strategy 1993–94 to 1995–96*. Canberra: Australian Government Publishing Service.

Northern Territory Department of Health. (1986). *Health Indicators in the Northern Territory*. Canberra: Northern Territory Department of Health.

Thomson, N. & Merrifield, P. (1988). *Aboriginal Health, an Annotated Bibliography*. Canberra: Australian Institute of Health.

World Health Organization. (1980). *Classification of Impairments, Disabilities and Handicaps*. Geneva: WHO.

BRAZIL

José Carvalho de Noronha and Eduardo Levcovitz

GENERAL INFORMATION

Brazil is the fifth largest country in the world, occupying a surface of 8,547,403 square kilometers. It borders all the countries in South America with the exception of Chile and Ecuador, and it has a coastline 7,367 kilometers long bathed by the Atlantic Ocean. It is inhabited by 155,589,212 (est. 1994, last census 1991) persons, most of them concentrated in the Southeastern region (42.6 percent), composed of the states of São Paulo, Rio de Janeiro, Minas Gerais, and Espírito Santo (FIBGE 1992). The Brazilian population is a mixture of various cultural and racial groups, and peoples of mixed races increase their share. African influence along the coast to the north, multicultural European influence (Italian, German, and Spanish) to the south, and more recently, Japanese influence in the state of São Paulo give to the basic Portuguese and native Indians the multicultural face of Brazilian people. Portuguese is spoken all over the country.

The majority of populated Brazil is under a humid tropical (temperatures over 20°C and 1,000 to 1,500 millimeters precipitation) and subtropical climate (mean temperatures under 20°C), except for a semiarid region in the Northeast. The legal Amazon, about 5 million square kilometers large, has an equatorial climate (mean temperatures between 23° and 26°C and over 2,500 millimeters of precipitation per year) (Editora Abril 1995).

Brazil is a federal republic divided into 26 states and one federal district. A president is directly elected every four years and governs assisted by ministers of state, freely designated. Legislative power is exercised by the National Congress, composed of the Chamber of Deputies and the Federal Senate. The deputies are directly and proportionally elected every four years, and three senators

Figure 1
Structure of Production Share of Gross National Product, Brazil, 1970, 1975, 1980, 1985

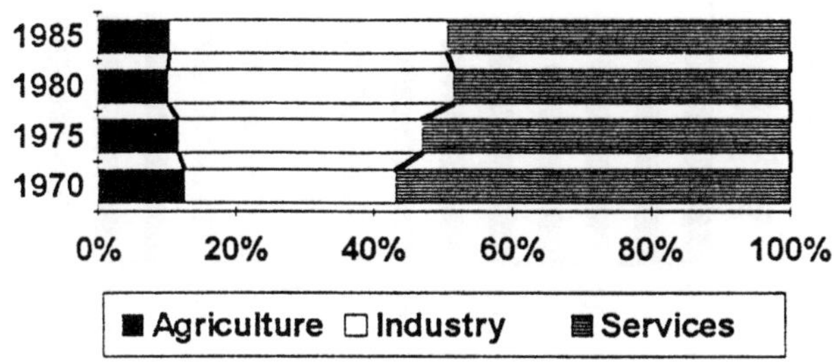

Source: FIBGE 1992.

are directly elected by state every eight years (two and one, alternatively, every four years). Each state is governed by a governor and a legislative assembly elected every four years. The states are divided into municipalities administered by a mayor (*prefeito*) and a local council. The judiciary is composed of several institutions. At the federal level, the highest court is the Federal Supreme Court, named by the president with approval of the Senate.

At the end of the military regime (1985), political parties became free to organize. Today the main political parties are, from the Right to the Left, the Republican Popular Party (PPR), the Party of the Liberal Front (PFL), the Party of the Brazilian Democratic Movement (PMDB), the Labor Democratic Party (PDT), and the Laborers Party (PT).

Economy

Brazil has a very diversified economy. It evolved from a primary producer and exporter until the middle of this century to a fairly industrialized country (Figure 1). In the recent past, during the late 1960s and 1970s, until the oil crisis, it experienced a very high rate of growth, industrial production rising at an average of 10 percent per annum. Agriculture's share in the gross national product (GNP) declined, and coffee, which accounted for 44 percent of Brazil's exports in 1965, was substituted for industrial goods as the main group of exports—67 percent in 1985.

After the oil and debt crises around 1980, the country underwent a period of stagnation and inflation that only very recently, 1993, commenced to subside (Figure 2). In 1994, the country underwent a deep monetary reform that brought down inflation from 40 percent a month to around 2 percent at the beginning of 1995.

In spite of having the tenth largest gross national product in the world (U.S.$456 billion in 1993), the strength of its industrial basis, and its capacity

Figure 2
Gross National Product, Brazil, 1980–1993

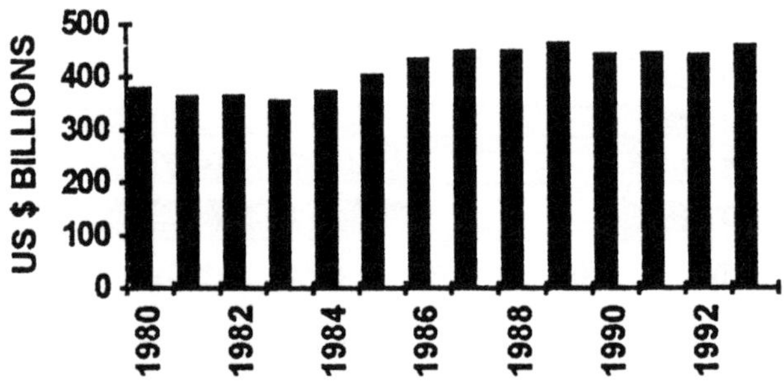

Source: Editora Abril 1995.

to overcome the big crises of the world economy in the 1980s and early 1990s, Brazil has been unable to find a way to reduce its huge inequities. About 30 percent of the population, or 45 million persons, earn less than twice the minimum wage, or R$140.00, equivalent to U.S. $164.00, per month (FIBGE 1992). The Gini coefficients were 0.5644 in 1980 and 0.6024 in 1990. In 1991, the wealthiest 10 percent appropriated 48.1 percent of the national income, while the poorest 50 percent participated with 12.1 percent. There are regional differences, the Northeast concentrating the greater part of the country's poor (Tavares and Monteiro 1994) (Figure 3).

Population

Brazil is facing a slow but steady decrease in its rate of population growth. From 1950 to 1960, its population grew 34.9 percent; from 1960 to 1970, 32.9 percent; from 1970 to 1980, 27.8 percent, and 23.5 percent from 1980 to 1991, the year of the last census. Recent projections estimate that the population will stabilize around 250 million around 2045. The fertility rate (number of children per woman in childbearing age) decreased from 6.16 in 1940 to 2.70 in 1990 (Editora Abril 1995). The age structure reveals a young population but already in a transitional stage (Table 1).

During the last 50 years, Brazil saw a large shift in the distribution of the population to urban areas. In 1940, only 30.24 percent lived in cities, as compared to 75.47 percent in 1991. The nine metropolitan regions of the country—Belém, Belo Horizonte, Curitiba, Fortaleza, Porto Alegre, Recife, Rio de Janeiro, Salvador, and São Paulo—accounted for 29.04 percent of the Brazilian population (Editora Abril 1995). More recently, there has been a decrease in rates of growth of the large metropolitan areas and a movement toward middle-sized (200,000 to 500,000 population) cities.

Figure 3
Income Distribution per Region: Up to 2 and More Than 20 Minimum Wages, Brazil, 1990

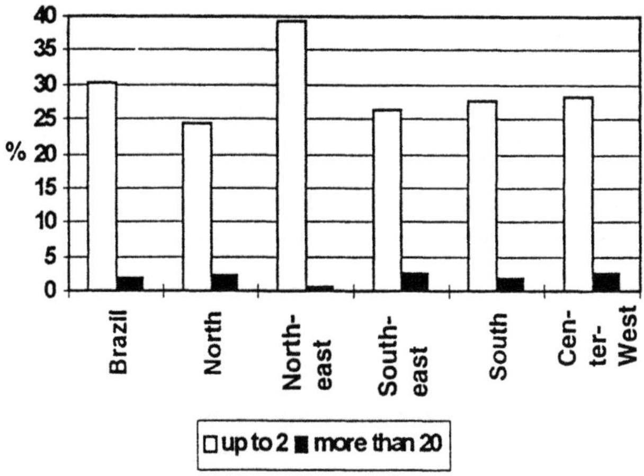

Source: FIBGE 1992.

MAJOR HEALTH PROBLEMS FACING THE COUNTRY

During the second half of this century, Brazil started to show a reduction in both natality and mortality rates (Figure 4). Life expectancy at birth rose from 52.7 years in 1970 to 60.1 in 1980 and 65.6 in 1990 (Tavares and Monteiro 1994). Infant mortality rates also showed a decrease in the 1980s—they dropped from 82 per 1,000 live births in 1980 to 59 in 1989. These improvements can be attributed to a decrease in birthrates, to a general improvement in sanitary conditions (mainly water supply), an increase in immunization coverage, and better education of women in childbearing age. In spite of these reductions, the regional differences are still very striking. In the Northeast the rates were 92 per 1,000 live births, as compared to 35 in the Southeast region in 1989 (Szwarcwald, Oliveira and Sabroza 1992). There are municipalities with rates as low as 10 and others as high as 135.

The developed world faced an epidemiological transition during this century, with the infectious diseases associated with poverty, undernourishment, and lack of sanitation giving way to chronic degenerative conditions. More recently, developed countries began to face new problems, mainly in their urban areas, with an increase of pollution-associated diseases and trauma as a result of urban violence (called *urban malaria* by Berlinguer in 1976). Brazil, like similar countries with delayed industrialization, did not follow the same patterns. Actually, it presents a sort of juxtaposition of mortality and morbidity patterns of different

Table 1
Age Structure of Brazilian Population, 1970, 1980, 1991

Age Group	1970	1980	1991
0 to 14 yr.	41.9%	38.2%	34.7%
14 to 60 yr.	52.9%	55.5%	57.8%
More than 60 yr.	5.0%	6.2%	7.3%
Ignored	0.2%	0.1%	0.2%

Source: Editora Abril 1995.

epochs. One can find coexisting side by side health problems of three kinds—homicides, acute coronary disease, and tuberculosis, for example—at similar high rates. It is true that nowadays cardiovascular diseases and trauma lead the causes of death, but infectious diseases are still present among the main groups of causes of death (Table 2).

The age structure of mortality also improved in the last years, although there is a high proportion of deaths in younger age groups (Figure 5).

The main causes of death, by age group, are:

Less than 5 years	Diarrheal diseases and lower respiratory infections
5 to 14 years	Transport accident, drowning, and pneumonia
5 to 39 years	Homicides, transport accidents, and ischemic heart disease
40 to 69 years	Cerebrovascular, ischemic heart disease, and neoplasms
More than 70 years	Ischemic heart disease, cerebrovascular, and respiratory

Morbidity

Poliomyelitis has been eradicated from the country after national immunization campaigns (Table 3). Measles, which used to be a big killer of children under five, is now being put under control. Diphtheria, pertussis, and tetanus also show an important reduction in the last years, but their incidence is still high. Leprosy and tuberculosis are endemic in many areas of the country, and malaria is highly endemic in the Amazonian region. In 1992 the country faced an epidemic of cholera that came through the Amazon basin from Peru. The state of Rio de Janeiro and four other states presented with an epidemic outburst of dengue in 1992. In 1995, Rio was facing another one of less magnitude. AIDS (acquired immunodeficiency syndrome) is a growing epidemic.

Figure 4
Crude Birth- and Death Rates per 1,000 Persons, Brazil, 1890–1990

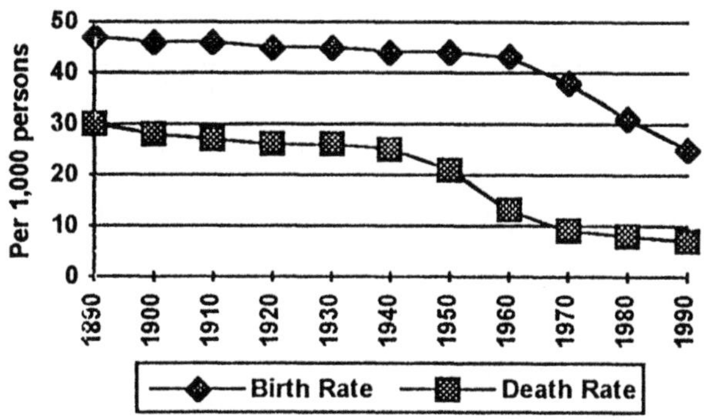

Source: Tavares and Monteiro 1994.

HEALTH CARE DELIVERY

The beginnings of the development of health care in Brazil are centers in the liberal practice of physicians and in the organization of charitable institutions, namely the Holy Houses of Mercy and the Beneficent Hospitals, directed to the care of the poor (Tavares and Monteiro 1994). The first House of Mercy was founded in 1543 in São Vicente. In 1741, a lazaretto was created in Rio de Janeiro, and several military hospitals were inaugurated in barracks and in Jesuitical schools after they were banished in 1759. Public hospitals were dedicated to the treatment of lepers and later to shelter lunatics, phthisics, and fever patients. The first general care public hospital was established only in 1920 in the city of Rio de Janeiro. Public health actions were directed mainly to specific problems, such as the fight against yellow fever or malaria. After independence from Portugal (1822), the first laws ordering the functioning of local councils (1828) established the first structured program of public hygiene. This movement gained strong support with the foundation of the Society of Medicine and Surgery in 1829. In 1808 the first School of Surgery in Salvador (Goncalves 1982) was created.

One has to wait until the beginnings of the twentieth century to find a structured policy of the central government regarding medical care. In an attempt to organize and expand the coverage of care provided by the friendly societies founded in the 1890s, a law was passed in 1923, known as Lei Elói Chaves, to regulate the functioning of the Caixas de Aposentadorias e Pensões (CAPs) (the friendly societies that provided retirement and health benefits, among others). This law and subsequent decrees determined, on the health side, that every caixa should provide inpatient care and drug prescription coverage. In 1933 the federal

Table 2
Main Groups of Cause of Death

Rates per 100,000 inhabitants, Brazil 1981, 1985, 1989

Group of Cause ICD-9	*1981* Number	*1981* Rates	*1985* Number	*1985* Rates	*1989* Number	*1989* Rates
Circulatory System	192,272	159.02	214,193	164.11	228,790	162.39
External Causes	71,833	59.41	85,845	65.77	102,252	72.58
Infectious Diseases	64,163	53.07	49,946	38.27	45,023	31.96
Neoplasms	62,947	52.06	71,023	54.42	80,614	57.22
Respiratory System	58,545	48.42	62,329	47.75	66,024	46.86
Perinatal Causes	54,898	45.40	46,419	35.57	41,191	29.24

Source: Ministry of Health 1994.

government (Getúlio Vargas was the president) created an Instituto de Aposentadoria e Pensões dos Marítimos—IAPM (literally Institute of Retirement and Pensions of Seamen) that inaugurated a series of similar institutes (IAPs) for other professional groups. These institutes had a tripartite management—workers, employers, and government representatives—and were funded by payroll taxes equally collected from employers and employees and coverage of ''administrative costs'' by the federal government (Oliveira and Teixeira 1986). These initiatives followed the emergence of a new urban-industrial pattern in Brazilian society.

From 1946 until the military coup d'état in 1964, the country lived a democratic experience and a period of economic development. The IAPs rapidly expanded their medical coverage schemes, some of them building hospitals and outpatient facilities, others contracting services to the private sector. States and municipalities also invested in health services, mainly in emergency services, covering the population that was not formally employed and therefore could not utilize the health services provided by the IAPs.

The military regime brought into power a new elite of technobureaucrats who—in an attempt to compensate the hard economic policies put into force to control the growth of inflation and to place the banners of social reform in the hands of the Left (the structure of free political parties was banned in 1965, and only two parties were allowed to function, with severe restrictions on the activities of the opposition)—started a reform in the social security institutions. The IAPs were amalgamated into a single national institute—the Instituto Nacional de Previdência Social (INPS) (National Institute of Social Security)—in 1966, and every regularly employed worker could obtain the benefits formerly available only to some professional groups. The tripartite administration was abol-

Figure 5
Death Rates by Age Group, Brazil, 1977, 1989

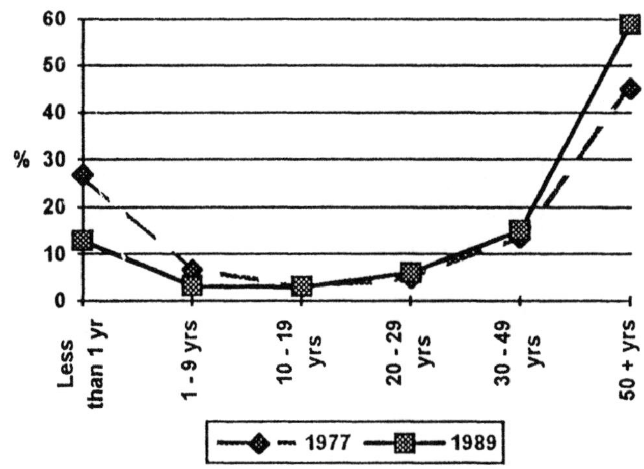

Sources: Tavares and Monteiro 1994; Ministry of Health 1993.

ished and a very centralized institution, as many others created during the military period, established. The authoritarian policies put into practice with very little debate by the universities and political world led to the development of a model of medical care very much centered in the delivery of individual medical acts. This model, mainly during the second period of the military regime, called the *abertura* (''opening''—the gradual and slow process of redemocratization commenced in 1974 and concluded in 1985 with the first civil government since 1964), facilitated the increase in the number of medical facilities throughout the country (Figures 6, 7, 8). At this time, about 80 percent of inpatient care and 50 percent of outpatient care were delivered by private facilities paid by social security.

This period of *abertura* assisted the progressive decline of legitimacy and loosening of the governing coalition that supported the military regime. The elections to the National Congress in 1974 marked the first victory of the opposition party. The new institutional scene allowed the emergence of many proposals of health reform, including ''a health reform project with strong authoritarian and modernising character.''

During the Geisel government (1974–1979), the INPS that belonged to the Ministry of Labor and Social Security was transferred to the newly created Ministry of Social Security and Assistance, and a specific agency for medical care was created: the Instituto Nacional de Assistência Médica da Previdência Social (INAMPS) (National Institute of Medical Care of the Social Security). Public health matters remained in the Ministry of Health. New policies were

Table 3
Number of Cases of Infectious Diseases Notified, Brazil, 1992

Disease	Number of cases
Malaria	577,098
Leprosy	228,775
Tuberculosis	85,955
Cholera	33,284
Meningitis	27,630
Leishmaniasis	20,857
AIDS	9,945
Measles	7,887
Pertussis	5,155
Dengue	3,215
Leptospirosis	2,083
Tetanus	1,551

Source: Ministry of Health 1993.

instituted that ensured the progressive inclusion of segments of the population in the benefits of social security, namely, access to medical care. Reductions in bureaucratic requirements for access to hospital care, an increase in the number of facilities available for care, and consequent federal funding led to a substantial increase in the proportion of the population covered.

The 1980s commenced with an important financial crisis within social security as a result of the economic crisis already mentioned that provoked the adoption of strong recessive measures. The expansion of social policies was refrained from in spite of the fact that they were needed for the recomposition of the eroding political basis of the authoritarian government. Criticism against the official health policies originated both from the popular and political opposition and from some bureaucrats inside the government. Some academic circles within some universities (Rio de Janeiro, São Paulo, and Campinas, namely) and the National School of Public Health promoted a deep review of these policies and initiated the development of proposals for their reorientation. These proposals would constitute the axis of the reformist movement that would take place after the return of the civil regime in 1985. They were centered in the recognition of health as a universal right; emphasis on active and permanent health promotion, both at individual and at societal levels; and the creation of a single national health system to be organized in a decentralized way, strengthening state and municipal levels of government and prioritization of basic health care.

Some of these ideas were taken by a council created by presidential decree

Figure 6
Number of Beds per Inhabitant, Brazil, 1900–1990

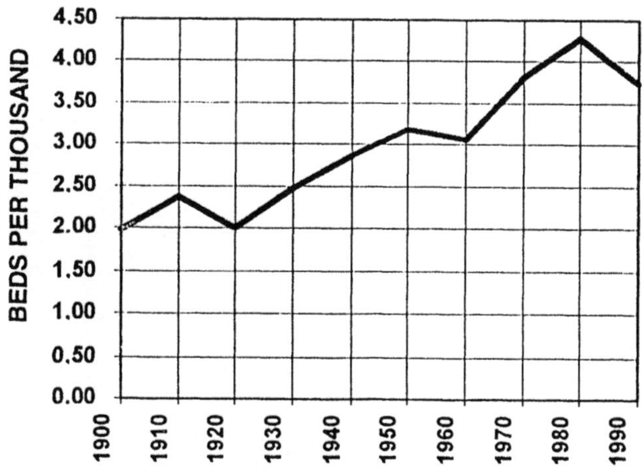

Sources: FIBGE 1984, 1990.

in 1981—called the Conselho Consulativo da Administração da Saúde Previdenciária (CONASP) (Consultative Council for the Administration of the Social Security Health)—that set a national plan for the reorientation of the main financing agency for medical care in Brazil, the INAMPS. One of its main features was a program called Ações Integradas de Saúde (AIS) (Integrated Health Actions) that allowed the transfer of federal funds to state and municipal governments for the development of basic health actions. This program was considered by the private sector to give disproportionate emphasis to the public sector. The reformists believed it to be an important step toward universal coverage and a significant measure to diminish the frauds observed in some contracts of private hospitals and the INAMPS. Another important feature of the plan was the introduction of a system of prospective payment for the reimbursement of care provided by private hospitals based on averaged reimbursement rates for groups of medical procedures (this system was later extended to teaching, charitable, and public hospitals).

In 1985, the civilians came back to government and a period called the New Republic was inaugurated. The Ministries of Health and Social Security were occupied by persons linked to the universalizing ideals of the reformist movement in the health sector. The AIS program was rapidly extended to more than 2,500 municipalities throughout the country. Soon afterward, in 1987, a national program for the building of unified and decentralized health systems (Sistemas Unificados e Descentralizados de Saúde [SUDS]) was launched. The main scope of this program was to put under unified control the three tiers—federal, state,

Figure 7
Number of Medical Attendances Provided by INAMPS, Brazil, 1970–1980

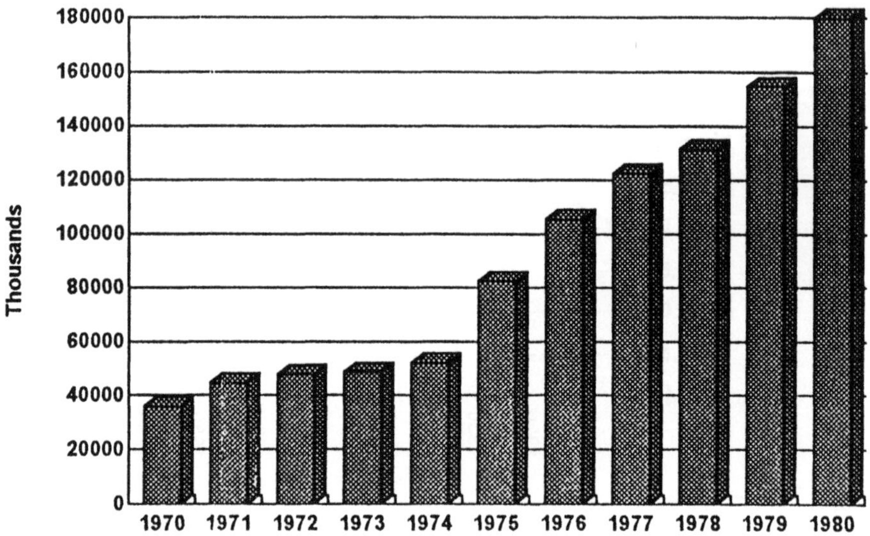

Source: Lima and Pucú 1981.

and municipal—of the Brazilian health system, with basic operative coordination in the hands of state governments. There was a significant increase in the amount of federal funding. The consequence of these policies was an important growth in the number of facilities administered by local governments, mainly primary care units as health posts and centers (Figure 9). The medical consultations delivered in public facilities increased from 157 million in 1985 to 198 million in 1990 (Figure 10). The emphasis on basic health care was felt also within the private sector, which showed an increase from 165 million medical consultations in 1985 to 182 million in 1990.

A National Constituent Assembly was elected in 1986 to elaborate a new constitution—the last one being elaborated by the military in 1969—which was promulgated in 1988. The chapter on health consecrates health as a basic right. Article 196 states: ''Health is a right of everyone and a duty of State, guaranteed by economic and social policies aimed to the reduction of the risks of illnesses and by the universal and egalitarian access to actions and services delivered for its promotion, protection and recovery.''

As compared with other countries, Brazil spends a low share of its gross national product on health. During 1989, the year of greater federal expenditure, it reached about 4.5 percent of GNP, with a per capita of about U.S.$100.00. Private expenditures are estimated to account for about one third of total spend-

Figure 8
Number of Hospital Admissions Provided by INAMPS, Brazil, 1970–1980

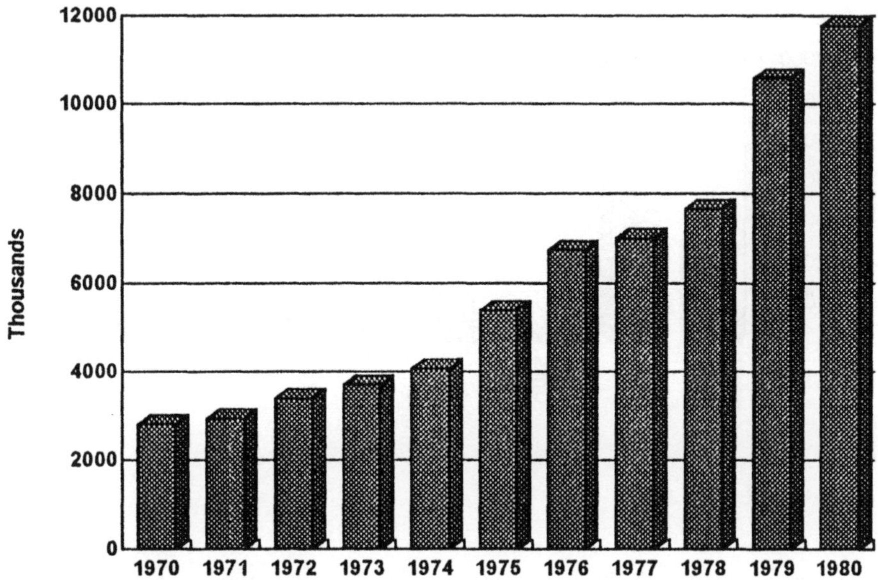

Source: Lima and Pucú 1981.

ing. Two thirds come from the public sector, with approximately two thirds from federal sources. Most of the federal funding until the end of the 1980s came from social contributions for social security. State and local government funds are derived from general taxation specific to them (states mainly through a sort of value-added tax and municipalities through property and services taxes) (Table 4).

At the end of 1989 the INAMPS was transferred from the Ministry of Social Security to the Ministry of Health. Some people celebrated this fact as a victory of the movement that proposed unification of federal actions in a single ministry. Others feared that far from the financial sources of social security the health care system could undergo a funding crisis. In 1990, the first directly elected president in 29 years—since the beginning of the military regime—came to power, Fernando Collor de Mello. In an attempt to diminish the strength of the governors of the states, Collor de Mello insisted that federal actions should be developed directly with the municipalities. In the health sector, there was a move toward so-called *municipalization.* The National Congress approved Law 8080, known as the Organic Law of Health, which detailed the mandates of the Constitution of 1988. In 1992, the minister of health was dismissed under charges of corruption that would eventually spread to other sectors of the federal gov-

Figure 9
Number of Municipal Facilities, Brazil, 1985, 1990

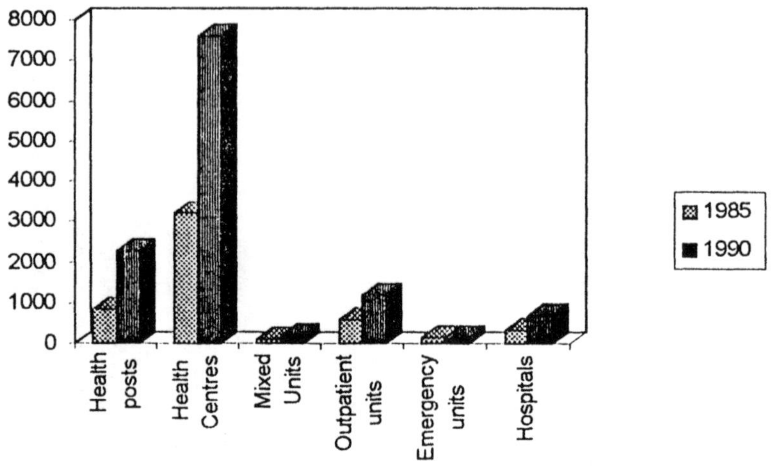

Source: FIBGE 1985, 1990.

ernment and end with the impeachment of Collor de Mello in September. The consequences were an increase in the pulverization of health actions and an important weakening of the capacities of management and control by the central government. Many local governments fought for more autonomy and tried to have federal funds directly transferred to them. In 1993, the Ninth National Health Conference was realized, having the empowerment of the municipalities as the central theme. By July the Ministry of Social Security interrupted the financial transfers of the Ministry of Health, and federal funding dropped to about U.S.$6 billion. The consequences were immediately felt, and public services underwent a deep crisis. The first half of the 1990s, therefore, was characterized by a multiplicity of local initiatives, some of them very successful, and a partial disintegration of the efforts directed to ensure the basic principles of universality and equity needed to transform the health system.

Privately Financed Services

There is no reliable information concerning the coverage of privately financed health care. Some studies estimate that some figure between 20 and 25 percent of the population represents the proportion covered by the different types of schemes. Four major forms of financing exist: prepaid group practice, medical cooperatives, company health plans, and health indemnity plans. The persons covered are usually upper class or employees of major industrial or commercial

Figure 10
Number of Medical Consultations, Brazil, 1981–1990

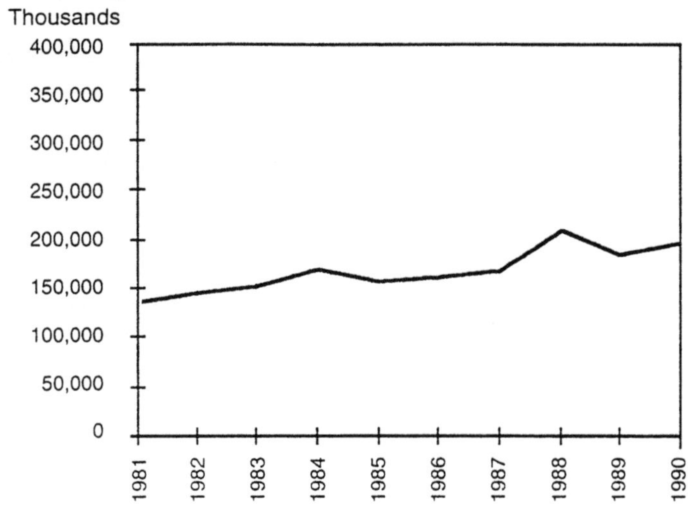

Source: FIBGE 1990.

enterprises. The average cost of these plans is estimated at U.S.$444 per person annually.

Public Health Services

As mentioned earlier, the public health services were directed mainly to specific problems and were organized as national "campaigns." At the beginning of the century, these campaigns were centrally administered by the federal government and mainly directed against yellow fever and malaria. Later on, federal structures were created to fight against tuberculosis, leprosy, mental diseases, and other endemic problems, such as trypanosomiasis (Chagas disease), schistosomiasis, leishmaniasis, and plague, among others. State and local governments began to have a role in public health by the 1920s when the first mother and child health programs were established. Immunization programs were later implemented by states and municipalities but federally conceived and funded. Vital statistics were regularly collected only in the capitals of the states, and only very recently have they acquired a national coverage (1976). Nowadays there is a national foundation—Fundação Nacional de Saúde (FUNASA) (National Health Foundation)—that takes care of public health activities at the federal level.

Table 4
Distribution of Health Expenditures Across Levels of Government, Brazil, 1980–1990

Year	Total	Federal	States	Municipalities
1980	9,784.1	7,336.5	1,743.5	704.1
1981	9,241.2	6,826.8	1,710.0	704.4
1982	9,580.4	7,126.1	1,649.6	804.7
1983	7,874.6	5,697.1	1,506.9	670.6
1984	7,959.7	5,938.6	1,429.3	591.8
1985	9,541.2	6,836.5	1,799.4	905.3
1986	10,924.8	2,212.8	2,212.8	1,111.8
1987	12,749.1	10,590.0	1,130.5	1,028.6
1988	10,924.8	9,979.0	-	1,614.3
1989	14,543.4	11,264.6	1,668.1	1,590.7
1990	12,930.7	9,404.8	1,995.9	1,530.0

Source: Medici 1993.

Drug surveillance and licensing are conducted by a special department at the federal level within the Ministry of Health. Food inspection is conducted by the Ministry of Agriculture in the production sites and by state and/or municipal departments of health at retail stores.

Training and research in public health are realized mainly in the Departments of Social and Preventive Medicine of medical schools; in autonomous institutes, such as the Institute of Social Medicine of the State University of Rio de Janeiro; and in the National School of Public Health, linked to the Oswaldo Cruz Foundation of the Ministry of Health. Some states have established schools of public health within state universities, as in São Paulo, or independent units, as in Rio Grande do Sul. There are training programs at all levels, from basic courses to doctoral degrees. Research activities increased in the mid-1970s, and the national congresses of the Brazilian Association of Graduate Programs in Collective Health (ABRASCO) has gathered over 2,000 people. ABRASCO, since it was founded in the early 1980s, has been one of the most important leading organizations in the debate of alternatives and perspectives of the health care system in Brazil.

MAJOR CHALLENGES FOR THE HEALTH SERVICES

Poverty

It is impossible to face the main health problems that afflict Brazil without finding a way to overcome stagnation. The current perspectives, in 1995, seem to point to a new wave of economic growth. However, recent Latin American experiences of structural adjustment following the mandates of the so-called "Washington consensus"—market deregulation, financial and commercial opening, and reduction of the size and role of the state (to reach the minimal state)—demonstrated the inability to reach a sustainable development and presented serious worsening of social conditions (Tavares and Monteiro 1994). How an emerging country can surpass underdevelopment in a world where the concentration of power and wealth reached such an enormous degree is the most difficult challenge.

Inequality

Unevenness of income distribution is followed by the unevenness in the allocation of resources that greatly influence health. Poor families eat badly and live badly. They lack sanitation, their schools are worse equipped and located with less places for their children to study, the roads and rails they have to commute and cross are more dangerous, and the shantytowns—*favelas*—where they live are also the places where drug dealers recruit their soldiers and hide themselves. To find an equitable way of developing and pursuing economic policies that benefit the poor and reduce inequalities, and expanding investment in social infrastructure (sanitation, education, transportation), constitute the most urgent tasks (World Bank 1993).

Three Epoch Health Problems

Brazil has to design and develop health policies that address at the same time "three epoch" health problems. Primary, secondary, and tertiary care are needed at the same time and with the same intensity. General preventive measures are required for basic health problems as for complex health situations. Oral rehydration therapy is as needed as coronary bypass surgery or intensive care for trauma patients. How to prioritize health problems and public investments is a very hard job. As the underdevelopment problems affect mainly the poor, there is tremendous pressure to allocate the scarce resources on hospitals and more sophisticated and expensive facilities instead of basic health units or general preventive programs. Research and technological developments have to be made in all fields and have to be prioritized. Cost-effective procedures must be identified, developed, and put into practice as quickly as possible.

Lack of Public Resources

Current economic adjustment policies are exerting enormous pressure upon social expenditures. Payment of internal and external interests precedes payment of social programs, mainly those oriented to the poorer sections of society. Tax evasion and uncovered fiscal subsidies make public financing very difficult. Brazil is one of the middle-income countries with the lowest proportion of GNP allocated to health care. Private social investment is negligible. Brazilian society has to reverse this pattern if a democratic country is to be built.

Consolidation of Institutional Reform

The institutional reform starting in the mid-1980s has to be completed. The roles of the different levels of government—federal, state, and municipal—are not very clear yet. Federal rules must be flexible enough to allow the setting of different policies in the various states. Health needs are quite diverse across the country. The concept of social security established in the Constitution of 1988 that included health and social assistance together with retirement and pensions benefits with common funding is not consolidated. Actually, recent federal policies seem to put it under attack.

Social Control

In order to fight against inequities, it is necessary to enable people to control public policies. Empowerment of nongovernmental organizations is crucial. Public and private health providers must be accountable to society.

Building a Policy Formulation Capacity

A recent report by the World Bank emphasized the need for building a policy formulation capacity. Most of recent policy reform is not based on sound considerations regarding performance and impact of health investments. Problems are identified and solutions outlined based on personal experiences and judgments.

Improvement of Managerial Capabilities

Civil service has also been under attack following the neoliberal adjustment policies. There is little professionalization among public health administrators. Social policies administrators are very badly paid, and there is no incentive for career development. Only very recently, even in the private sector, has the need for development and improvement of managerial capabilities in the health sector been acknowledged.

Improving and Enforcing Regulations

Regulations exist almost only for the construction of health facilities. Recently, professional organizations (such as the Federal Council of Medicine, responsible for the licensing of practicing physicians) began to set some standards of practice, but they are very poorly enforced. There is no accreditation program for health care facilities and organizations. Medical schools also need to be subjected to some sort of permanent evaluation. Measures for consumer protection need to be set in the health sector. Private insurance and other prepaid medical coverage are not regulated at all.

Cost Control

The available resources are inadequately allocated besides their evident insufficiency. There is tremendous need to implement appropriate evaluation of current costs of services. There are many cases of overprovision of care in spite of the general scarcity of resources. The choice of the most cost-effective technologies is most urgent. Discussions on the package of benefits to be provided to every citizen are still to be set. There are many incentives to the utilization of expensive technologies that need to be revised.

Monitoring and Improving Quality of Care

The development of standards for clinical care, administrative and financial services and physical plant and equipment, and the placement of quality on the policy research agenda were stressed in a recent World Bank report. The application of quality management tools is very scarce among the health care providers and needs to be stimulated.

Controlling Fraud and Abuse

Finally, there is a need to enhance administrative and legal measures to prevent and combat many situations of fraud and abuse by public and private providers.

Brazil is a country with enormous potential to reenter an era of development. It has proved during the last decades that social development can be attained in spite of economic difficulties. If it survives the attempts to demolish the very beginnings of its welfare structures, one can be hopeful of building a country for all its inhabitants. If discriminatory policies overwhelm it, its destiny will be of a lacerated country with growing social injustices and unrest.

REFERENCES

Berlinguer, G. (1976). *Malaria urbana—patologia delle metropoli.* Milan: Feltrinelli.

Brasil, Ministério da Saúde. (1993). Distribuição de casos e agravos e doenças infecciosas e parasitárias notificados em 1992. *Informe Epidemiológico do SUS*, 2, no. 3. Brazil: Ministério da Saúde.

Editora Abril. (1995). *Almanaque Abril—1995.* São Paulo: Abril.

Fundação Instituto Brasileiro de Geografia e Estatística (FIBGE). (1984). *Estatísticas da saúde, assistência médico-sanitária.* Vols. 5, 15, and 19. Rio de Janeiro: FIBGE.

Fundação Instituto Brasileiro de Geografia e Estatística (FIBGE). (1990). *Estatísticas da saúde, assistência médico-sanitária.* Vols. 15 and 19. Rio de Janeiro: FIBGE.

Fundação Instituto Brasileiro de Geografia e Estatística (FIBGE). (1992). *Anuário estatístico do Brasil—1992.* Rio de Janeiro: FIBGE.

Goncalves, E. L. (1982). Avaliação crítica do sistema assistencial brasileiro. Goncalves, E. L. (Coord.). *Administração de saúde no Brasil.* São Paulo: Pioneira.

Lima, L. F. M. & Pucú, A. S. S. (1981). *Doze anos de assistência médica na previdência social 1968–1980.* Revista Saúde em Debate no. 13. Rio de Janeiro: DEBES.

Machado, R., Rodriguez, R. H. & Tavares, R. (1978). *Danação da norma.* Rio de Janeiro: Graal.

Medici, A. (1993). *Aspectos federativos das políticas de saúde no Brasil.* São Paulo: IESP/FUNDAP. (mimeographed)

Ministry of Health. (1993). *Population Estimated by the Institute of Social Medicine.* Rio de Janeiro: Ministry of Health.

Ministry of Health. (1994). *Population Estimated by the Institute of Social Medicine.* Rio de Janeiro: Ministry of Health.

Oliveira, J. A. O. & Teixeira, S. M. F. (1986). *(Im)previdência social—60 anos de história da previdência social.* Petrópolis: Vozes.

Szwarcwald, C. L., Oliveira, J. A. A. & Sabroza, R. C. (1992). Tendências da mortalidade infantil no Brasil nos anos 80. *Informe Epidemiológico do SUS*, 1, no. 2. Brazil: FNS, CENEPI.

Tavares, R. & Monteiro, M. F. G. (1994). População e condições de vida. In: Guimarães, R. & Tavares, R. (Eds.), *Saúde e sociedade no Brasil.* Vol. 80. Rio de Janeiro: Relume-Dumará. 43–47.

World Bank. (1993). *Investing in Health. World Development Report.* Washington, D.C.: World Bank.

CANADA

Robert A. Spasoff

THE COUNTRY

Canada is a federal state with ten provinces, ranging in population from 130,000 to 10 million, and two territories. Eight provinces are primarily English speaking, Québec (population 7 million) is primarily French speaking, and New Brunswick is officially bilingual. Although the country is one of the most decentralized federal states, most provinces are demanding and receiving greater autonomy. The population of 28 million is thinly spread over a vast area, for a population density of 3.0 persons per square kilometer (5.0 excluding the northern territories). Three quarters of the population live in urban centers. About 4 percent are aboriginals, half of them living on reservations. Although 45 percent of adults have graduated from secondary schools (roughly 12 years of education), 16 percent of adults are functionally illiterate. The economy is a mixture of private and (decreasingly) public enterprise and is based on primary industries: forestry, agriculture, mining, and (formerly) the fishery. Manufacturing has developed primarily in the two central provinces, Ontario and Québec. The average per capita wealth is about U.S.$17,500, but the country's relative position among nations is declining. The top income decile of families receives 22 percent of all family income, while the bottom decile receives 2.9 percent. The 1990s brought a major economic crisis, with unemployment stuck at over 10 percent and uncontrollable government deficits. The level of taxation is higher than in the United States, making it unacceptable to many Canadians, over half of whom live within 80 kilometers of the border. Canada's proximity to the United States, which has ten times the population and more than ten times the wealth, and which speaks the same language as most Canadians, has made it difficult to maintain a separate Canadian identity. The economy is foreign owned to a greater extent than that of any other developed country.

MAJOR HEALTH PROBLEMS FACING THE COUNTRY

Overview of Health Status

The health status and health problems of the Canadian population are similar to those of other developed countries. Life expectancy in 1990 was 80 for females (of which 81 percent is disability free) and 74 for males (of which 84 percent is disability-free). Infant mortality was 6.8/1,000 live births in 1991. Sixty-one percent of Canadians describe their own health status as excellent or very good, and another 26 percent as good (Health and Welfare Canada 1993). Most indices are improving.

Infectious Diseases

Vaccine-preventable diseases are well controlled (e.g., 1,033 cases of measles in 1990), consistent with the high immunization rates (around 75 to 80 percent of two-year-olds and 95 percent of children at school entry have been adequately immunized). Tuberculosis has remained fairly common (1,964 new cases of tuberculosis in 1990), especially among some immigrant groups and the aboriginal population; there is very little multiple-drug-resistant tuberculosis. Just over 10,000 cases of AIDS (acquired immunodeficiency syndrome) have been reported, most of them in homosexual males, intravenous drug abusers, immigrants from high-prevalence countries, and sexual partners of these groups; the incidence rate is now decreasing. The prevalence of HIV (human immunodeficiency virus) infection is not accurately known but is estimated to be around 32,000, or 0.12 percent. Chlamydial infection has become the most common sexually transmitted disease, while gonorrhea rates are falling rapidly. Hepatitis B is a problem among intravenous drug users and some immigrant groups.

Chronic Diseases

Noncommunicable diseases and injuries are the major causes of morbidity and mortality. Cardiovascular causes account for 39 percent of all deaths; cancer, 27 percent; respiratory diseases, 8 percent; and injuries and poisoning, 7 percent. The leading causes of potential years of life lost (PYLL) before age 75 are ischemic heart disease, motor vehicle injuries, suicide, and lung cancer in males, and breast cancer, motor vehicle injuries, ischemic heart disease, and congenital anomalies in females. Age-adjusted mortality from ischemic heart disease and stroke has fallen by nearly half since 1965. Cancer mortality is fairly stable overall, with lung cancer increasing and most other cancers stable or falling. The leading causes of cancer deaths in males are lung (now stabilizing), followed by colorectal and prostate; in females, lung cancer mortality continues to rise dramatically and has just passed breast cancer. There is an unexplained rise in asthma mortality. Mortality from motor vehicle crashes has dropped with reductions in speed limits and introduction of seat belt legislation. Leading causes of morbidity are mental, cardiovascular, respiratory, and musculoskeletal diseases. Overall age-adjusted cancer incidence rates are rising, especially lung, prostate, colorectal (only in males), and breast cancers and melanoma.

Mental Health

Many chronic psychiatric patients who would previously have been institutionalized are now homeless on the streets. Canada has relatively high suicide rates (around 3,500 deaths per year), especially in the aboriginal population; the impact on PYLL is high, because young people are especially affected. Although 81 percent of adults drink alcohol, only 6 percent of drinkers drink more than 14 drinks per week. Average alcohol consumption is around 8 liters per year. Five percent of Canadians report using marijuana or hashish and 1 percent cocaine or crack during the previous year.

Age, Gender, and Social Class Effects

There are the expected health gradients by age. All-causes mortality is higher in males, but morbidity is higher in females. There are substantial inequalities in health by income group; for example, life expectancy is 6.3 years less among males in the lowest-income quintile than among those in the highest-income quintile; the discrepancy for disability-free life expectancy is 14.3 years (Wilkins and Adams 1983). There is a fairly marked geographic gradient in mortality, being higher in the East and lower in the West (Statistics Canada 1991). Although the exact causes are unknown, the pattern is parallel to patterns for income and certain risk behaviors (e.g., smoking). Aboriginals present by far the most notable inequalities in health. Canadian aboriginals are disadvantaged in almost every way: education, employment, income, housing, and health. Infant mortality is around 17 per 1,000 live births, over twice that in the general population, and life expectancy is almost 10 years lower. Rates of substance abuse (alcohol, illicit drugs, glue and gasoline sniffing) are high, and mortality from injuries and violence correspondingly elevated. Suicide among youth is up to six times that in the general population.

Health Situation of Immigrants and Refugees

The various waves of immigrants have brought their health problems with them, but these have been fairly quickly controlled. Immigrants have been a major focus of tuberculosis for decades, most recently among the recent influx of Somalis. About one quarter of immigrants are refugees, many of whom bear the scars of war and torture. In the past, most immigrants have been economically disadvantaged for only a generation, but with the recent economic depression, it is much harder to become established, and many must live on welfare.

Population Development

The founding peoples of the modern state were French and English, but their numbers have been equaled by massive immigration from Europe and more recently from Asia; 16 percent of the 1991 population was born outside of Canada. The Canadian population is relatively young for a developed country, with 12 percent above age 65, but is aging fairly rapidly. Fertility is below replacement level at around 1.8 live births per woman but is supplemented by about 250,000 immigrants per year. Six percent of all births are to women aged less than 20. Contraception is widely available and used, mainly in the form of the contraceptive pill, although condoms have been widely promoted since the arrival of AIDS. Since the law regulating it was struck down by the courts in 1992, abortion is treated much like any other surgical procedure. It is available in many hospitals and in free-standing clinics but is highly controversial. There were 17.5 therapeutic abortions per 100 live births in 1990.

Nutritional Problems

Until recently, the main nutritional problem was overeating: 87 percent of the population derive more than 30 percent of their dietary calories from fat, and 42 percent have a body mass index above 25 (Ontario data). Despite major improvements, half the population remains sedentary. It is estimated that up to one quarter of all children now live in poverty, and undernutrition among these children has become a major concern.

Environmental Hazards

Few adverse effects of the environment have been confirmed in the general population, although there are many in occupational groups (e.g., lung cancer in uranium miners, injuries in farmers) and in wildlife. Air pollution is a concern in the industrialized east (Canada claims that most of its pollution comes from the United States, while the United States makes similar claims about Canada) but is minor by international standards. Indoor air pollution is increasingly recognized (volatile organic compounds, molds) and may be a factor in the rising rates of asthma. Exposure to ultraviolet radiation is increasing with the thinning of the ozone layer. Natural radon levels are high in parts of western Canada and explain a small proportion of lung cancer cases. The most important pollutant to which most Canadians are exposed is tobacco smoke—either through smoking or indirectly. About 31 percent of men and 28 percent of women smoke cigarettes regularly; smoking is most prevalent among lower-income groups. Smoking rates are falling in general but rising in young girls.

PROVISION, UTILIZATION, AND IMPACT OF HEALTH SERVICES

Organization of Health Services

Canadian health services are mainly private (nongovernmental). The major professions are self-regulating, under the authority of the provincial governments. Most doctors and dentists are independent professionals, working alone or in small groups. Community health centers sponsored by community groups care for less than 5 percent of the population. Allopathic physicians are almost the only portal of entry to the formal health care system, since most other practitioners are either forbidden to practice medicine or are not reimbursed by the health care payment program. The supply of physicians is around 1 per 514 population, counting interns and residents; a high proportion of physicians are immigrants. In general, physicians are allowed to practice wherever they wish, although the need for hospital admitting privileges limits the concentration of specialists in attractive areas. The geographic distribution of physicians is accordingly very uneven, despite many government programs to lure them to rural areas. Nearly half of all doctors are general practitioners or (certified) family physicians. Family medicine is strong and will become stronger with a recent change in making certification in family medicine or a specialty a requirement for licensing.

Chiropractors and osteopaths and optometrists have limited ability to bill the health care payment program, but nurses, psychologists, and social workers do not. There were no midwives until the 1990s, and almost no nurse practitioners.

Most hospitals are owned by charities (religious or secular) or municipalities. The provinces own the (much-reduced) chronic psychiatric hospitals, and the federal government owns hospitals for the military and for aboriginals. There are practically no for-profit hospitals, although there are many for-profit nursing homes. There are about 4.7 hospital beds per 1,000 population, 3.6 acute and 1.1 chronic. Overall, there are 135 hospital separations and 1,530 days of hospital care per 1,000 population per year, for an average length of stay of 11.3 days. The health care system has always emphasized institutional care but is now moving toward shorter lengths of stay, outpatient care, and day surgery. Nearly all births occur in hospitals, many of which are now developing birthing centers to offer a more natural childbirth.

Public and Private Health Insurance

Because health is primarily a provincial responsibility under the constitution, the national health care program actually comprises ten provincial programs and two territorial programs. It is the dominant feature of the system and so popular as to be regarded as a defining feature of the country. When the program was introduced in the 1960s, the federal government agreed to pay one half the cost of provincial programs that met certain conditions (Crichton, Hsu, and Tsang 1990). The resulting program left the existing delivery system essentially unchanged, confining itself to paying bills. In 1977 the 50-50 cost sharing was replaced by an arrangement in which the federal government's contributions were based on population and economic growth rather than on the costs of the program. The Canada Health Act of 1984 restated the conditions as universality (at least 95 percent of the population must be covered), comprehensiveness (all medically necessary hospital and physicians' services must be covered), accessibility (user charges are prohibited), portability across provincial boundaries, and public administration. Only hospital and physicians' services are covered (although some provinces have added some dental and drug coverage), and the program does not replace income lost due to illness. The net effect of the conditions is the existence of a single-tiered system in which the provincial governments are the sole payers for covered health services; private insurance is permitted only for extra services not covered by the public program (e.g., drugs, dentistry, private ward accommodation). In 1991 the federal government announced the gradual withdrawal of its cash contributions, leading to concern that it would then be unable to enforce the conditions of the Canada Health Act.

Health Care Financing

Premiums are charged in only two provinces; the remainder support the program from general revenues (mainly personal income taxes), and a few charge payroll taxes to employers.

Hospitals are on global budgets, based on the previous year's budget plus whatever increment the provincial government offers. Most physicians are paid by fee-for-service, a few by capitation, and perhaps a third are salaried (trainees, academics, specialists in pathology, radiology, and public health, and physicians working in various health centers). Dentists, psychologists, and pharmacists are paid directly by their patients or by private insurance plans.

Just over 70 percent of all health care expenditures are made by governments, down from 75 percent a few years ago. Health care costs amount to about 10 percent of the gross domestic product (GDP), or U.S.$1,650 per capita per year. When per capita expenditures are plotted against per capita wealth among developed nations, Canada is either on or slightly above the regression line (Rachlis and Kushner 1994). Cost control has been achieved through limitation of hospitals' capital and operating budgets and physicians' fee schedules and through restricting the numbers of hospital beds and (less successfully) physicians and the growth of expensive technology (e.g., imaging). After a period of rapid growth soon after introduction of the program (especially of the hospital sector), costs stabilized at around 7 percent of GDP in the 1970s and 9 percent in the 1980s, reaching 10 percent in the 1990s. Because of the economic recession, these costs can no longer be afforded. Drugs are the fastest-growing component and are mostly not covered by the program.

Relation Between Ambulatory and Hospital Health Care

Neither physicians nor hospitals are responsible for the care of defined groups of patients. Large hospitals operate specialized outpatient clinics. Most physicians are private practitioners, who apply to hospitals for hospital admitting privileges. Family doctors and general practitioners can obtain such privileges but increasingly do not do so, finding that they cannot afford the time to visit inpatients. They are withdrawing from obstetrics for similar reasons and because of the growing costs of malpractice insurance (although litigation is much less common than in the United States).

Preventive Health Care

Preventive services are provided both by public health services (described below) and by private practitioners. Immunization is provided by public health services in some provinces, by private practitioners in some, and by a mix in others. The Task Force on the Periodic Health Examination has developed excellent practice guidelines for scientifically based preventive medicine (Canadian Task Force on the Periodic Health Examination 1994), but there has been no systematic implementation program. Private practitioner services are variably covered by the provincial programs. Routine physical examinations have been "delisted" by some provinces, and health education can only be billed as counseling—and to a limited extent. Cervical and breast cancer screening are covered, although physicians are not always adequately remunerated for same. Most provincial governments have recently introduced specialized breast screening clinics, and all have mounted heart health promotion programs. Half of known hypertensives have their hypertension adequately controlled, 70 percent of women have had a cervical smear within the past three years, and 40 percent of women aged 50 to 69 have had mammography within the past two years.

Rehabilitation Services

This sector is probably underdeveloped and underfunded. Physical medicine and rehabilitation is a recognized medical specialty, although not a prestigious one. There are rehabilitation hospitals in the larger cities and specialized Workers' Compensation facilities in most provinces. Health spas do not exist.

Public Health Services

Public health accounts for roughly 3 percent of health expenditures. Like other health services, public health is mainly a provincial responsibility. Federal government involvement is limited to regulation of food and drugs, surveillance of health and disease (through Statistics Canada and the Laboratory Centre for Disease Control), and policy leadership in health promotion and to some extent in prevention. In seven provinces, public health services are provided directly by the Ministry of Health through regional health units (except that larger cities have their own health departments), two provinces have local boards of health, and Québec assigns community services to regional boards and individual services to local community services centers (CLSCs), which also provide primary care (Pineault et al. 1993). Except for the CLSCs, public health services are quite separate from personal health services. Ontario has dealt with the challenge of maintaining standards in a decentralized system by legislating Mandatory Programs that all health units must provide (Public Health Branch 1989). The Medical Officer of Health is chief executive officer of the health units in most provinces. Because of reluctance to pay adequately, most provinces have difficulty recruiting public health physicians, and many posts are vacant or filled by general practitioners. Public health nurses are the most numerous public health profession, followed by public health inspectors.

Major responsibilities include communicable disease control, maternal and child health, environmental health, health promotion, and often provision of organized home care. Canada helped to develop the "New Public Health" (e.g., the 1984 "Beyond Health Care" conference sponsored by the Toronto Department of Public Health introduced the concepts of healthy public policy and healthy cities) (Hancock, 1985), and Canadian public health has been much influenced by it. One effect (somewhat resisted by front-line workers) is a trend away from provision of services for individuals to population-level interventions.

The Canadian Public Health Association (2,000 members) with its provincial branches is a strong focus for public health, holding annual conferences, publishing a journal, advocating for public health, and taking on projects for governments.

Self-Help Organizations

There are many voluntary organizations, some of which receive some public funding. In addition to providing mutual support, these organizations advocate for their members, attempting to influence public policy. AIDS-related organizations are especially strong and have often come into conflict with public health agencies.

Accessibility and Equity of Services

Financial barriers to obtaining medical services have been generally removed, although indirect costs remain, for example, travel. The existence of a single tier of health services means that the rich do not enjoy a deluxe service relative to the poor. There are much larger inequalities in utilization of uncovered services, like dentistry. Rural-urban maldistribution of resources limits accessibility in many rural and northern areas. Rural people claim that the closing of many small hospitals has aggravated the problem and rarely accept the idea that a health center can meet their needs.

THE INFRASTRUCTURE OF TRAINING AND RESEARCH IN PUBLIC HEALTH

Undergraduate training in public health is limited mainly to the modest introduction received by medical and nursing students; an exception are the programs for public health inspectors. There are no Schools of Public Health functioning under that name, but the Universities of Toronto and Montreal have well-established Divisions of Community Health within their medical schools, offering professional and research degrees. Many other universities offer M.Sc. degrees in epidemiology and related disciplines, and a few offer Ph.D. and professional master's degrees. There is a fairly well-developed specialty of community medicine (formerly public health and preventive medicine), requiring five years of training beyond the medical degree. There are ten training programs and about 300 certified specialists, but most provinces are yet to require their Medical Officers of Health to have this certification. The federal government's Laboratory Center for Disease Control offers a two-year Field Epidemiology program providing practical training mainly to physicians.

There is no national institute for public health, but the Laboratory Center for Disease Control has an active research program in applied epidemiology. Ontario has supported eight teaching health units, based on the concept of the teaching hospital and intended to strengthen teaching, research, and practice in public health (Spasoff et al. 1988). The federal and several provincial governments support university-based research units in health promotion and community health. The federal government provides research project funds to academic researchers and (through the Health Promotion Contributions Fund) to community groups. The Population Health program of the Canadian Institute for Advanced Research has been active in conceptualizing and promulgating research on the social determinants of health (Evans, Barer, and Marmor 1994). An attempt to develop public health practice guidelines parallel to the report of the Task Force on the Periodic Health Examination yielded the Community Health Practice Guidelines, which so far cover three interventions: STD (sexually transmitted disease) partner notification, immunization delivery, and restaurant inspection (Community Health Practice Guidelines Working Group 1994).

Although Canada is a member of the Pan-American Health Organization, it has very strong links to the European Office of the World Health Organization because of the interest of that office in developed countries. Many Canadians have worked in its Office of Health Promotion.

MAJOR CHALLENGES FOR THE HEALTH SERVICES

The major challenge for the health care system is to maintain the level of service as the economy declines. Canada has built a fairly elaborate "welfare safety net" to protect its citizens in times of economic disadvantage, a factor in its repeated ranking by the United Nations among the most desirable countries in which to live. This safety net can no longer be sustained in the face of rising government debts, insistence from international financiers that governments cut their expenditures, and citizen resistance to higher taxes. Furthermore, many of these programs are seen as unfair subsidies by the United States, Canada's biggest trading partner, and are becoming harder to defend. A very specific challenge is presented by the 1987 North American Free Trade Agreement: U.S. insurance and hospital companies are seeking access to the Canadian market, but providing that access would fundamentally change the program.

The demand by Québec (and to a lesser extent, by other provinces) for greater autonomy is leading to devolution of more and more power from the federal government. Since the provinces have very unequal wealth (the Atlantic provinces are historically poorer than the rest of the country), it will be increasingly difficult to ensure any sort of uniformity of benefits across the country.

Preserving the system will require more effective planning and greater emphasis on effectiveness and efficiency of services. The country's historic dependence upon institutional care is becoming less viable as the population ages. A way will have to be found to allocate health care resources in relation to need; at present, health professionals locate where they would like to live, and health care dollars follow them. Greater accountability will have to be built into the system—for example, by making hospitals and professionals responsible for the care of defined populations. It is widely believed that responsibility for planning and even for funding health services would be better handled by local communities than by central ministries, but only Québec and Saskatchewan have actually given financial authority to such bodies. Ontario introduced regional health planning councils 25 years ago but has failed to provide them with resources adequate to handle their mandate or with more than an advisory role. Hospitals tend to act rather independently, and it is difficult to achieve coordination of their actions. Twenty years after the suggestion was first made, the boards of all the hospitals in several cities have been merged so that the hospitals become a single administrative entity.

Although health services research is fairly strong, it must be better linked to services and administration. The vast majority of the (inadequate) research funding goes to biomedical research, with relatively little going to research on injuries, social factors in health, or health services research. Only a few provinces have capitalized on the automatic data collection provided by fee-for-service payment of physicians and have developed data systems able to support planning and research. Other provinces must follow the lead of Manitoba and Saskatchewan in making these databases linkable to sociodemographic, mortality, and other health data. Government departments of health need more policy expertise and a stronger population health orientation, which should lead to greater emphasis on prevention, equity, and cost-effectiveness of health services.

Achieving these ends will require greater dedication to strategic planning for health. Canada has only very recently made any move toward developing national health goals, although several provinces have proceeded to develop goals and objectives. Absence of such goals has probably contributed to the excessive emphasis upon health services, as distinct from the broader determinants of health, and lack of explicit goals for health services has made planning difficult. Several provinces have developed intersectoral councils in an effort to facilitate intersectoral coordination and development of healthy public policy (Spasoff 1992).

Canada has been active in developing the international health promotion movement, going back to the publication by the then–Minister of National Health and Welfare of *A New Perspective on the Health of Canadians* (Lalonde 1974). The First International Conference on Health Promotion was held in Canada and led to publication of the Ottawa Charter for Health Promotion. At the same conference, a Canadian discussion paper was released (Epp 1986) and has formed the intellectual basis for a considerable amount of health programming (Pederson, O'Neill, and Rootman 1994). But the document was not accompanied by budgetary allocations, and government has not backed up its rhetoric with substantial action. Meanwhile, disadvantaged groups (e.g., poor children, single mothers) are at particular risk as the social safety net is restructured (critics say dismantled).

The health of the aboriginal populations should be a top priority. It is widely acknowledged that their health problems are founded in social disintegration and can be resolved only through regaining of their self-esteem. Devolution of much political authority to aboriginal communities is under way, and many bands have taken over responsibility for their own health services.

REFERENCES

Canadian Task Force on the Periodic Health Examination. (1994). *The Canadian Guide to Clinical Preventive Health Care.* Ottawa: Supply and Services Canada.

Community Health Practice Guidelines Working Group. (1994). Community Health Practice Guidelines. *Canadian Journal of Public Health,* 85 (Supp. 1), 5–70.

Crichton, A., Hsu, D. & Tsang S. (1990). *Canada's Health Care System: Its Funding and Organization.* Ottawa: Canadian Hospital Association Press.

Epp, J. (1986). *Achieving Health for All: A Framework for Health Promotion.* Ottawa: Health and Welfare Canada.

Evans, R. G., Barer, M. L. & Marmor, T. R. (Eds). (1994). *Why Are Some People Healthy and Others Not? The Determinants of Populations.* New York: Aldine de Gruyter.

Hancock, T. (1985). Beyond health care: From public health policy to healthy public policy. In: Beyond Health Care: Proceedings of a Conference on Healthy Public Policy. *Canadian Journal of Public Health,* 76 (Supp. 1), 9–11.

Health and Welfare Canada. (1983). *Canada's Health Promotion Survey 1990: Technical Report.* Ottawa: Minister of Supply and Services Canada.

Lalonde, M. (1974). *A New Perspective on the Health of Canadians.* Ottawa: Information Canada.

Pederson, A., O'Neill, M. & Rootman, I. (1994). *Health Promotion in Canada: Provincial, National and International Perspectives.* Toronto: W. B. Saunders.

Pineault, R., Lamarche, P. A., Champagne, F., Contandriopoulos, A.-P. & Denis, J.-L. (1993). The reform of the Quebec health care system: Potential for innovation. *Journal of Public Health Policy*, 14, 198–219.

Public Health Branch. (1989). *Mandatory Health Programs and Services Guidelines.* Toronto: Ontario Ministry of Health.

Rachlis, M. & Kushner, C. (1994). *Strong Medicine: How to Save Canada's Health Care System.* Toronto: HarperCollins.

Spasoff, R. A. (1992). A new approach to health promotion in Ontario. *Health Promotion International*, 7, 129–133.

Spasoff, R. A., Corber, S. J., McGee, M., & Keys, C. (1988). The Teaching Health Unit: The Ottawa experience. *Canadian Journal of Public Health,* 79, 420–42.

Statistics Canada. (1991). *Mortality Atlas of Canada. Volume 4: General Mortality Patterns and Recent Trends.* Ottawa: Health and Welfare Canada and Statistics Canada.

Wilkins, R. & Adams, O. (1983). *Healthfulness of Life.* Montreal: Institute for Research on Public Policy.

CHINA

Keyou Ge and Xudong Yang

China is a developing country with a population of more than 1.1 billion. Its territory is 9.6 million square kilometers, accounting for about 7 percent of the world's total. It has 30 provinces, municipalities, and autonomous regions in the mainland of China, plus the province of Taiwan. Since the founding of the People's Republic of China in 1949, China has pursued policies on socialist revolution and construction, and the superiority of the social practice has been fully reflected in the improvement of the health status of the Chinese people.

MAJOR HEALTH PROBLEMS FACING THE COUNTRY

Infectious Diseases

The Chinese health authority always emphasizes the principle of ''Put Prevention First.'' As early as the 1950s, smallpox, plague, kala-azar, typhoid, recurrent fever, and venereal disease had been eradicated. The total number of cases of measles, poliomyelitis, diphtheria, and whooping cough have been reduced by 98.4 percent in four decades, from 11.83 million in early the 1950s to 130,000 in 1991. The morbidity of acute infectious diseases has been reduced from 20,000 per 100,000 to less than 284 per 100,000 during the same period. In the order of causes of death, infectious disease has dropped from first to ninth.

However, there are still more than 3 million people suffering from acute infectious diseases every year in China, 80 percent of them enterogastric disorders. The total prevalence of infectious diseases in 1992 was 235.1 per 100,000, and AIDS (acquired immunodeficiency syndrome) has entered China recently. Therefore, infectious diseases will remain as a major problem endangering people's health in China for a fairly long period of time.

Chronic Diseases

With rapid economic development and a massive decrease in the death rate from infective and parasitic diseases, life expectancy has risen from 35 in the early 1950s to 71 in 1988. Now, the proportion of the elderly population is growing with a speed of 2 percent per year. The expansion of the aged population, the change of lifestyle and the aggravation of environmental pollution are making chronic disease a more and more serious problem in China.

According to a report from the Ministry of Health (1992), noninfectious diseases account for more than 70 percent of all deaths. About 13,000 deaths per day are caused by noninfectious disease. The mortalities of cancer, stroke, and heart disease in the urban areas are 141.34, 120.07, and 78.10 per 100,000, respectively. A national survey in 1985 indicated that the prevalence of chronic disease in urban inhabitants was as high as 25.1 percent, and in rural people, 9 percent. It was estimated that about 60 million people suffered from hypertension, 15 million from diabetes, and 5 million from stroke in that year. The "early death" caused by chronic diseases accounted for 63 percent of the loss of the potential life expectancy.

Mental Health

With social reform, economic development, and the changes in family and population structure, the morbidity of mental diseases is showing a tendency to increase. According to an epidemiological survey of 12 main areas of China in 1982, the prevalence of mental disease is 12.69 per 1,000. It is estimated that there are 13.95 million mental disease patients in the country; among them, schizophrenia and mental retardation are the main causes of disability. The highest morbidity of schizophrenia is 5.69 per 1,000, and mental retardation is 2.88 per 1,000. In addition, the increase in life expectancy causes a concomitant increase in the percentage suffering senile dementia, which is the common mental disease in the elderly population. The morbidity of moderate and severe senile dementia is 1.82 percent in the age group over 65; it is 10 percent in the age group above 80.

Preventive work on mental disease started late in China. In the 1950s, there were only about 1,000 hospital beds for mental disease patients; doctors numbered less than 100 in the whole country. With the efforts made over 40 years, hospital beds increased to 84,000 and doctors to 11,570. Though the manpower and facilities have risen significantly, the shortage remains serious. In the late 1980s, the government began to pay more attention to mental health. The Second National Conference on Mental Health held in 1993 advocated development of a community preventive system and efforts to increase hospital beds for mental diseases. The community prevention system would rely on the existing preventive health care network. It emphasizes the training of health care staff and members of suffering families to enable them to effectively care for patients at home. This new concept in care management needs to be further developed.

Age and Social Class Effects

According to the 1992 *Annual Report on Chinese Diseases Surveillance* (Department of Health 1993), in the urban population, cardiovascular disease, cancer, and respiratory diseases are the three top causes of death. In the rural population, however, respiratory disease ranks first, while cardiovascular disease takes second place. There are few differences found between male and female groups. For statistical purposes, all the diseases are categorized into (1) communicable, maternal, and pediatric diseases; (2) chronic diseases; and (3) injuries. In group 1, the mortality in rural areas is several times higher than in urban areas. Communicable diseases are the main cause of death both in children below 4 and the elderly over 60. In group 2, the morbidity of cardiovascular disease is the highest in the elderly over 60. Cancer is the main killer in the population aged 35 to 59, accounting for 27.06 percent of total deaths. The morbidity of lung cancer is increasing, at 10 percent annually in the rural area and predominantly in males over 45 years of age. The mortality of rheumatic heart disease is highest in rural females. Chronic obstructive lung disease causes most of the deaths in the elderly over 60 years of age; the mortality in rural areas is twice as much as the urban area.

Population Development

China has made obvious strides in the implementation of population control policy and family planning. However, the huge population is still the most important problem in China. In 1953, the population was 0.58 billion. Then two birth peaks followed: the first was in 1953–1958, the second in 1962–1972. The total population increase was 304.28 million in 19 years. The annual growth rate during each peak was 23 per 1,000 and 25.5 per 1,000. The natural growth rate has dramatically decreased to 17.48 and 11.61 per 1,000 in 1974 and 1979. In the 1980s, the natural increase rate was no more than 15 per 1,000. It dropped to 10.81 per 1,000 in 1984, the lowest point in the country's history, and has remained at less than 14 per 1,000 since 1986. According to the Fourth Population Census of People's Republic of China in 1990, the total population of China's mainland is 1,133,682,501. Now China is facing a third birth peak in the 1990s and will reach 1.3 billion in the year 2000.

Nutrition Problems

With the development of the economy, great progress has been made in alleviating malnutrition and improving the nutritional status of the Chinese people.

The third national nutrition survey in 1992 showed that the average energy intake was 2,328 kilocalories, protein intake was 68 grams, and fat was 58.3 grams per reference man per day. So the food security problem has been solved nationally. But because of the uneven development of the economy, and the influence of factors such as geography, environment, culture, and lifestyle, there are notable differences between rural and urban and high-income and low-income populations.

Nutritional deficiency diseases are still regarded as the main nutritional concern. About 19.8 percent of urban children and 35.7 percent of rural children below six years old were short of stature; 9.9 percent and 19.6 percent of urban and rural subjects were underweight. The prevalence of nutritional anemia in children under three years is 11 to 22 percent in urban areas and 16 to 29 percent in rural areas. The average daily per capita intake of vitamin A was 476 μg retinal equivalent (RE), accounting for only 61.7 percent of the RDA (recommended daily allowance). The average prevalence of rickets was 40.7 percent in children under three years. There are still 6 million cases of endemic goiter and 0.2 million cases of cretinism. But in some relatively developed areas, overnutrition problems are becoming more and more obvious. Almost 1 percent of urban children from zero to seven years old are suffering from obesity. The prevalence of overweight and obesity among middle-aged and elderly women was as high as 50 percent in Beijing, the capital of China.

Environmental Hazards

The most serious environmental hygiene problem is air pollution. Now the two main sources of air pollution are industrial emissions and the burning of coal, and the two most significant air pollutants are suspended particulate matter and sulfur dioxide. The Chinese National Environmental Protection Agency (NEPA) reported that the annual average of total suspended particulate (TSP) was 403 $\mu g/m^3$ in southern cities. For sulfer dioxide, NEPA reports an annual average of 95 $\mu g/m^3$ in large urban areas of China. The southern cities suffer frequent acid rain because of the sulfur dioxide emissions. The air inside households is significantly worse than the air outside. One study measured levels of sulfur dioxide as high as 860 $\mu g/m^3$ in urban households.

Water pollution is another problem. Most cities and villages do not have sophisticated sewage treatment facilities, so water supplies often become contaminated with bacteria and viruses. Industrial discharges further contaminate water supplies. The common pollutants are ammonia nitrogen, volatile phenols, heavy metals, arsenic, cyanide, petrol pollutants, and oxygen-causing organic matter. NEPA noted that nearly 2 million pounds of arsenic and 130 million pounds of "petrol pollutants" were discharged into rivers in 1992. In freshwater lakes, pollution by heavy metals such as mercury and hexavalent chromium is rather serious.

PROVISION, UTILIZATION, AND IMPACT OF HEALTH SERVICES

Public and Private Health Insurance

China is now providing employee medical care insurance service that includes free medical care insurance service and labor insurance service. The former is enjoyed mainly by functionaries of governments, parties and nongovernmental organizations (NGOs), personnel of institutions of culture, education, science, and health at various levels, and army men with disability of B grade second class and above, as well as university/college students. The medical care cost is allocated by the Ministry of Finance according to the annual quota per capita. By the end of 1991, the number of people enjoying free medical care insurance service was 28 million. The latter is enjoyed mainly by workers in state enterprises. The cost is covered by the welfare funds drawn from individual enterprises according to a certain proportion of the total wages. By the end of 1991, the number of people enjoying labor insurance service was 137 million. The two services make basic medical care service available to all of the staff and workers in various organizations, institutions, and enterprises and has played an important role in promoting economic development and social security.

The employee medical care insurance service was formulated in the early 1950s and was designed to fit the socioeconomic situation at that time. But in recent years, many problems have emerged along with the increasing number of people enjoying the services and the accelerating growth of medical care expenditures. In 1991, the Chinese government incorporated the reform of medical care insurance service into the Ten Years Plan for National Development and launched a pilot project in some cities. Now the project is under further development.

Health Care Financing

Since the implementation of the policy of reform and opening to the outside in the late 1970s, the mechanism of financing health services through diversified channels and at different levels has been gradually established. The main sources are (1) input by the central and local governments, including health service budget, capital construction investment, and subsidy for special services; (2) imput by the medical care insurance system, including free medical care insurance service, labor insurance service, and various kinds of cooperative medical service in rural areas; (3) payment by patients; (4) input by other government sectors (such as agricultural, forest and water conservancy sectors, etc.) and contribution of organizations and individuals; and (5) donation and loans from foreign governments and international organizations. Among the above-mentioned sources, the input by the government and various medical care insurance systems constitutes the major source for the total health care finance in China.

Preliminary estimation showed China's total health care expenditure was 64.5 billion yuan, representing 3.6 percent of gross national product (GNP) in 1990, which averaged 56 yuan per capita. Among the total expenditure, government input amounts to 12.5 billion yuan, accounting for 19.4 percent; medical care insurance amounts to 28.3 billion yuan, representing 43.9 percent; patient fee payment amounts to 23.3 billion yuan, making up 36.1 percent; and foreign loan amounts to 420 million yuan, accounting for only 0.6 percent.

The funds have been mainly utilized for the following purposes: (1) to develop health services including institutions and personnel; (2) to maintain normal operation of medical and health institutions; and (3) to increase health service delivery capability.

Preventive Health Care

Preventive health care has been rapidly developed in the last ten years. In 1992, there were 8,359 professional preventive health care units, 25 percent more than in 1980, at county level and above. Of these, 3,673 units majored in sanitary and epidemic control, and 2,841 were maternal and child health care centers. Furthermore, a three-stage network (county, township, and village) of primary health care has been set up in rural China. Each town or village clinic usually has a group of professionals specializing in prevention health services. Some towns have even set up independent prevention health stations. At the end of 1988, there were 53,153 grassroots preventive health care units in the urban area of the country. At the end of 1992, 88.5 percent of the villages had set up health services units, the total number being 796,523. These widespread local health care networks have provided the basic health care services for the vast population.

The manpower of preventive health care has also been greatly strengthened. There are 320,000 health professionals working in the preventive health institutions at various levels in the country, of which more than 190,000 are in sanitary and epidemic prevention stations, 72,000 are in maternal and child health care centers, and 58,000 are in specific prevention clinics or stations. The professionals with high, middle, and primary titles accounted for 51.8 percent, 34.9 percent, and 13.3 percent, respectively. The total number of health professionals has been increased 1.3 times more in the last ten years.

The expenditure for preventive health care in the national budget in 1988 was 1.2 million yuan, 1.7 times more than that in 1978. The average expenditure for preventive health service was 1.12 yuan per capita per year. It is still very low, though it has increased greatly during recent years.

There were 85,000 beds in preventive health institutions, of which 53,000 belonged to the maternal and child health care centers.

Public Health Services

In 1949, when the People's Republic of China was founded, there were only 3,670 health institutions, 80,000 hospital beds, and 541,000 professional health workers including 505,000 technical personnel. By 1992, medical and health institutions had grown to some 204,787 in number, an increase of over 56 times, including 61,352 hospitals, 126,512 outpatient departments and clinics, 3,673 sanitary and epidemic prevention stations, and 2,841 maternal and child health care centers. Thus, a nationwide medical and health service network from the central down to the grassroots level has taken shape. Hospital beds have been increased by 37.4 times, with a total of 2.99 million, averaging 2.35 beds per 1,000 population. The number of professional health workers of all categories has grown to 5.025 million, an increase of 9.3 times, of which technical personnel make up 3.985 million, an increase of 7.9 times; doctors (including doctors and assistant doctors of both Western and traditional Chinese medicine) number up to 1.78 million, an increase of 4.9 times, averaging 1.56 per 1,000 population.

A multitude of forms and approaches has been employed to develop China's health services. Efforts have been made to energetically promote the development of the collective-run health institution and encourage private practice, while developing the state-run health institutions. There are now about 62,000 private practitioners. Among the existing medical and health institutions, the majority of big and medium-sized ones at county level and above are under state ownership, the majority of those at grassroots levels are under collective ownership, and private practice serves as a supplement to the state and collective-run institutions.

Since about 80 percent of the population live in the rural areas, diseases prevention and control for the 800 million rural people constitute a top priority in China's medical and health work. There are 2,199 general hospitals, 1,893 sanitary and epidemic prevention stations, and 1,722 maternal and child health care centers in a total of 1,986 counties. Health centers have also been set up at the township level. There are 38,248 health centers with 432,452 beds averaging 11.3 per center and 560,000 professional health workers averaging 14.8 per center in the whole country. Some 88.5 percent of the administrative villages have set up village health organizations in diverse forms. The village doctors are responsible for medical care, sanitation and epidemic prevention, technical guidance, and so on. The number of village doctors (used to be called *barefoot doctors*) has reached 1.253 million, of which 777,000 village doctors have gone through training to a level equivalent to that of a vocational medical school graduate.

Traditional Chinese Medicine

Traditional Chinese medicine has a history of thousands of years and has its unique theories with rich practical experience. Traditional Chinese medicine has played an important role in protecting people from illness. Proceeding from the longtime coexistence of traditional Chinese medicine with Western medicine in this country and actual needs of its people, the government has explicitly pointed out that both traditional Chinese medicine and Western medicine should be developed in China. ''Development of traditional Chinese medicine and pharmacology'' is stipulated in the constitution, with a series of principles and policies laid down and various effective measures taken to promote the development of traditional Chinese medicine and pharmacology. The State Administration of Traditional Chinese Medicine was officially established in July 1986.

In the field of traditional Chinese medicine, there are now more than 500,000 professionals and 2,222 hospitals of traditional Chinese medicine at and above county level with 195,000 beds; and units of traditional Chinese medicine have been set up in 95 percent of hospitals of Western medicine at and above county level. Most of the 1.3 million trained village doctors can use medicinal herbs and acupuncture in preventing and treating diseases. There are 31 colleges of traditional Chinese medicine and pharmacology with 73,000 undergraduate students and 1,200 graduate students of doctoral or master's degrees, in addition to the 57 research institutions of traditional Chinese medicine in the country.

Accessibility and Equity of Services

In the urban areas of China, most of the people equally enjoy the free medical care service and labor insurance medical service. In rural areas, various forms have been adopted on a voluntary basis in running medical services for the population to ensure the availability of doctors and medicine for disease prevention and treatment. With regard to the rural medical care insurance system, all localities will continue to introduce and implement comprehensive or unitary medical insurance schemes such as health insurance, cooperative medical service, and contractual insurance services for preventive care, prenatal care, and child immunization by adopting diversified forms covering different items of services with different premiums according to local conditions.

At present, the government has taken the implementation of primary health care, improvement of people's health conditions, and attainment of the strategic goal of ''Health for All by the Year 2000'' as one of the objectives of social development.

THE INFRASTRUCTURE OF TRAINING AND RESEARCH IN PUBLIC HEALTH

Medical training has occupied an important place in education and health services in China. A relatively complete education system with its distinct characteristics has been established. In 1991, there were 122 medical universities and colleges with 198,000 undergraduate students, accounting for one tenth of the total undergraduate students of universities and colleges in China. Postgraduate training is available in 85 medical universities and colleges and 30 research institutions with 11,658 graduate students. There are 563 vocational medical schools with 240,000 students, representing 13.7 percent of the total students of vocational schools. In addition, there are about 300 vocational health schools in the country. With a view to further improving quality of professional health personnel, the country has vigorously developed adult medical education. There are now 41 adult medical universities and colleges with 11,000 students. Medical and health personnel have been trained in a systematic way through correspondence training programs, evening university, and self-study training programs. There are 330 middle-level in-service training schools for medical and health professionals, and 1,128 county health schools. More than 460,000 medical and health personnel have been trained every year through short-term training programs and postgraduate training programs of various forms conducted by medical education institutions and medical and health institutions at all levels.

As for the research work on medical sciences, there are 1,403 independent and affiliated medical and health research institutions with 90,000 staff professionals. Seventeen Advisory Committees of Medical Sciences and Technology with 437 experts appointed as their members have been set up in the Ministry of Health to provide the ministry with advice and recommendations on all aspects of guiding nationwide scientific research work in health. The Chinese Academy of Medical Sciences, the Chinese Academy of Traditional Chinese Medicine, and the Chinese Academy of Preventive Medicine are among the biggest medical and health research institutions in China.

MAJOR CHALLENGES FOR THE HEALTH SERVICES

Campaign on Food Hazards

Since 1978, economic reform and an open policy have been carried out in China. The rural "People's Commune" system was abolished. The rural household production responsibility system effectively overcame the previous overcentralized management of production, authoritarian abuse of management, and egalitarianism in income distribution and set agricultural production on the right tract of steady development. The government has implemented a series of policies such as raising the purchase price for agroproducts and reducing the agriculture tax to promote grain production. By the end of 1984, grain yield reached 407.3 million tons, for the first time breaking the historical record of 400 million tons, and per capita grain availability reached 396 kilograms, approaching the worldwide average level. The grain output further increased to 446.24 million tons in 1990, but per capita grain availability was only 384 kilograms because of the population growth.

The Policy of Family Planning

China has a big population base and rapid population growth. Although the total amount of many important natural resources in China ranks high in the world, per capita resources are low. Most of the newly increased national income was used to satisfy the needs of new population. So if there are no effective measures for controlling population growth, the living conditions of the people cannot be improved.

Before the 1970s, the government was lacking clear guidelines and consistent policies on population control. The impact of the Cultural Revolution also caused family planning to fluctuate. Since the 1970s, the policy of family planning has become widely accepted and has made great progress. Now ''one couple with one child'' has been well accepted by the urban population, but in rural areas, one couple still has two or three children. From about 35 per 1,000 in the 1950s and 1960s, the birthrate had declined to 20.83 per 1,000 by 1989.

The purpose of family planning in China is not only to control population growth but also to improve the quality of the population. China has included ''healthy birth and upbringing'' as the core issue under the policy of family planning to improve the health, culture, and morals of the population. The law of marriage stipulates that marriage between people having direct blood relationship and indirect blood relationship within three generations is prohibited. This regulation plays an active role in the healthy reproduction of the population. The state attaches importance not only to healthy birth but also to healthy upbringing; it widely propagates scientific knowledge about bringing up children by every means available, enforces services of maternal and child health care, and develops educational opportunities.

Health Inspection and Supervision System

The health inspection and supervision system has been established since the 1950s. Following the implementation of ''Provisional Law on Food Hygiene of the People's Republic of China'' in 1983, health inspection and supervision services have been greatly promoted in the country. The State Council has approved series of regulations on health management in public places, pneumococcis control, health inspection of cosmetics, protection from radioactive isotope and X-ray apparatus, school hygiene, and so on, thus making health management turn from general administrative to legal management. In 1989, a Department of Health Inspection and Supervision was set up in the Ministry of Health. According to existing laws and regulations, sanitation and epidemic prevention stations at all levels were to be monitored by health authorities on food hygiene, nutrition, environmental health, occupational health, radiation health, and school health. Up to the end of 1990, there were about 70,000 health inspectors at and above county level, in addition to a large number of health inspectors working at township level.

The national qualified rate of food hygiene increased from 61.5 percent in 1982 to 82 percent in 1990; the quality of environmental health has been greatly improved through monitoring drinking water and air pollution, issuing hygiene licenses for public places, and so on. No less than 615,427 million people, or

70.3 percent of the total rural population, had access to improved drinking water. The attainment rate of dust and poisoning standards increased from 50 percent in 1986 to over 60 percent in 1991 at working places. In addition to instituting a health license issuance system for radioactive isotopes in nuclear installations and actinoapparatus, health inspection and monitoring have been carried out on radiation levels and radioactive contamination of food, drinking water, milk, fertilizer, daily necessities, and building materials. ''Regulation on school health work'' has provided a legal guarantee for the protection of the mental and physical health of 200 million teenagers. At present, a student health care system closely coordinated between health and education sectors has been basically established in the country, with the incidence of infectious and common diseases among the students reduced greatly.

A Patriotic Health Campaign

The Patriotic Health Campaign is a uniquely Chinese undertaking calling for full participation of the masses. The national Patriotic Health Campaign committee was set up in 1952 but was slack in function during the Cultural Revolution. In 1978, the state rebuilt the central committee of the campaign and so did each province and autonomous region. The campaign emphasizes the integration of public education and social participation, with regular performance review and appraisal in order to improve the health habits of individuals and the health knowledge and self-care ability of the people. The campaign mobilizes the masses to focus their efforts on solving such difficult problems as the elimination of water-snails and schistosomiasis; cleaning up dust, rubbish, and litter; wiping out flies, mosquitoes, and rats; and fostering the ideas of ''promoting hygiene and cleanliness.'' Over the past 40 years, this nationwide health movement of the masses has contributed enormously to the prevention of infectious diseases and has played an important role in eliminating parasitic diseases, improving environmental hygiene, and fostering maternal and child health care.

Developing Primary Health Care

In recent decades, the government has placed great emphasis on developing the basic health care network throughout the country. The nationwide spread of rural and urban services is built on a solid foundation of huge numbers of primary health care workers at the village and urban street levels. Above this grassroots level, well-organized supervisory and referral services have evolved at the township, county, district, and city or provincial levels. These not only play an important role in the prevention and control of diseases but also reflect the goals of equity and health care for all social classes.

To ensure women and children's health is one of the important tasks of the health services. Now that over 90 percent of lying-in women have their babies delivered with sterile methods, the maternal mortality rate has been reduced from

150 per 10,000 in the early days of the founding of the People's Republic of China to 9.47 per 10,000 at present. The national monitoring center and dynamic surveillance network for birth defects has been set up. In the work of the promulgation of *Regulation on Labor Protection for Female Workers* and *Provisional Regulation on Health Care of Female Employees*, female employees have been provided with better care and protection during menstruation, pregnancy, maternity, lactation, and menopause.

The government has attached great importance to the protection of children's health and has signed two important documents: *The World Declaration on the Survival, Protection and Development of Children* and *Plan of Action on the Implementation of the World Declaration on the Survival, Protection and Development of Children* expressed that the Chinese government will fulfill its due obligations. The infant mortality rate had been reduced from 200 per 1,000 before 1949 to 35 per 1,000 in 1990. Thanks to the successful implementation of the Expanded Program on Immunization, a number of acute infectious diseases seriously threatening children's lives has been brought under control. Children's nutritional status has constantly improved, and severe malnutrition is rarely seen in most parts of China.

REFERENCES

Department of Health and Epidemic Prevention of Ministry of Health, Chinese Academy of Preventive Medicine. (1993). *Annual Reports on Chinese Diseases Surveillance.* A Series of Reports on Chinese Diseases Surveillance. Beijing: Hua Xia Publishing House.

Editorial Committee of Health Yearbook of China. (1994). *1993 Health Yearbook of China.* Beijing: Publishing House of People's Health.

Editorial Committee of Statistical Yearbook. (1994). *1993 Statistical Yearbook of China.* Beijing: Chinese Statistical Publishing House.

Ministry of Health. (1992). *A Brief Introduction to China's Medical and Health Services.* Beijing.

Research Team for Developing the Strategy and Goal of Preventive Health Care by the Year 2000 in China. (1991a). *Prevention of Non-infectious Diseases, Background Material on Developing the Strategy and Goal of Preventive Health Care by the Year 2000 in China.* Beijing. 55–66.

Research Team for Developing the Strategy and Goal of Preventive Health Care by the Year 2000 in China (1991b). *Rational Nutrition, Background Material on Developing the Strategy and Goal of Preventive Health Care by the Year 2000 in China.* Beijing. 114–127.

FRANCE

D. Philippe Duprat

INTRODUCTION

Among industrialized countries, France presents a total population of 57 million inhabitants, with an average age of 37 years and steadily growing. The country has an average gross national product (GNP) per inhabitant slightly exceeding U.S.$24,000 (January 1995 exchange rate), of which health-related expenses represent more than U.S.$2,200 (9.4 percent in 1993), placing France at the first rank in European Economic Community (EEC) countries. Despite health information systems that can be described as quite weak, a good range of information is available to evaluate the various aspects of public health and health systems in France. The French citizen benefits from what can be defined as wide coverage in terms of health services and in theory in the context of quasi-universal access. As in many other countries, cost containment issues and various question marks about health system efficiency are pushing for further changes in a country where the state still intends to keep the leading role in the control of health matters and health care expenses. Next to these facts, the perception of the situation by French citizens is globally favorable. In recent surveys, more than half of French citizens consider that the health of the population has improved over the last ten years.

MAJOR HEALTH PROBLEMS FACING THE COUNTRY

Sources of Information

Since 1960, national health surveys provide a description of the morbidity of the French population. The last one was performed in 1991 and 1992 by INSEE

(Institut National de la Statistique), CREDES (Centre de Recherche et de Documentation en Economie Sociale), and SESI (Service d'Etudes et de Statistiques du Ministère de la Santé), and it includes data on medical services used. Hospital morbidity is assessed through a specific national survey for public and private hospitals. A recent change in legal requirements about hospitals' acute care activity reporting is gradually enriching the available information. Selected long-term diseases and professional diseases can be analyzed through specific reporting systems, mostly quantitative. Some diseases are described through dedicated processes or registries. This is the case for the list of the so-called diseases with compulsory declaration. For cancer cases, a permanent survey covers the institutions specialized in cancer treatment, but cancer registries also provide information. Among other special projects, a national surveillance system has been organized for AIDS (acquired immunodeficiency syndrome) cases, completed with a twice-a-year hospital survey. A telesystem network provides reports on the evaluation of the incidence of influenza nationwide.

Deaths certificates contain some medical information of uneven quality that is collected regionally and treated on a national basis.

Accidents benefit from a more rigorous reporting, at least quantitatively. Major work injuries are published annually by the two main insurance funds. Traffic accident figures are systematically registered and annually published by the police and safety forces. Other accidental injuries (domestic, school, leisure) are studied mainly through two sources. The first one is a systematic yearly retrospective survey performed by the National Health Insurance Fund (CNAMTS, Caisse Nationale d'Assurance Maladie des Travailleurs Salaries). The second is related to the participation of France in the European observation system, implemented in the emergency department of selected hospitals.

Alcohol consumption data are available through the taxation system information and treated by INSEE, which also publishes the tobacco sales data. More precise and context-related information on alcohol use, tobacco, and other toxicomanias can be obtained from the national health survey mentioned earlier. A specific yearly survey, including information on treatments, is also available for toxicomanias, and a national observatory on this matter has recently been set up.

Health in France

With a global average life expectancy at birth of 77.7 years in 1991, following continuous improvements over the century, France is a leading country in the European Union. But this figure is mostly explained by the average life expectancy observed for women (81.1 years), the number of 72.9 for men ranking only in eighth position for Western European countries. The life expectancy without handicap has improved more rapidly and was estimated in 1991 at 63.8 for men and 68.5 years for women.

For some diseases and population groups, the national situation appears quite favorable. Cardiovascular diseases are the leading cause of death, but at a lower rate than in other European Union countries (200/100,000). This is true both for cardiac ischemia and for cerebrovascular diseases. The negative trend of these causes of death has been observed since the 1970s and is also observed for premature deaths. However, the prevalence of cardiovascular diseases increased in the last decade, probably under the combined effect of better reporting and screening improvements. Looking at other causes of mortality showing improvement in the last ten years, the key facts are: a decrease of 34 percent for alcohol-related and cirrhosis deaths (age group: 15–64), of 14 percent for traffic accidents deaths (age group: 5–65), and of 19 percent for deaths linked to aerodigestive cancers among men. For the observed morbidity, only two disease groups have declined: digestive diseases and mouth and teeth diseases.

Three population groups are remarkable for the progress recently observed. The French women life expectancy mentioned earlier is only surpassed in Japan. However, no satisfactory explanation has been found among the various possible factors involved (biology, sociology, etc.), and the topic is still a research area. Next to that, specific problems are obviously generated by the feminization of elderly.

Elderly are also per se a group of interest, as the decrease of mortality in their age group explains most of the gain in life expectancy from 1980 to 1990. This correlates also to the improvement of life expectancy without handicap among people over 65 years of age. It is clear that the growing importance of this age group creates new needs in terms of care, housing, and psychosocial support.

Newborns and children can be considered as well as groups with improved health situation. Perinatal mortality, estimated at 7.2 per 1,000 in 1990, does not compare favorably to most other Western countries (tenth rank), but its improvement was sustained in recent years. Sudden infant death syndrome kills 1,500 each year, and prematurity and hypotrophia are targets for the coming years.

Various factors can obviously be analyzed for explaining these facts: standards of living (the "French paradox"), social cohesion, demographic patterns, GNP, good level of education, food, and housing. The increase in health care consumption in the last 20 years must be quoted as well, its potential role in health improvement deserving further evaluation.

Next to these "good" performances, several negative facts must be pointed out. Premature deaths are high, and their main causes are known. Accidents and violent deaths (including suicide) explain about 20 percent of these deaths. Lung cancers and aerodigestive cancers are playing an important role—alcoholic cirrhosis also. The emergence of AIDS has provoked up to now over 4,000 premature deaths, with high incidence of disease.

It is estimated that more than 50 percent of premature deaths are avoidable, about two thirds through potential modifications of risk-taking behaviors, and one third through better care and prevention. Alcohol, tobacco, and other toxic substances use and abuse play a central role in this situation.

A social "malaise" is said to have grown in the country, as suggested by the place among morbidity causes of mental disorders such as depressive syndromes, anxiety, and sleep disorders. As a mirror, psychotropic drugs consumption is significantly higher than in neighboring countries. Suicides take more than 11,000 lives, and their trend is higher compared with neighboring countries. Violence toward children is also a significant and persistent problem. Unemployment and the so-called new poverty impacts are still to be assessed. Chronic diseases patterns are obviously shaping many of the features of the French health system.

Following the same pattern as in most industrialized countries, three factors today are important contributors to chronic diseases: the partial control of previously rapidly lethal diseases, the increase of life span for chronic disease patients, and the aging process of the population with more comorbidities in the last years of life.

Cardiovascular diseases have already been mentioned. Cancers are better known for figures of mortality than for their figures of incidence and prevalence. The most recent sources suggest about 220,000 new cases every year. Lung, upper aerodigestive tract, prostate, and colorectum are the most frequent cancers in men; breast, colorectum, and uterus are the most frequent among women.

AIDS is a major public health problem in France, with a cumulative number of more than 30,000 identified cases, causing 17,500 deaths. Sixty percent of the cases are identified in three regions: the Paris area, Antilles, and Guyana, South-East. The pattern of patient groups has changed with 39 percent homosexuals, 28 percent toxicomaniacs, 16 percent tranfused persons, and 1 percent newborns, the remaining 16 percent being attributed to heterosexuality.

Diabetes has a prevalence close to 2 percent, with 85 percent of non-insulin-dependent forms. The disease tends to be more frequent as a result of the higher proportion of aging and some improvement in life expectancy among insulin-dependent patients through diagnostic and therapeutic improvements.

Among the other most frequently seen chronic diseases, some are increasing. A first category is the osteoarticular disease group, with a predominance among women. Rheumatoid arthritis concerns 1 percent of the population, striking people at an active age, causing severe handicaps and social difficulties. Lumbar disease prevalence is only indirectly assessed but is responsible for 13 percent of work accidents and 7 percent of work cessation. While direct statistics on osteoporosis are scant, the frequency of hip fractures among women after menopause is quite high (50,000 a year), causing death in the following year for 15 percent of cases and affecting autonomy for 50 percent of victims. Asthma appears to be more frequent, with mortality increasing since the early 1980s. Several epidemiologic studies suggest increases among young subjects.

Iatrogenic diseases are responsible for significant shares of morbidity and mortality. Drug-related problems are usually considered as important, but recently the greatest emphasis was given to nosocomial infections, which appear to be present in about 7.4 percent of hospitalized patients. However, data on iatrogeny and nonquality are still rare. Several major therapy-related dramas (transfusion-induced human immunodeficiency virus [HIV] contamination of hemophiliacs, hepatitis among blood receivers, Creutzfeld-Jacob disease in children treated with human pituitary extract) are contributing to greater emphasis on therapeutic safety.

ORGANIZATION, PROVISION, UTILIZATION, AND IMPACT OF HEALTH SERVICES

The Ministry of Health is the leading public authority on health affairs. Created in 1920, its responsibilities have frequently changed. Up to June 1995, the ministry was responsible for health services, social affairs, and urban policy. It has been reorganized under the new government and is now called the Ministry of Health and Social Security, this change reflecting a political will to improve the coordination of delivery, financing, and control for health. Medical research matters are placed mainly under the supervision of the Research Ministry. Health issues and health care services organization are systematically discussed with the Finance Ministry. The Health Ministry also plays with the Finance Ministry a key role in the control of social security. The ministry has direct responsibilities over a wide range of technical areas, but recent debates and policy options have favored the creation of several specialized agencies (pharmaceutical products [Agence du Médicament], blood and derivates [Agence du Sang], development of medical evaluation [Agence Nationale pour le Développement de l'Evaluation Médicale], public health surveillance [Reseau National de Santé Publique]). The general organization can be described as vertical, most key decisions being made at the central level. Administration and control are left to peripheral structures. At the regional level, regional health and social affairs offices (DRASS, Direction Regional de l'Action Sanitaire et Sociale) are in charge of facilities planning but also are involved in occupational health and prevention of accidents. Recent changes in hospital budgeting may give to this regional level a key role in hospital budgeting. At the regional level, regional health observatories (Observatoires Regionaux de Santé) are now in charge of developing health information systems. At the department level (each region being constituted of several departments), departmental health and social affairs offices are in charge of controlling the various health institutions and activities, including the budget control of public hospitals. They also are in charge of implementing various risk-oriented programs and collecting epidemiological data. They manage some special programs, such as the "minimal income for insertion" (Revenu Minimum d'Insertion) fund. Social security also has a regional and departmental administration system, completing the national structure.

In France, despite the existence of a national health insurance system, two sectors coexist for the organization of health care delivery. The public sector concerns mostly hospital care, where two thirds of acute care beds are directly managed by the public administration. The private sector is based on liberal practice and serves the larger part of ambulatory care.

Various types of health care institutions are encountered in the French system: public institutions, private not-for-profit institutions, and private for-profit institutions. More than 540,000 beds exist, employing a number close to 1 million persons. The public sector represents 64 percent of beds. Acute care beds numbered 284,718 in 1993, among which more than 100,000 beds were managed by the private sector. Roughly, the repartition of acute care beds is: 50 percent medicine and medical specialties, 40 percent surgery, 10 percent gynecology and obstetrics. Three different hospital categories exist. Thirty-one regional hospital centers offer a full range of simple to complex diagnostic and treatment services and play a key role for teaching and research in medicine. General hospital centers also offer a wide range of services but usually exclude human graft programs, burn units, and very high-tech care processes. The rest of the hospitals are sector and local hospitals aiming at providing a network of basic hospital services with easy geographic access. Several years of efforts to control overcapacities (still estimated at about 50,000 beds) have led to continuous reductions of medical and obstetrical beds since the early 1980s.

Hospital activities are currently only described through classical indicators. The number of admissions was 13,519,305 for the year 1992, of which acute care represents 91 percent. The number of admissions follows a regular positive trend. The number of inpatient days amounts to 158,646,982 days, of which close to 100 million days are produced by the public sector. There is a declining trend for this figure, which is reflected in declining lengths of stay (LOS) (average LOS of 6.4 days for acute care in 1992). Occupancy rates have increased, with a national average at 75.2 percent for acute care. Some 734,830 births occurred in 1992, among which 15 percent were performed with cesarian section. A medicalized information system is being implemented and will provide an exhaustive description of care episodes through standardized hospitalization summaries coded with the International Classification of Diseases. The recent hospital law of July 31, 1991, redefines the framework of missions, activities, and obligations for each type, developing the concept of "Health Institutions." These structures usually provide mostly inpatient care, but day care (31,000 places, 6,551,000 care episodes), night care (452,000 care episodes), and home care (164,000 hospitalized patients) are taking a growing share of the activities. Ambulatory surgery is only emerging but should have a strong expansion in the coming years. All Health Institutions are subject to the control of the state, aiming at improving safety, improving the health care service, and adapting it to the changes of technologies and needs. Professional organizations have only a secondary say on these matters. The traditional, and unequally enforced, central planning system for beds and major equipment (*carte sanitaire* created in 1970) is being enriched by national or regional health organization schemes (*schéma régional d'orientation sanitaire*), aiming at a more decentralized, detailed, and need-oriented approach for the regulation of health care services.

The operational management of public health institutions under the new law is now more flexible, as state control (through its departmental and regional inspections) is now performed a posteriori. However, strategic planning, the budgeting process, and physician recruitment are still under a strict a priori control. Various legal possibilities allow institutions, both public and private, to share resources and/or to cooperate. Important differences characterize the public and private sector, which can be summarized as follows: In public and not-for-profit institutions, most personnel, including physicians, are paid by salary. Teaching and research are the exclusive domain of the public sector, which is playing the key role not only in emergency care and resource-intensive and complex treatments but also in long-term care and psychiatric care. The private sector has focused its activity on surgery and obstetrics, relying mostly on liberal practitioners.

A major reform of the resources allocation process, based on a regionalized approach and taking into account the level of activity, is being implemented in an attempt to improve the budgeting process, which has been organized for the public through a yearly rate-adjusted global budget since 1983. Currently, 75 percent of beds are financed through the global budget, the remaining 25 percent being paid on a rate-set daily price.

Emergency services have an original organization. Next to the traditional role of liberal physicians, a national system of urgent medical help (SAMU, Service d'Aide Médicale Urgente) regulates, in coordination with police and firemen, the response to health emergency calls requiring on-site interventions. According to initial assessment, the departmental regulation centers can request the intervention of specialized medical mobile units (SMUR, Service Mobile d'Urgente et de Reanimation) or the most appropriate service. This organization also plays a role in disaster plans and major catastrophes. A new law has recently called for the implementation of a single unique number (18) for health emergency calls, a system jointly managed by administration, public hospitals, and private physicians.

Mental health services are organized in a specific manner. The French territory is divided into 788 sectors connected with a referral hospital center. This organization has encouraged the development of ambulatory services and multidisciplinary approaches. Next to this organization, a vast restructuring of psychiatric hospitals has been ongoing since 1980, with bed number reduction using a specific planning methodology. Private practice psychiatrists provide a significant share of ambulatory care. Funding for all such services is provided by social security.

Most health professions are regulated by the public health code, both for graduation and registration and practice, involving maintenance of professional lists in each administrative departmental area. Included are physicians, dentists, midwives, and pharmacists, each having a professional order that delivers professional cards and maintains a monopoly of practice.

In 1994, the number of licensed physicians in France was 160,235, a 60 percent increase since 1980. However, a "numerus clausus" policy has now reduced the number of students, limiting the number of new practitioners every year. The number of physicians per inhabitant is now 278 per 100,000. One physician out of 2 is a general practitioner; 27 percent are specialists and 12 percent surgeons, the remaining 11 percent being psychiatrists, biologists, or public health physicians. France also counts over 10,000 psychiatrists. It should be pointed out that 68 percent of physicians work as liberal professionals, 100,000 of these in their own private practice. Most of the physicians paid by salary are working in the hospital setting (35,140 practitioners in 1993). The national average revenue per physician is 740,000 francs (U.S.$180,000), with an average increase of 3.4 percent from 1989 to 1992.

The activity of physicians is estimated through the figures found in CNAMTS reimbursements. From 1975 to 1993, the number of physician contacts more than doubled, with 242 million consultations and 64 million home visits. Upon their own decision, liberal physicians can practice under a fully controlled price system (patient reimbursement being maximum) or under a more flexible pricing system (which is the case for many specialists).

The number of dentists has been stable since the beginning of the 1990s, at 38,000. Midwives numbered 11,479 in 1993. The number of pharmacists is given later in this chapter.

Other health professionals are practicing under the same type of regulation, with monopoly of practice, but they do not have official professional orders. More than 320,000 persons hold a nursing degree; among these, 261,525 hold a state nursing degree, the rest being psychiatry nurses. Physiotherapists number 41,858, and other paramedical specialties gather about 20,000 professionals.

The production and distribution of drugs are strictly regulated. Any marketed product must obtain an authorization for market use. Approval, previously granted by a specialized committee of the Health Ministry, is now granted by a national agency (Agence du Médicament). Ethical drug prices, reimbursement rates, and acceptance on the social security list are defined through legal decrees. If the price setting of such products is tightly controlled, over-the-counter drug prices are not controlled by the government. Pharmaceutical products are distributed to pharmacies through wholesalers; hospital supplies are directly purchased from companies through public tenders. Delivery of drugs is under strict supervision of pharmacists. Pharmacists numbered 56,289 in 1993, with a majority holding retail private pharmacies (26,099 pharmacists in 22,377 sites, a number under a strict authorization process by the state) and controlling the delivery to the public. Alternative delivery systems are not developed in France. Total sales of pharmaceutical products amounted to 123,987 million francs in 1993. The French pharmaceutical industry is in a period of concentration through various mergers and acquisitions and confronted with the new challenges of the single European Common Market. Pharmaceutical products constitute the health area of most concern by the new European regulations.

Biological laboratories are dependent on government regulation under the public health law, every liberal laboratory being submitted to approval. The number of laboratories in 1993 was close to 4,000. A system of codification is defined by law, mentioning the nature of tests and their relative value through a system of key letters. An important reform of codification started in December 1989, and currently, annual objectives of activity are negotiated with social security, with incentives for volume control. The national drug agency has recently been commissioned for the quality control of biology practice.

For many years, the French blood transfusion system has been a state monopoly. Up until recently, blood transfusion public institutions coordinated by a national transfusion center were in charge of collecting, manufacturing, controlling, and distributing blood, blood components, and blood derivatives. The most important feature of this system is that it relies exclusively on a volunteer system, excluding any payment to donors. In 1992, a total of 3,567,200 donations were registered. Important dysfunctions in the last decade, linked to inefficient decision making and causing serious public health damages among exposed patient groups, have led to a profound reform of the French transfusion system, with major restructuring and the creation of a national blood agency in charge of improving safety, efficiency, and control of human blood product use.

The French health system is only a part of the social protection system, a complex set of seven different subsystems covering five major areas: health, work accidents, family, retirement, and unemployment. The basic concept of French social security is solidarity among individuals and among generations. Since 1989, health expenses, though higher than in most Western countries, are showing a slowing of growth. This can be explained both by a set of cost-containment measures and by the difficulties of economic activities. The main expenses are financed through the social security system, but the coverage by social security has decreased from 76.5 percent in 1980 to 73.9 percent in 1993, one of the lowest figures among Western European countries. The main objectives of health insurance, covering disease and pregnancy, are to pay, totally or partially, for the costs generated by health care services delivery but also to compensate partially the loss of revenues of citizens in cases of disease or pregnancy. Social security payments are compulsory both for workers and for employers.

Mutual insurances are not-for-profit institutions aiming at the provision of additional reimbursements. Registration is voluntary and usually linked to professional branches. Regulated by a special code, under the legal and financial control of the state, they bear a growing share of expenses (6.3 percent in 1993). Private insurers still play a modest role with 3 to 4 percent of reimbursements. State and other public institutions, despite their key role in regulation and administration, are directly financing only 0.8 percent of the expenses. The major fact is the constant increase in out-of-pocket expenses, directly paid for by individuals and families.

National health budgets reporting complies with the rules of national public accounting. They describe the totality of health expenses. Social security budgets specifically describe direct benefits in each category of risk covered, and correlation with health budgets requires several retreatments. As an example, the total amount of about 730,000 million francs spent in 1993 as total current health expenses included 632,525 million francs of direct medical services and goods but also 50,000 million francs for monetary patient benefits, 17,000 million francs for preventive services, and about 30,000 million francs for research, education, and administrative costs.

Closely linked to health care service activities, specific approaches for child health, aging, handicap, and poverty are characteristic of the French public health system. Maternal and Child Protection was established with social security in 1945 and aims to protect the health of mothers and children up to the age of six. The responsibility of this program was centralized in 1983 and transferred to departmental services. Despite such efforts, with a natality rate of over 13 per 1,000 maintained, the program has shown a modest performance for infant mortality, in contrast with programs and technologies available. Recently, a new perinatal program was implemented in an attempt to improve the performance of the system. Communal development programs organize the services for young children in day care. Handicapped children can be cared for in specialized education institutions after orientation by departmental special education committees. In 1992, a total number of 1,934 registered specialized institutions hosted 107,946 children with various major physical and/or mental handicaps. In case of major social difficulties and/or danger, or when the family cannot secure its role, the Aide Sociale à l'Enfance program organizes the placement of children in a specialized institution or in a welcoming family, a function placed under the responsibility of departments.

The family support policy is also a tradition in the French system, managed by the national fund for family subsidies. Some benefits are not linked to resources (familial subsidy for family with two children or more, young children subsidy); others are linked to income level (schooling, housing, etc.) or support families in which both parents are working. In 1993, this complex system distributed more than 155 billion francs to 5.8 million families, benefiting over 12 million children.

The aging process is one of the most salient features of the French population. The last national census in 1990 confirms the aging process with 20 percent of citizens aged 60 years and more. There is a population of 540,000 institutionalized elderly, more than 60 percent of them having partial or total loss of autonomy, but 94 percent of old people live at home. Two categories of institutions welcome elderly. Social and medicosocial institutions are retirement homes, which may have a medicalized section. They are under the control of departments and in 1992 offered 527,287 places. Long-term care beds, which numbered 73,852 in 1992, are more oriented toward persons with permanent medical needs and are usually connected or included in the hospital system.

Next to the pension funds, which provide only an average monthly revenue of U.S.$1,200, various systems are providing additional benefits to the most needy, such as the Minimal Revenue Fund for Elderly (*minimum vieillesse*), or social help for elderly (daily support, housing).

Concerning handicapped persons, the law of 1975 recognizes their rights to health, education, and social and professional life and operates mainly through decentralized departments, with specialized commissions in charge of taking decisions for each case. Their role is to supervise the use of two types of benefits: services and financial supports. For young handicapped persons, departmental committees for specialized education evaluate the level of disability and provide the corresponding status, support, and orientation. Physical support can be performed in specialized institutions or through ambulatory and home services. The adult situation is reviewed by a more complex system of specialized committees, with two levels of decision: ability to work and evaluation of handicap and related needs. Various institutions and services provide special working environments, programs for rehabilitation, and housing. Since 1987 a law requires that a business having more than 20 workers must hire at least 6 percent handicapped persons.

In addition to these components of the health and social system, support systems are offered to the citizen with great social difficulty, a group of growing importance within the frame of growing unemployment the last ten years. Two programs exist, both decentralized. The first one is the Social Help system, which can provide services and support to orphans, handicapped, elderly, and families and includes a special medical help program giving access to free services. Since 1988, a second program has been established: The RMI (minimal revenue for insertion) is a financial benefit provided to French residents aged 25 or more, providing funds for securing a minimal resources level, which was set for 1994 at U.S.$460 per month per person. Various requirements exist, taking into account other resources, number of dependent relatives, and participation in reinsertion programs. However, much controversy persists about the social efficacy of the program and its impact on the unemployment problem. The RMI program is financed by the state and served 792,944 persons in 1993, providing an average 1,837 francs per month to beneficiaries.

Altogether, health and social sectors in France represent important amounts of funds and sophisticated services and constitute both a major source of activities/employment as well as an important economic burden to the country.

THE INFRASTRUCTURE OF TRAINING AND RESEARCH IN PUBLIC HEALTH

Today, the French health system is not built around public health concerns but represents historically more a heritage of arbitration between political imperatives, social progress, and professional and/or industrial lobbies pressure, with a fragmented scene and multiple actors. It is only recently that public health has started to gain a more visible place. This is measurable through the analysis of public health as a professional activity. Professionals, experts, and researchers specialized in public health are still few and, in many cases, are in charge of inspection and control, rather than dealing with operational health problems. Among the 160,000 licensed physicians, only 2,755 are qualified in public health. Nationwide, public health physicians inspectors number about 400; public health pharmacist inspectors, 121; and sanitary engineers, 185. The training system is usually described as poorly structured, but the main difficulties reside in the lack of political priorities and resources that were devoted to this field in the past.

A leading role is played by the National School of Public Health, created 50 years ago. Directly depending on the Health Ministry, the school performs the initial training of all the public administration health executives. It also offers various continuing education programs. Activities include training programs, research, and expertise, both at the national level and in various international projects. University public health activities have also been developed, and most medicine faculties have created departments of public health with teaching and research. For historical reasons, the level of development of these structures is still highly variable. In 1982, a specific public health track for physicians was created but requires further development (only 94 positions opened nationwide in 1994, and problems of employment/career track for such graduates). The training of physicians is still lacking emphasis on the public health dimensions of health care.

Despite a rich history in public health, especially in hygiene and control of infectious diseases, France still lacks the critical mass of public health influence that may have positive effects on health care services organization and impact more clearly on population health. This situation is also reflected by the relatively low volume of public health research and publications, despite the existence of some specialized research units and information production institutions. Various reasons have been suggested for explaining the situation, beyond the lack of priority of the matter in health policy up to recent years. It is quite clear that this heritage is multifactorial, involving historical, structural, sociological, and political mechanisms.

Recently, legislative changes, status improvements, and creation of new structures and institutions have led to the emergence of a more public health–oriented vision of the health system. Several examples can be taken: the creation of the High Committee of Public Health (Haut Comité de la Santé Publique), of the National Network of Public Health, and of specialized agencies; the strengthening of the health administration structure and human resources; the undertaking of global programs (perinatality, anesthesiologic safety, emergencies, etc.), and networks of care for target groups (AIDS patients, alcoholism, toxicomania).

MAJOR CHALLENGES FOR THE HEALTH SERVICES

The main objectives proposed for the coming years by the High Committee of Public Health are derived from four major goals: reduce avoidable deaths, reduce avoidable handicaps, improve quality of life for patients and disabled persons, and reduce inequities in health. Specific objectives focus on key health problems representing the main identified priorities in terms of severity, frequency, economic impact, and feasibility. Main targets include traffic accidents, domestic accidents, work accidents, cancer prevention, and most other topics that reflect the main areas listed earlier (aging, mental health, toxicomania, pain control, perinatality). Special attention should be paid to HIV infection. Some health determinants are also considered as key objectives because of their established detrimental impact on health. Alcohol intake is decreasing, but France is still ranked first in Europe. Further diminution is sought from the current 17 liters of alcohol per inhabitant in 1989 through the focus on target groups and regions especially exposed. Tobacco usage, linked to one death out of five among men aged 35 to 64, should also be reduced, with priority on young smokers.

But overall the reduction of system inequities is also a major challenge. Social security coverage was 99.3 percent in 1991, leaving only 0.3 percent without coverage and 0.4 percent accepted in the free medical access program described earlier. Despite an appearance of universality, social disparities in the use of health care services, paralleling with differences in mortality, are persistent (differences are clear for lower-class and lower-income categories). About 20 percent of low-income households do not use ambulatory services for economical reasons.

A last issue is also a great concern: environmental health and pollution control. In Paris hospitals, children consultations for respiratory diseases are linked to air pollution in one case out of three. Waste elimination, water control, and toxic agents exposure reduction are also still to be improved.

The general report on health provides a list of these priorities, with an attempt to set quantified objectives and key actions. However, the program, the budget, and the implementation of such goals are the main challenges, which still deserve further elaboration. These public health thematic objectives are also mainly dependent on the implementation of structural reforms in the French health system and of the improvement of resources use. Several topics are of prime importance in this respect.

The main politically visible priority for 15 years has been to control the growth of health expenses, with little success until recently. Such focus on economic control may have delayed the emergence of other aspects necessary for health system efficiency such as quality of practice, elaboration of standards, and fairness of resources allocation. The improvement of structure, processes, and performances of the major health institutional and professional actors requires a vast range of reforms. The hospital system is already engaged in such attempts at modernization: optimization of resources and budget, coherence of the offer, harmonization of rules for the public and the private sector, restructuring of services organization, and increased development of ambulatory care. The organization of better links of hospitals with other health institutions and health professionals is also to be encouraged to avoid the tradition of hospital-ocentrism. The past years have shown that the task is not easy and requires firm political will conjugated with sustained efforts of all players. Changes in private ambulatory services are also inescapable, as they represent a first level of care that currently has few incentives for efficiency. Several areas should be worked out, such as the improvement of professional practices (a new system of medical references is being implemented), the development of the coordination of care with tools for better follow-up of patient episodes at the various levels of the system, the shift of lone-player individual mentality to group practices, and synergies among practitioners.

These points are prerequisites for developing integrated health services approaches and promoting preventive health concern at the professional level.

As in any change process, the educational requirements are important and time-consuming. The integration of new domains and tools are essential for a revisited professionalization of providers. As an example, the implementation of a culture of evaluation and quality is currently requiring important efforts. Sensibilization and responsibility on the economical implications of medical decision making are also at the center of debates. However, it is quite clear that the design and use of incentives, which have been lacking in the past, are required for improving efficiency.

Another characteristic of the French health system is the low level of visibility of citizens as health consumers. This can be analyzed both from the fact that most French health consumers feel that they are happy with a system of ''easy access'' and ''nonvisible'' financing and from the reluctance of professionals to share power and lose autonomy. Most active representations stem from patients and families iteratively confronted with some services (diabetes, AIDS, hemodialysis). Encouraging better representation of health consumers and taking more into account directly expressed needs are tracks that deserve more attention to shift toward a more ''client-oriented'' approach, giving better opportunity to citizens to be responsible for their health.

Finally, the implementation of a stronger public health approach (public health as a problem-solving activity) in the French health system is the immediate challenge for France. This would require a mechanism to structure and grade a coordinated national public health program, with sufficient resources to have a rapid and measurable impact. The development of public health in professional practices and among the public is part of this challenge, like the development of training and research. Special attention should also be paid to areas that are frequently neglected in the field: follow-up, evaluation, and information systems development.

Like most Western countries, France is confronted with a vast process of change in order to improve public health while controlling costs. However, French reformism is facing various obstacles. Some are specific to the health sector; others are shared by most of the economic sectors. It is quite clear that further modernization of the health system is on the way and will continue. But the intensity of resistance to change will most probably require a wider public debate and possibly national consultations.

REFERENCES

Haut comité de la santé publique. La documentation française. (1994). *La santé en France.* Paris. (general report)

INSEE. (1994). *La société française. Données sociales 1993.* Paris.

Serie études de politique de santé. (1993). *Les systèmes de santé des pays de l'O.C.D.E.* No. 3. 2 vols. Paris: OCDE.

SESI, Ministère des Affaires Sociales de la Santé et de la Ville. (June 1994). *Comptes nationaux de la santé.* (report)

SESI, Ministère des Affaires Sociales de la Santé et de la Ville. (1995). *Annuaire des statistiques sanitaires et sociales.* Paris.

Solidarité santé, Etudes statistiques. (1994). *Les français et leur santé, enquête santé 1991–1992.* No. 1 (January–March).

Soubie, R. Commissariat général du Plan. La documentation française. (January 1995). *Livre blanc sur le système de santé et d'assurance maladie.* Paris.

GERMANY

Jürgen von Troschke, Axel Hoffmann-Markwald, and Ulrich Stößel

INTRODUCTION

Germany is located in central Europe, sharing borders with the Netherlands, Belgium, Luxembourg, France, Switzerland, Austria, the Czech Republic, Poland, and Denmark. The Federal Republic of Germany (FRG) was founded after World War II on May 23, 1949, in the area controlled by the American, the British, and the French occupying forces. In 1950, the Soviet-occupied zones became the German Democratic Republic (GDR). Both states were unified under the Unification-Contract on October 3, 1990. The FRG is a federally governed country with 16 states and has membership in the European Union (EU), the United Nations (UN), and the World Health Organization (WHO).

After reunification, there were 81.19 million people living in Germany in June 1993 on a territory of 356,959 square kilometers (228 people per square kilometer). Its demographic structure has changed considerably during the last 20 years. The characteristics are as follows:

- The mortality rate is low (1991: 11.4 per 1,000) with a high average life expectancy (1992: 73.2 years of age for men and 79.6 for women).
- The birthrate is in decline at a low level (1991: 10.4 per 1,000).
- While emigration is insignificant, the immigration rate is higher due to the repatriation of ethnic Germans from central and eastern Europe, immigration from other European countries, and refugees.

A further population decrease is predicted for the future, combined with an absolute and relative increase in the elderly population.

The age structure of the population is a result of a declining birthrate during economic recessions and a high mortality rate during the world wars (Figure 1).

Figure 1
The Pyramidal Distribution of the German Population (data for 1992; prognosis for 2015)

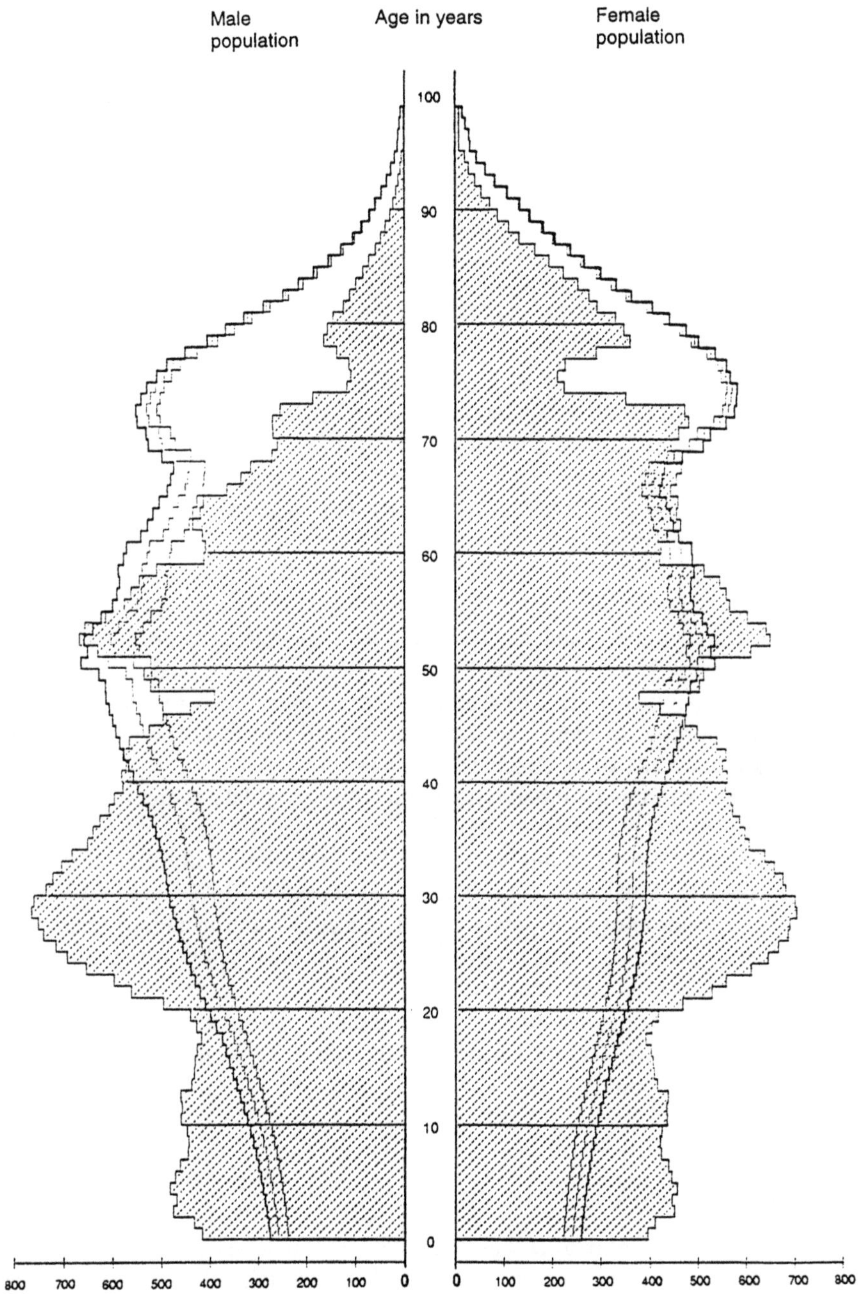

Source: Statistisches Bundesamt 1994.

MAJOR HEALTH PROBLEMS FACING THE COUNTRY

During the last decade, Germany has undertaken considerable efforts to improve its epidemiological database to describe and evaluate principal health problems. The memorandum of the German Research Association (Deutsche Forschungsgemeinschaft [DFG] 1995) about ''Health System Research in Germany'' defines (in particular, in the chapters on public health reporting and evaluation research) the demand for a theoretical foundation and methodological transfer. The goal is to have uniform standards in the differential analysis and assessment of primary health problems among the population. A second problem in this respect is the merging of two different health reporting systems after the reunification of Germany. Trend analyses and trend developments do not always assume the same basic figures. Consequently, two federal ministries—the Ministry of Education, Science, Research and Technology (BMBF) and the Ministry of Health (BMG)—commissioned a research project at the National Office for Statistics. Its aim is to develop a reporting system within three years that is equally suitable for public health politics, the public, and the science. The planned 100 chapters can be attributed to the following fields: framework, state of public health, health behavior and health hazards, illnesses, resources of health provision, benefits of the health care system, expenses, cost, and financing of the health care system.

The part illnesses will compose about 30 percent of the report, that is, the largest share. Apart from public health reporting on a national level, several initiatives, pilot projects, and newly developed concepts exist on the state, regional, and local levels (e.g., IDIS 1993). Beske, Brecht, and Reinkemeier (1993) have examined over 270 data sources on their value for public health reporting. According to them, the data that should give insight into the health of the population still show considerable flaws.

Despite the mentioned imperfections, the following data sources have been utilized: statistics of registered illnesses, microcensus questions concerning health, national statistics of the handicapped and the chronically ill, statistics of traffic and occupational accidents, statistics of reported AIDS (acquired immunodeficiency syndrome) cases, state cancer register, health insurance data, data from pension insurance funds, statistics of public health physicians, and data from physician boards and associations.

Apart from the evaluation of the ''routine data,'' also data from larger population studies will be included because they allow for projections on specific parts of the population.

Infectious Diseases

According to the National Disease Legislation (Bundesseuchengesetz) and the changes that have gone into action since 1962, certain illnesses have to be reported. The reports of new cases, however, depend on a lot of factors. Estimated trends about the spread of a communicable disease among the population, consequently, have to be taken with caution.

Among the notifiable diseases, intestinal diseases are in the majority. They are summarized under the category of "Enteritis Infectiosa" (in 1992 about 300 per 100,000 persons; BMG 1993). Illnesses protectable by vaccinations (diphtheria, tetanus, polio, measles, mumps, rubella) have to be reported only in certain cases. Studies about the rate of immunization among the population and the immunization behavior of the private practice physicians suggest a possible increase of these illnesses unless the immunization rate rises considerably (currently 40 to 50 percent).

Since October 1, 1987, human immunodeficiency virus (HIV) infections and illnesses have been registered anonymously. In 1993, about 70 percent of the total of 60,000 reports concern men, with a somewhat increasing share of women. Among infected women, the largest share can clearly be found between the ages of 20 and 40. Every sixth infected man, however, still belongs to the 40- to 50-year-olds. Most outbreaks of the disease, accordingly, fall into these age brackets as well. Till June 30, 1994, there were in total 11,497 reported AIDS cases (since 1982); 1,739 between July 1993 and June 1994 (BMG 1994).

For virus hepatitis, the annual number of cases is 18.9 per 100,000; for tuberculosis 17.4 per 100,000 (BMG 1994). For illnesses that are nonnotifiable, only scattered data exist from often regionally limited studies. A study with data from pediatricians mentions a prevalence of 6.8 percent for scarlet fever, 5.6 percent for chickenpox, and 4.9 percent for whooping cough among the total number of patients.

Chronic Illnesses

No new statistics exist about the share of the chronically ill among the total sick population. The last microcensus of this issue dates from 1980. Among children and adolescents (up to age 15), the rate is 767 (per 100,000 of the same age group). Looking at the share of chronically ill among all sick persons of all age groups and in trend analysis, the percentage of chronically ill has increased in all groups between 1974 and 1982. Women, much more often than men, contact their physician because of their chronic disease (60 percent versus 40 percent).

The last time the state of the population's health was surveyed was in the microcensus of May 1992. It shows an average of 11.7 percent of ill or injured persons among the population as a whole. As can be expected, the highest percentage, that is, 27 percent, occurs among the group of 75 years or older. The age group of 10- to 15-year-olds, instead, shows the smallest illness rate of 5 percent (see Figure 2).

The Disabled

According to the microcensus of April 1989, 6.39 million officially recognized handicapped persons lived in the FRG. The majority of them were severely

Figure 2
Health of the German Population

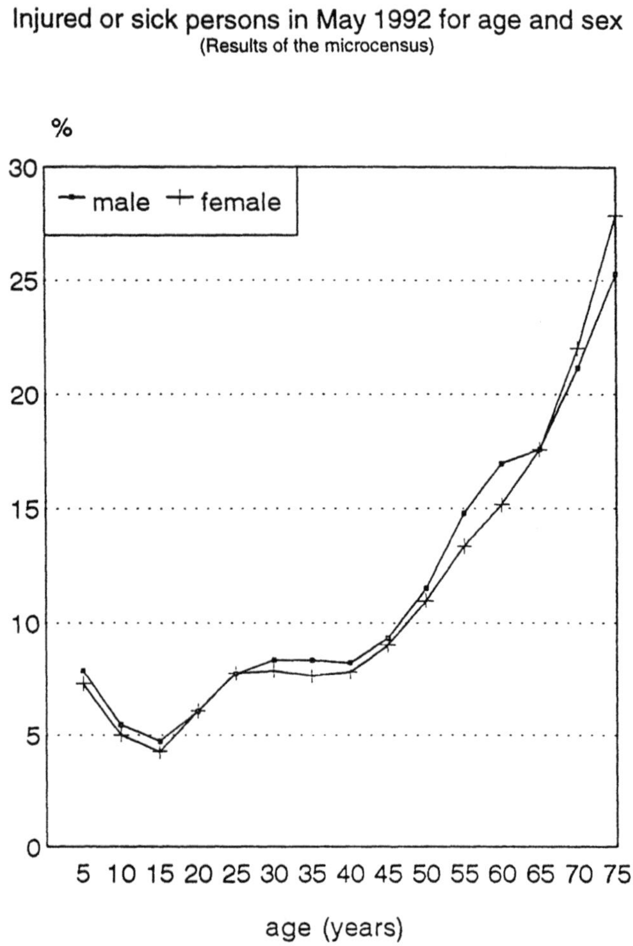

Source: Statistisches Bundesamt 1994.

handicapped (55.7 percent men). Seventy percent of the handicapped fall into the age group of the 55-year-old and older. Every fourth handicapped person lives alone; two thirds of the handicapped do not earn any salary.

Mental Health

The microcensus of 1982 shows an occurrence of 76 per 100,000 inhabitants for mental illnesses, mental retardation, and illnesses of the nervous system. An

Figure 3
Selected Causes of Death in Germany, 1993, for Age and Death (in % of the population of same age)

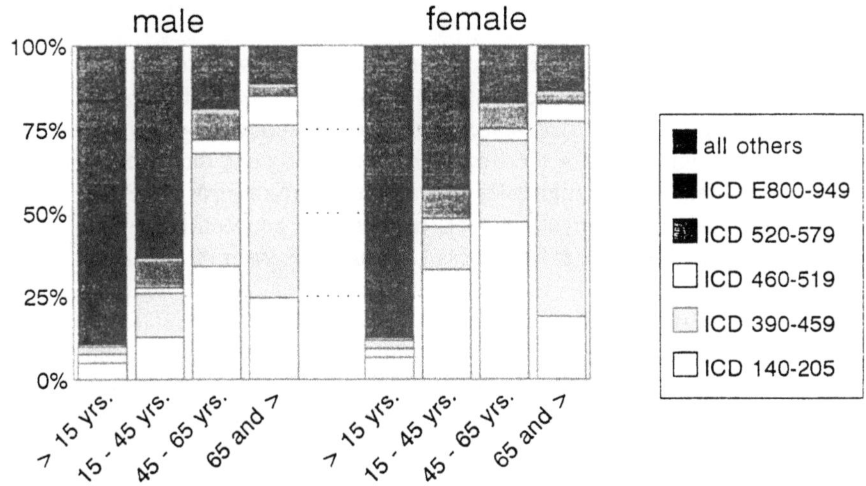

ICD 140-205 = malignant neoplasms; ICD 390-459 = cardiovascular diseases
ICD 460-519 = respiratory diseases; ICD 520-579 = digestive
ICD E800-949 = accidents

Source: Bundesministerium für Gesundheit 1994.

evident rise of the prevalence rate among these diseases occurs with increasing age, with a steeper slope for women than for men. Psychological problems constitute the main diagnosis among general practitioners and privately practicing internists in 3 to 4 percent of all cases. These data have been confirmed by the national health surveys. They show that, according to age group, between 1.8 percent and 3.9 percent among men and 1.3 percent and 2.9 percent among women reported to have consulted a physician because of mental disorders during the last four weeks. The national surveys are limited to residents between the ages of 25 and 69. Fundamentally, the epidemiology of mental illnesses faces a number of methodological problems. Therefore, underreporting may be possible.

Considering the mortality spectrum in Germany, about 53 percent of all deaths fall into the group of cardiovascular diseases (ICD 390–459), and cancer (ICD 140–205) with 23 percent (see Figure 3).

Age, Gender, and Social Class

Health and illness correlate in numerous ways with age and gender. The morbidity rates, for example, show an obvious correlation for children in the age group 0 to 5 years. Their morbidity risk is as high as in the age group of 30- to under 35-year-olds. The risk of illness is smallest among the 10- to 15-year-olds (about 5 percent). An apparent increase is noticeable after the age of 40. The morbidity rate for women after the age of 45 is rather below average. After the age of 65, however, it exceeds the rate of men (compare microcensus 1992).

Morbidity and mortality are, as demonstrated by all statistics, not only different between men and women but also with respect to location of residence. Relatively major regional differences exist for the frequency of illness and injury. A correlation exists for the size of the community and the illness rate: The larger the community, the higher the prevalence rate (Schwartz and Busse 1995). Female and male unemployed persons, in particular between the ages of 40 to 65, face a much higher risk for illness or injury. Higher risk for illness exists among workers.

A number of studies exist in Germany that deal with the correlation of social injustice and illness (*Sozial- und Präventivmedizin* 1993). They confirm that illness and health are linked to the social position of people. This concerns diagnoses that show a causal correlation with occupational stress, as well as occupational health hazards, risky exposure, and subjective accounts of illness. Numerous studies also allude to the relationship between unequal social opportunity and different use of screening offers among the population. With the intensification of the equity debate, a new methodological discussion of theoretical concepts of social-epidemiological equity research also emerged.

Health Situation of Immigrants and Refugees

Some 6.5 million of Germany's more than 80 million inhabitants are from abroad (Turks, citizens of the former Yugoslavia, Italians, Greeks, Polish, and others). Only singular studies deal with the health situation and health care provision of specific ethnic groups. Comparable data (as, for example, for infant mortality between 1982 and 1986) show a higher risk for foreign children. Also, the mortality rate among children between 1 and 4 years is higher for foreign children of either gender. Among the 5- to 14-year-olds, however, the mortality rate does adjust to the rate among German children. In the age bracket of the 15- to 24-year-olds, the mortality rate among German males exceeds the mortality rate among foreign males by 100 percent. The statistics of the injury insurance funds show that foreigners face a higher risk of work-related injury among the insured employees than their German colleagues.

Population Development

The observation of morbidity and mortality in the context of demographic development points to the special challenge for the German health care system. Due to a longer life expectancy and an increasing birthrate, the urn-shaped population development more and more approaches a pillar shape (Schwartz and Busse 1995). The demographic development, however, is not the sole variable in the demand assessment for health care. One also has to consider the development of the illness spectrum away from mostly infectious illnesses toward chronic and nontreatable diseases, which do not immediately lead to death. Furthermore, the technological progress in medicine signifies another variant of this issue. Forecasts about future demand also have to include the value society and politicians assign to which measures of primary, secondary, and tertiary health care.

Nutrition

Several diseases are considered to be precipitated by nutrition that may cause a deficiency as well as an excess supply of nutritional elements. According to Henke (1986), general malnutrition can account for 27 percent of all illness costs. The share of the obese population increases with the age. Among women of 65 or older, 30 percent can be considered heavily overweight (calculated according to body mass index [BMI]).

Environmental Hazards

During the last ten years, increasingly, an environmental-epidemiological perspective has developed. The effects can be found, for example, in the creation of chairs for Environmental Health at universities. Even though an unequivocal definition of environmental medicine is still lacking, the correlation of the environment and health has increasingly received public attention. Large population studies, however, are still missing in parts because of a research methodology that lacks sophistication. Individual studies exist, for example, about the chemical solvents problem, carcinogenic compounds, and the effects of climate change and traffic emissions. Also, pollutants in consumption goods and generated by waste treatment (toxic waste processing and waste transportation) increasingly become part of scientific research. As listed by Wemmer and Korczak (1993) in an overview of ecological destruction, multiple efforts will be necessary to scientifically examine the possible environmental influences on health.

PROVISION, UTILIZATION, AND IMPACT OF HEALTH SERVICES

Germany's social security system has a long history, and its efficiency is legend. Social benefits and services account for nearly 30 percent of the gross national product and in 1992 exceeded DM900 billion. Today's Public Health Offices evolved out of the institution of the "town physici." In the Middle

Ages, miners had set up joint funds to support needy colleagues after accidents at work.

With the strengthening of the cities and their increasing independence, a sense of responsibility grew for the poor. Early on, the dangers of the emergence and spread of epidemics caused cities to organize quarantine and hygienic measures. In the eighteenth and nineteenth centuries, a multitude of organizations and government initiatives sprang up to provide public health education to the population. A politically committed social medicine and public hygiene developed toward the end of the nineteenth century. Names of scientists like Virchow, Neumann, Mosse, Tugendreich, and others are associated with this period.

The gradual implementation of a statutory social insurance system through the German government laid the groundwork for a comprehensive social safety net, that is:

- Statutory health insurance (SHI) since 1883,
- Statutory accident insurance since 1884,
- Statutory pension insurance since 1889, and
- Statutory unemployment insurance since 1911.

Therefore, according to its constitution, the FRG considers itself as a democratic social welfare state.

Organization of Health Services

In agreement with its federal structure, the FRG is organized on a national, state, and regional or community level. The principle of competing legislation lets the states decide on issues of health and education unless federal laws exist (i.e., the final decision lies with the Upper House of Parliament as the assembly of the state representatives).

On the federal level, the Ministry of Health (BMG) and its departments are in charge (in 1994, the National Public Health Office [BGA] was transformed into four independent institutes). In the 16 states, the responsibility lies with the state ministries and the state public health offices. Communities and cities have local public health and welfare offices.

One can distinguish three pillars of the German health system: (1) ambulatory medical care through private practices; (2) inpatient medical care in hospitals; and (3) public health services. During the last 20 years, a fourth column has developed that comprises a comprehensive system of self-help groups.

Apart from the state, nongovernmental organizations are also responsible for institutions in the health system (Table 1). They are mostly summarized in the Independent Welfare Associations (Freie Wohlfahrtsverbaende).

In ambulatory medical care, private practices play a decisive role. Nonprofit organizations constitute the central backers for public nursing homes. Finally,

Table 1
Principal Backers of Medical Service Institutions

Medical Service Providers	*Public Institutions –State –Region –Communes*	*Nonprofit, Nongovernmental Institutions DCV[1)] DW[2)] DPWV[3)] AWO[4)] ZWST[5)]*	*Private Backers*	*N=*	*Institution per Inhabitant*
Private practices	—	—	***100%***	77,276	1:1,048
Acute care hospitals	45%	39%	16%	2,145	1:37,762
Old-age nursing units	—	***100%***	—	3,069	1:26,392
Prevention and rehabilitation institutions	20%	19%	***60%***	1,209	1:66,997
Public health offices	***100%***	—	—	512	1:158,203
Medical schools	***97%***	—	3%	36	—
Schools of public health	***100%***	—	—	8	—

[1]DCV = German Caritas Association (Deutscher Caritasverband).
[2]DW = Lutheran Institute of the Protestant Church (Diakonisches Werk der Evangelischen Kirche).
[3]DPWV = German Welfare Association (Deutscher Paritaetischer Wohlfahrtsverband).
[4]AWO = Workers Welfare (Arbeiterwohlfahrt).
[5]ZWST = Central Association of Jews in German (Zentralwohlfahrtsstelle der Juden in Deutschland).

Source: Beske, Brecht, and Reinkemeier 1993.

the government bears the main responsibility for medical school training; public health offices report to it.

In 1995, Germany had 3,600 hospitals with 810,000 beds; statistically, there was one hospital bed for every 100 inhabitants. Eighty-one percent of the physicians in ambulatory care work in private practices, either alone or with colleagues (usually in groups of two). Inpatient and ambulatory care are separate. The share of physicians with hospital privileges is small. Only 656 of the 105,013 specialized physicians are "physicians for public health," of which the overwhelming majority work as chiefs of public health offices. In 1992, statistically, there was one privately practicing physician for every 1,000 inhabitants. Table 2 provides insight into the relative numbers of various medical professionals in the health system.

The responsibility for outpatient medical care was shifted from the government to the Associations of SHI-Authorized Physicians (organized in National and Regional Associations) and the SHI funds as corporations under public law and the principle of self-administration.

Table 2
Employees in the Field of Health in 1990

Professional Fields	*Number*
Physicians	195,254
Dentists	43,167
Pharmacists	36,474
Nonmedical practitioners, herbalists	7,000
Nurses and midwives	574,000
Dietitians, pharmaceutical-medical assistants	29,000
Physical therapists and chiropractors	83,000
Medical laboratory workers	72,000
Medical assistants	300,000
Total	1,339,895

Source: Beske, Brecht, and Reinkemeier 1993, 173.

Drugs are supplied through 20,648 public pharmacies (1993) that work as independent businesses. For every 3,500 inhabitants, there is 1 pharmacy.

Public and Private Health Insurance

The German Social Insurance System is based on social legislation that was founded toward the end of the nineteenth century. In 1881, Chancellor Otto von Bismarck read an "imperial message" before the Parliament (Deutscher Reichstag) that is considered the birth of the German social insurance scheme. The most significant elements that are valid today are:

- A statutory insurance for employees under a certain level of income,
- The right of the insured to benefits,
- Mandatory employer contributions, and
- Self-governing insurance companies.

The relationship between the health care providers (for example, hospitals and private practice physicians), the insured, and the cost bearers (health insurance funds, pension funds, employment agencies, welfare agencies) has been summarized in the Social Code Legislation (Sozialgesetzbuch [SGB]), which consists of ten volumes. The declared goal is the "realization of social justice and social security." Through social benefits the following should be achieved: ensure a humane existence; create equal opportunities for personal development, in particular for the young; support and promote the family; permit for a freely

Table 3
Population According to Type of Health Insurance

Local health insurance funds	271	40.9%
Professional health insurance funds	741	4.4%
Company health insurance funds	173	10.7%
Bundesknappschaft (Miners fund)		2.2%
Agricultural health insurance funds	21	1.7%
Substitute health insurance funds	15	29.0%
Private health insurance funds		8.9%
Other insurances		2.0%
No insurance coverage		0.3%
Total	1,221	100.0%

Source: Bundesministerium für Gesundheit 1994.

chosen job to support a living; allow for a resort to self-help in times of special life crises to overcome these.

Of particular significance for public health are the benefits of statutory health, injury, and pension insurance. They are defined in detail. Benefits of the statutory health insurance according to SGB V are the following:

1. Benefits to promote health, to prevent and detect illness early
2. In case of illness
   a) Medical and dental care
   b) Medicine, bandage, and health aids
   c) Home care and household help
   d) Hospital care
   e) Medical and supplementary benefits for rehabilitation
   f) Work assistance for farmers
   g) Illness allowances
3. Home nurse in case of a need for permanent care
4. In case of pregnancy and motherhood: medical care, midwife, inpatient delivery, household assistance, maternity allowance, delivery allowance
5. Death allowance

The majority of the German population is enrolled in the statutory health insurance (Gesetzliche Krankenversicherung [GKV]), and only 0.3 percent are not insured (Table 3).

Since World War II, health insurance legislation has been altered several times in order to include or limit new benefits. In the late 1980s, fundamental structural changes in the health system were prepared. On January 1, 1989, the primary parts of the Health Care Reform Legislation (Gesundheitsreformgesetz [GRG]) were enacted. On January 1, 1993, they were complemented by a law to ensure and structurally improve the statutory health insurance (health care structure legislation—[Gesundheitsstrukturgesetz (GSG)]).

In the comprehensive social welfare system of Germany, additional assistance such as an additional child-raising allowance, rent subsidies, and grants to allow for the integration of handicapped persons are paid if needed. Among the social benefits are assistance to meet subsistence level, assistance in special situations, assistance to establish or maintain subsistence level, preventive health aids, aid to integrate handicapped persons, assistance for the blind, assistance in social emergency situations, aid to the elderly, counseling for handicapped persons, and assistance in finding and maintaining housing.

The professional associations are in charge of rehabilitation benefits in case of accidents and disability payments. The social insurance protection covers all citizens. Some 88.8 percent of the inhabitants are enrolled in statutory health insurance, and 8.9 percent are privately insured. One hundred percent of employees are enrolled in the ''statutory accident insurance,'' in the statutory pension insurance, and in the statutory unemployment insurance. According to social aid legislation, in cases lacking insurance protection, the costs are usually taken care of by the local welfare office.

Health Care Financing

The taxes that employers have to pay are accordingly high. Table 4 shows the increase of social spending for different benefits for the states of former West Germany.

Medical services are financed through different sources: premiums of the statutory social insurance, additional private expenditures and insurances, employers' benefits (e.g., sickness money), and government payments (e.g., investment in hospitals, universities, etc.) that are financed through taxes.

Relation Between Ambulatory and Hospital Health Care

The medical care system is organized in a graded fashion. Upon exhaustion of the aid possibilities in the so-called lay system (self-treatment and self-medication with drugs from the pharmacies), privately practicing physicians are responsible for primary care (86 percent of all citizens claim to have a family physician that they consult first in case of illness).

If needed, the primary care physicians refer to specialists for ambulatory care or to hospitals for inpatient care. Rehabilitation therapy is offered by specialized institutions, both as outpatient and inpatient treatment. The average duration of stay in hospital decreased from 19.6 to 15.6 days in 1992.

Table 4
Social Budget of the FRG (Old States) in 1960 and 1992 (in billion DM)

	1960	1992	increase
Social spending overall	68.94	826.05	12.0-fold
of which:			
Pension insurance	19.59	241.22	12.3-fold
Health care insurance	9.6	177.18	18.5-fold
Accident insurance	1.75	15.47	8.8-fold
Unemployment insurance and assistance	1.2	55.19	46.0-fold
Civil servant pensions	6.78	48.22	7.1-fold
Pension for farmers	0.18	5.34	29.7-fold
Sickness benefits	3.00	42.89	14.3-fold
Children allowances	0.92	17.01	18.5-fold
Child raising allowances	-	6.45	-
War victims care	3.95	13.43	3.4-fold
Housing allowances	0.002	4.00	2.000.0-fold
Juvenile assistance	0.44	15.61	35.5-fold
Social assistance	1.32	40.18	30.4-fold
Social spending per capita in DM	1 235	12 738	10.3-fold
Social quota (Social spending as % of gross national product)	23	30.3	1.3-fold

Source: Bundesministerium für Gesundheit 1994.

Preventive Health Care

The preventive health care system is subdivided into different areas. Health education in kindergartens and schools is subject to the education jurisdiction of the states. Different organizations on the federal, state, and city level are engaged in health education through public media. They are usually joined at a national level:

- The Federal Office for Health Education in Köln (Bundeszentrale für gesundheitliche Aufklärung [BZgA]) is a subordinate office of the BMG.
- The Central Association for Health is in Bonn-Bad Godesberg (Bundesvereinigung für Gesundheit).
- The German Center of Public Health Care in Frankfurt (Deutsche Zentrale für Volksgesundheitspflege [DZV]) is an association of nongovernmental organizations in the field of prevention and health promotion.
- The German Center Against the Dangers of Addiction in Hagen (Deutsche Hauptstelle gegen die Suchtgefahren [DHS]) is engaged in prevention of addiction.

- The German Institute of Hygiene in Dresden continues with the tradition of health exhibitions.

On the state level, activities on prevention and health promotion are carried out by the Central State Associations (Landesvereinigungen). And there are associations on the regional and community levels. They are organized in working groups by the local public health offices. They arrange local health days and health campaigns.

The Health Insurance Legislation (SGB V) obliges physicians and health insurers to support health promotion and illness prevention. According to §1 of the SGB V, they have the duty "to maintain the health of the insured, to restore or improve their state of health." The health insurers have to inform them about healthy ways of living via education and counseling.

To allow for the early detection of illnesses, the insureds have a right to screening examinations, which are performed by privately practicing physicians (during pregnancy, for infants, and for several chronic and malign illnesses among women over 20 years of age and men over 45 years of age).

Rehabilitation Services

Germany has a rehabilitation system that can be considered unique due to history. The system is based on the three pillars of medical, professional, and educational rehabilitation. It relies on the support of several institutions (statutory pension and health insurance, the National Ministry for Labor, the Welfare Office, etc.).

The Pension-Insurance Law (SGB VI) governs the tasks of the pension funds to appropriate pension allowances, disability and invalidity payments, and inpatient measures to avoid early retirement. In 1990 about 850,000 medical rehabilitation measures were granted by the pension funds. About 75 percent of the medical rehabilitation measures are prescribed for illnesses that can be attributed to three or four categories of disease groups. This share has been constant over the last few years. With respect to the total statutory pension insurance, the main reasons for application among males were illnesses of the skeleton, muscles, and connective tissue (45 percent), followed by illnesses of the cardiovascular system (19 percent) and psychological illnesses including substance abuse (12 percent). Among women, the prevalent reasons for application for rehabilitation treatments are illnesses of the skeleton, muscles, and connective tissue (46 percent), followed by psychological illnesses including substance abuse (16 percent), malignant tumors (13 percent), and cardiovascular diseases.

With respect to the total number of all pension-insured employees in Germany, the share of administered rehabilitative medical measures lies between 2.6 and 3.2 percent. Apart from the concession of rehabilitation measures, the main responsibilities of the pension funds are the payment of disability and invalidity allowances and pension payments.

Worker pension insurance is organized on the state level by the State Insurance Fund for Workers (Landesversicherungsanstalt für Arbeiter [LVA]). For other employees, the Federal Insurance Fund for employees (Bundesversicherungsanstalt für Angestellte [BfA]) manages pension insurance.

Public Health Services

Among the tasks of the government with respect to the health care system are the following: (1) the national and state specific health administration, (2) the health administration of the statutory health and pension insurances, and (3) the public health offices of the states, communes, and the cities.

The German Ministry of Health (BMG) has comprehensive responsibilities. Among these are health insurance, nursing insurance, medical service of the health insurances, epidemiological statistics, hospital care, illness prevention, health professions, addiction and hygiene, health research, pharmaceutical issues and pharmacies, environmental health issues, nutritional education, and other public health issues. Different administrative bodies are assigned to the Ministry of Health: (1) Federal Office for Health Education (BZgA), (2) National Office for Vaccines and Serums, (3) German Institute for Medical Documentation and Information, (4) Robert-Koch-Institute for Infectious and Noninfectious Diseases, and (5) Max-von-Pettenkofen-Institute.

The Ministry for Labor and Social Relations (Bundesministerium für Arbeit und Sozialordnung [BMAS]) is, among others, responsible for pension and accident insurance. The Ministry for Environmental Protection and Nuclear Safety (Bunderministerium für Umwelt; BMU) has, among others, the responsibility for health protection in connection with environmental pollution. The Ministry for Education, Science, Research and Technology (Bundesministerium für Bildung, Wissenschaft, Forschung und Technologie [BMFT]) supports several research projects in the field of public health. They are incorporated in its program "Health Research 2000."

The federal states have far-reaching tasks and responsibilities. They are responsible for the execution of state laws, possess jurisdictive authority, and have technical supervision over public health. The Health Departments of the state ministries control not only the public health service but also social insurance (including health insurance), the private practice service, veterinary medicine, and food surveillance. The activities of the states are coordinated by a Permanent Conference of State Ministers and Senators of Health (GMK) and The Working Group of Executive State Health Officials (AGLMB).

Industrial inspection boards guard compliance to occupational protection laws. Offices of inquiry regulate the execution of health directions, in particular in the National Disease Legislation (Bundesseuchengesetz) and the Drug Legislation (Arztneimittelgesetz). At the lowest level of the administrative hierarchy, public health offices have been established in all districts and cities to standardize the management of public health services.

In 1991, there were 524 public health offices. The director is a public health physician, a physician who went through additional training in public health. Physicians that work in public health offices are civil servants and therefore are not subject to termination. Currently, about 5,100 physicians and 1,100 dentists work in public health offices. Public health offices are responsible for:

- Supervision and control of persons and equipment employed in the health professions.
- Prevention and combat of infectious diseases.
- Supervision of handling of food, pharmaceutical, and toxic substances.
- Health aid, that is, school health promotion, counseling of mothers and children.
- Medical care for patients affected by tuberculosis, sexually transmitted diseases, handicapped persons, addicts, and the disabled.
- Health education and counseling.
- Promotion of hygiene and sports.
- Medical consultation for public health offices, courts and health insurers.

Adolescent, family, elderly, and handicapped aid, public nursing wards, and counseling offices are organized either on a communal level with government subsidies or by nongovernmental welfare organizations (Freie Wohlfahrtsverbände).

Self-Help Organizations

The traditional measures of self-help in the familiy setting or through professional cooperatives and associations have increasingly lost their significance in the context of social structural change and the establishment of a comprehensive social insurance system. Linked to a growing public criticism of traditional medicine, different self-help groups of afflicted persons were established in the late 1960s. Modeled after the Alcoholics Anonymous groups, self-help circles also emerged that provided mutual support in coping with the illness. After initial resistance on the part of physicians, operational and referral structures developed. Today private practitioners and self-help groups and organizations cooperate closely. On a regional level, associations of self-help groups were founded to serve, on the one hand, as a representation of an interest group vis-à-vis the officials and, on the other hand, as a mediating role for interested citizens.

Accessibility and Equity of Services

On the basis of the comprehensive social insurance system in Germany, essentially all medically necessary services are freely available to all citizens. The insurance coverage usually refers to in-kind service. In the case of a lack of insurance coverage, and financial necessity, government aid measures are granted. In the social welfare system of the FRG, basic medical care and social security are granted for all citizens in the same way.

THE INFRASTRUCTURE OF TRAINING AND RESEARCH IN PUBLIC HEALTH

The educational system is the responsibility of the states. School attendance is obligatory between the ages of 6 and 16 years. Principally, there are three different high school degrees:

- Vocational high school with a subsequent apprenticeship,
- ''Practically'' oriented high school (degree: *Mittlere Reife*), and
- ''Academically'' oriented high school (degree: *Abitur*).

The *Abitur* qualifies one to attend university. There are also other paths to achieve entrance into university by gaining additional qualifications, for example, going to night school.

The education and training for the different public health professions vary. Medical school training encompasses six years plus a mandatory 18 months of residency. It takes place at 1 of the 35 departments of medicine at public universities (there is only one private medical school). Physicians' training is regulated through law. The final degree awarded is the medical license. The medical boards are corporations under public law and are responsible for additional training and postgraduate study programs for physicians.

The continued education to become a public health physician takes another 5.5 years. The theoretical part of the training takes six months of full-time study. It is administered by public academies in Duesseldorf, Munich, and Schwerin. These academies also offer training programs leading to a certificate in social medicine (for physicians working for the medical service of health insurances, pension funds, rehabilitation clinics, etc.). Furthermore, they conduct continued training for physicians working with adolescents, public health engineers, social workers, and social-medical assistants.

No programs existed in Germany until 1989 to receive the master of public health degree. Due to the increased demand for professionalism and high-quality work in this area, in the late 1980s the government established a program to promote public health training. The German Academic Exchange Service (Deutscher Akademischer Austauschdienst [DAAD]) offers scholarships for professional training programs in epidemiology and public health at a school of public health abroad.

The Ministry for Education and Science (it was merged with the Ministry for Research and Technology in 1994 and today is the Ministry for Education, Science, Research and Technology) cooperated with the state ministries in promoting the development of public health research structures at universities (Table 5). Currently eight public health postgraduate programs exist at universities.

At the University of Bielefeld, a new department for public health has been created. It offers nine areas of research: (1) social epidemiology and health care system design, (2) biomedical foundations and population medicine, (3) epidemiology and biostatistics, (4) prevention and health promotion, (5) public health management, (6) nursing sciences, (7) rehabilitation and social gerontology (in progress), (8) environmental health (in progress), and (9) social psychiatry (in progress). At the Technical University of Berlin, an Institute for Public Health Sciences has been established.

In total, there are 220 places available for public health students in Germany a year. Nevertheless, it should be considered that a university degree in a health-related field is an entry requirement for these postgraduate programs. A primary basic university program is currently not available in this area. Training and continued education programs in different public health areas are also increasingly offered by technical colleges. The University of Magdeburg established a degree program in public health promotion. Simultaneously, a fundamental move has been made to make the professional training of nurses more of an academic education and include different programs concerning the pedagogy of nursing and management of nursing. Similarly, possibilities exist for economists to receive additional training in hospital and health insurance management. An attempt is made to develop the area of health economics in the university setting.

As a result of the federal "Program for the Promotion of Public Health" currently at 17 universities in 13 German cities, new research structures are being created. The aim is the development of high-quality and efficient research centers in Germany. A German Consortium for the Health Sciences (Deutscher Verband für Gesundheitswissenschaften [DVGE]) is engaged in the promotion of professional interests. The German Research Association (DFG), as the largest research promoter in Germany, currently prepares a focal point of research in the area of health care system research. The Donors' Association for the Sciences and Humanities in Germany sponsors a focal point "Health Sciences/Public Health" with grants of the Fritz and Hildegard Berg Foundation. Accordingly, a Coordinating Agency for Public Health (Koordinierungsstelle Gesundheitswissenschaften/Public Health) was founded at the Department of Medical Sociology at the Albert-Ludwigs-University of Freiburg. Tasks of this coordinating agency are to document, evaluate, and support the process of institutionalization of public health in research, education, and practice in Germany. Therefore, the Coordinating Agency

- Organizes financial support for scientific meetings and symposiums,
- Publishes the journal *Public Health Forum* (four times a year),
- Publishes a book edition (so far four volumes, a "Who Is Who in Public Health"), and

Table 5
Schools of Public Health in Germany

	Berlin	*Bielefeld*	*Ulm*	*Dresden*	*Düsseldorf*	*Hannover*	*Heidelberg*	*Munich*
Responsible Body	Technical University of Berlin	School of Public Health, University of Bielefeld	Medical Department of University of Ulm	Medical Department of Technical University of Dresden	Medical Department of University of Düsseldorf & Academy for Public Health	Medical School Hannover	Institute for Tropical Hygiene and Public Health, University of Heidelberg	Medical Department of Ludwig-Maximilians-University
Name of Program	Public Health	Public Health and Public Health Promotion	Public Health	Public Health	Public Health and Social Medicine	Population Medicine and Public Health	Community Health and Health Management in Developing Countries	Public Health and Epidemiology
Start	October 1992	Spring 1989	October 1995	April 1991	April 1991	October 1990	July 1989	May 1993
Degree	M.P.H.	M.P.H.	M.P.H.	Diploma in Public Health (M.P.H. in planning)	M.San.	M.P.H.	M.Sc.	Certificate
Duration	2 years	2 years	2 years	2 years	2 years	1–2 years	1 year	2 years
Places	40 per semester	70 per semester	20 per semester	30 per semester	20 per year	20 per year	20 per semester	25 per semester

- Appoints a yearly award for the best examination paper in one of the postgraduate studies in public health.

In close cooperation with the scientific associations (German Society of Medical Sociology, German Society of Social Medicine and Prevention, German Association of Public Health), the Coordinating Agency is planning to establish a system for the evaluation of public health programs at universities and technical colleges to guarantee a high standard of quality in education.

MAJOR CHALLENGES FOR THE HEALTH SERVICES

Toward the end of the twentieth century, the historically tried and proven health and social insurance system of the FRG faces new challenges and a changed systemic environment. There are different reasons for this, which are mutually interdependent. During recent years, the public health discussion has been mainly determined by increasing costs for medical services and a corresponding rise in taxes and insurance premiums for citizens. Several political measures (conferences of representatives of the major organizations in the health system—Concerted Action) and legislative steps (Cost-Abatement Law, Health-Care Reform Law, Structural Health System Law) did not have any decisive impact on this development. The reasons are:

- The technological progress that features costly medical-technical innovations.
- The change of the demographic structure with an absolute and a relative increase of the elderly population.
- The changes of the societal measure of illness and discomfort. This is, among other reasons, linked to the orientation of "well-being" propelled by a consumerist society.
- The dwindling significance of religion and a corresponding disorientation and changed expectations in life.
- Disintegration and relativization of traditional social bonds (in particular, the family), a parallel increase of living expenses in a "single society" (more one-person households), and, therefore, a diminishing sense of solidarity with one's fellow citizen.
- Changes in disease patterns with an increase in age-related ailments and chronic illnesses.
- An increasing demand for sound public health reporting as a ground for public health planning.
- Increasing differences in the likelihood for health or illness according to class affiliation, in the sense of the "two-thirds society."

The critical issue is to what extent it will be possible to initiate a population-wide discussion about fundamental values and if it will lead to political action:

- How far should average life expectancy rise in Germany, in Europe, and among the global population as a whole?
- What illnesses do we want to die from—that is, what is considered a "good death" in our society?
- How much of malady, pain, handicaps, impairment, and discomfort is part of human life? Moreover, can psychosocial work—that is, the coping with the above—contribute to individual and collective orientation?
- What is the value of the health and social security insurance system in the eyes of the population? What is the share of income/gross national product that, according to the population, should be invested in it?
- To what extent should the health care system be organized by market forces, by medical service supply, or by public services?
- To what extent can personal data concerning health and illness be collected, saved, and used to direct the health care system?
- How can the population of the FRG, the population of Europe, and—last but not least—the governments of the world be propelled to develop a fundamental sense of responsibility for the natural environment and to subsequently make sacrifices?
- What significance will work have for the population of the postindustrial society?

Currently, there exist several initiatives in Germany to reform the health care system. Through the appropriate professional training and continued education, professionalization is promoted—in particular, in the areas of prevention and health promotion. The aim is an adequate qualification of the professionals in this field. In the context of a broad discussion regarding quality control of medical services—mostly under the system of professional self-administration—quality standards have been elaborated and rules to ensure quality have been analyzed (e.g., quality circles).

Supported by government funds, comprehensive public health reporting has been established. It will lead to an improvement in public health planning on a national, state, and community level.

NOTE

The authors wish to thank Beatrice Harnasch for translating this chapter.

REFERENCES

Beske, F., Brecht, J. G. & Reinkemeier, A.-M. (1993). *Das Gesundheitswesen in Deutschland.* Köln: Deutscher Ärzteverlag.

Bundesministerium für Gesundheit (BMG). (1993). *Daten des Gesundheitswesens.* Vol. 25. Baden-Baden: Nomos Verlagsgesellschaft.

Bundesministerium für Gesundheit (BMG). (1994). *Daten des Gesundheitswesens.* Vol. 26. Baden-Baden: Nomos Verlagsgesellschaft.

Deutsche Forschungsgemeinschaft (DFG). (1995). *Gesundheitssystemforschung in Deutschland.* Memorandum. (Ed.: F. W. Schwartz). Weinheim: VCH Verlag.

Deutscher Städtetag (Ed.). (1989). Bonner Manifest der deutschen Städte—Ohne Städte keine Zukunft. Vol. 58. Stuttgart: Kohlhammer Verlag.

Henke, K.-D. (1986). *Die Kosten ernährungsbedingter Krankheiten.* Stuttgart: Kohlhammer.

IDIS. (1993). *Gesundheitsberichterstattung: Beispiele für einen vereinheitlichten nationalen und internationalen Datensatz für die kommunale Gesundheitsberichterstattung in Nordrhein-Westfalen.* Bielefeld: IDIS (LÖGD).

Schwartz, F. W. & Busse, R. (1994). *Fünf Mythen zur Effizienzsteigerung im Gesundheitswesen: Zur aktuellen gesundheitspolitischen Diskussion in Deutschland.* Jahrbuch für kritische Medizin 23. Hamburg: Argument Verlag. 149–170.

Schwartz, F. W. & Busse, R. (1995). Morbidität, Demographie und technischer Fortschritt als Determinanten künftiger Entwicklungen im Gesundheitswesen. *Die Betriebskrankenkasse*, 83 (2), 80–85.

Sozial- und Präventivmedizin. (1993). Schwerpunktheft ''Soziale Ungleichheit und Krankheit.'' 38 (3).

Statistisches Bundesamt. (1994). Entwicklung der Bevölkerung bis 2040. In: *Wirtschaft und Statistik.* Vol. 7. Wiesbaden: Statistisches Bundesamt. 497–554.

Wemmer, U. & Korczak, D. (1993). *Gesundheit in Gefahr.* Daten-Report 1993/94. Frankfurt: Fischer Taschenbuch Verlag.

ISRAEL

Eitan F. Sabatello, David Chinitz,
Palti Hava, and Leon Epstein

DEMOGRAPHIC ASPECTS OF THE POPULATION RELATED TO MORTALITY

Population Growth and Migrations

In less than 50 years the population of Israel has vastly increased by almost sevenfold, and at mid-1995, it numbers close to 5.5 million people (versus about 800,000 in May 1948).

This growth, perhaps worldwide unique for a nation in the last two centuries, has been largely determined by immigrants and their descendants. Between 1882 and 1947, five different waves of immigrants, 500,000 in total, established the demographic base of the future State of Israel. After the abolishment in May 1948 of the restrictive policy of the British Government's Mandate (1922–1948) vis-à-vis the immigration of Jews to Palestine, and the establishment of a policy granting Jews everywhere the right to settle in Israel (Law of Return, 1950), 2.5 million immigrants arrived in the country, and 90 percent of them were integrated as permanent resident citizens. Five other large waves of immigrants can be identified in that period: The most numerous (close to 700,000 persons) and crucial (because it allowed Israel to be viable as a state) was that of 1948–1951, which gathered in almost equal parts displaced persons from post–World War II Europe and people from the Jewish communities in the Middle East Moslem countries. Since 1990, more than 600,000 new immigrants have joined Israel. Some 550,000 were from the former USSR and constitute in 1995 about 10 percent of the total Israeli population, close to 30,000 came from Ethiopia, and 50,000 arrived from other, mostly developed countries worldwide. Most of the immigrants to Israel have come with family rather than as unattached persons (Bachi 1976).

In addition to Jews (39 percent of whom are first-generation and 23 percent are second-generation migrants), there are in Israel also close to 900,000 Arabs and a few European-born citizens (16 percent of the total population), mostly Moslems but also Christians and Druzes, and other permanent Arab residents.

Aging and Fertility

This mosaic of people of different origins, creeds, and migratory experiences shows several demographic and social features that distinguish Israel from other developed countries (mostly in Europe and North America). Perhaps the most peculiar demographic aspects are aging and fertility patterns.

The immigrations not only contributed to a rapid increase of the population but also generated an age structure that has made, and in the medium range will keep, the population of Israel one of the youngest among the developed nations: In the 1990s, less than 10 percent of Israelis are 65 years old or above, and this share is expected to increase only slightly for the next 20 years; but by around 2015, Israel is expected to start experiencing an ''elderly boom''—just an unavoidable demographic echo effect of the high fertility and numerous babies of the many immigrants of 1948–1951; the aging effect will worsen around 2025 and also later when the baby-boomers of the 1950s will enter their middle seventies and the generations of the 1960s and the 1970s will reach 65 (Eizenbach and Sabatello 1991).

From the above observations, it is clear what has been the long-range effect of mass immigration at the beginning of Israel's independence. On the other side is the country's aging process, which started gaining momentum in the 1970s (5 percent elderly in 1960, 7 percent in 1970, and 9 percent in 1980). The aging process is mainly an effect of the numerous previous immigrants (those of the 1930s through the 1950s) as they reached 65 years, rather than of declining fertility, as has generally been the case in Western countries. In fact, total fertility rates (TFRs) in Israel are unusually high as compared to those prevailing in Europe, North America, and some developed Asian countries. Israeli Arabs and Jewish immigrants from the Middle East area both showed very high fertility rates in the past; rates have decreased over time, especially since the 1960s and more so for the ''Oriental'' Jews than for the local Arabs; since the early 1990s, TFRs for these two groups stand at 3 and 4.5 children per woman, respectively. With the exception of the new immigrants from the former USSR (whose TFR is significantly lower than 2), Jews of European origin have shown ''non-European'' fertility rates of well above 2.5 children per woman for the past 40 years; somewhat higher fertility rates have prevailed among the growing sector of Israeli Jewish women born in the country (now 70 percent of the female Jewish population in the childbearing ages). These patterns have resulted in a total fertility rate for the Israeli woman of around 3 for the last 15

Table 1
Crude Death Rates, IMR, and Life Expectancy in Israel: Values for the 1960s, 1975, and the 1990s and Relative Position Internationally

	1960s		*1975*		*1990s*	
	Value	*Position*	*Value*	*Position*	*Value*	*Position*
CDR, total	6.3		7.0		6.3	
Jews	6.2		7.2		7.0	
Arabs	6.4		5.5		3.4	
IMR, total	28.2	20	22.9	25	9.5	25
Jews	23.0		16.8		7.5	
Arabs	45.0		36.0		14.0	
Life expectancy						
Males	69.9	6	70.3	5	74.9	3
Females	72.8	16	73.9	19	78.4	20

Note: Values are averages for 1990–1992.

Sources: WHO Year Books, various years.

years—50 to 150 percent higher than those currently prevailing in the developed countries (UN 1993).

In total, the age-sex pyramid of the Israeli population (and to a somewhat lesser extent, that of its Jewish majority) is one of an expanding population and thus very different from those of the European countries; that of the Israeli Arabs is similar to those of many developing societies. However, its very large base (young ages) is not only due to high fertility but also to relatively low and decreasing infant and child mortality.

Mortality

Relatively high fertility, continuing sustained immigration and the resulting moderate aging have a special impact on the mortality trend in Israel. The most obvious one is comparatively low crude death rates (CDRs), slightly more than 6 per 1,000 inhabitants in the 1990s; no other developed country can show a lower CDR, as young age structure and sustained fertility clearly advantage Israel. In terms of more refined mortality measures, in 1993 Israel's infant mortality rate (IMR) was less than 8 countrywide, a level that puts Israel in the middle among European (and other developed) countries, though below practically all the Western and northern ones. In the 1960s the relative position of Israel was higher (see Table 1), but by the early 1990s, countries like Italy,

Spain, Greece, and Portugal seem to have obtained more conspicuous results in curbing infant mortality. Differences within Israel are still a matter of concern: Arabs' IMR (12 to 13 per 1,000 live births) was in 1993 about double that of the Jews; the same is true for poorly educated people versus postsecondary-trained people, "developing" peripheral towns versus metropolitan areas, and to a lesser extent, Jews of North African origin versus those of European or Asian origin (CBS 1993).

In terms of life expectancy, which currently averages 76 years nationwide and during the 1980s moved from eleventh to tenth place in Europe (WHO 1994), Israel presents an unusual pattern by sex: At any given age the difference between men and women is small—about half that prevailing in other developed countries. At birth, for instance, the gap is only 3.5 years (75 years for men and 78.5 for women). Therefore, life expectancy of Israeli men occupies one of the first five places among the developed countries, while that of Israeli women is only placed around the twentieth place. Though intriguing, the reasons for the relative supermortality of females in Israel vis-à-vis males are still unclear and perhaps have not been an object of sufficient research.

Causes of Death

A brief analysis of data on causes of death might, however, give a preliminary answer: Figure 1 reports age-sex standardized data for the last four decades; the data include the Jewish population only, since reliable data for the Israeli Arabs are available for a shorter period and their addition does not significantly change the countrywide picture.

After controlling for changes in the age structure of the population, it appears that only in one (but prevalent group—malignant neoplasms) out of six large groups of causes was there no significant change; therefore, since the early 1980s malignant neoplasms have composed the leading group of causes of death for women, and since the early 1990s, for men, too, instead of ischemic heart disease. Ischemic heart disease prevalence, which steadily increased until the early 1970s, decreased thereafter to less than half the top level; males' death rates by this group of causes are almost twice that of females, somewhat less than expected according to international experience.

The rates of external causes and of the ecological causes (infectious diseases, pneumonia) have been decreasing over time, about 50 percent in almost 40 years; also differences between sexes have diminished, with men still showing slightly higher rates.

The rates of cerebrovascular diseases, which oscillated somewhat during the 1950s through the mid-1970s, have also been curbed since then by 50 percent for males and even more for females. Death rates for women in this group seem very similar to those for men, an unusual feature in international perspective. Therefore, it is suggested that the relative low life expectancy of women in Israel (low compared to the life expectancy of Israeli men) is partly explained

Figure 1
Age-Standardized Mortality Rates, by Sex, for Selected Causes (Jews), 1950–1992

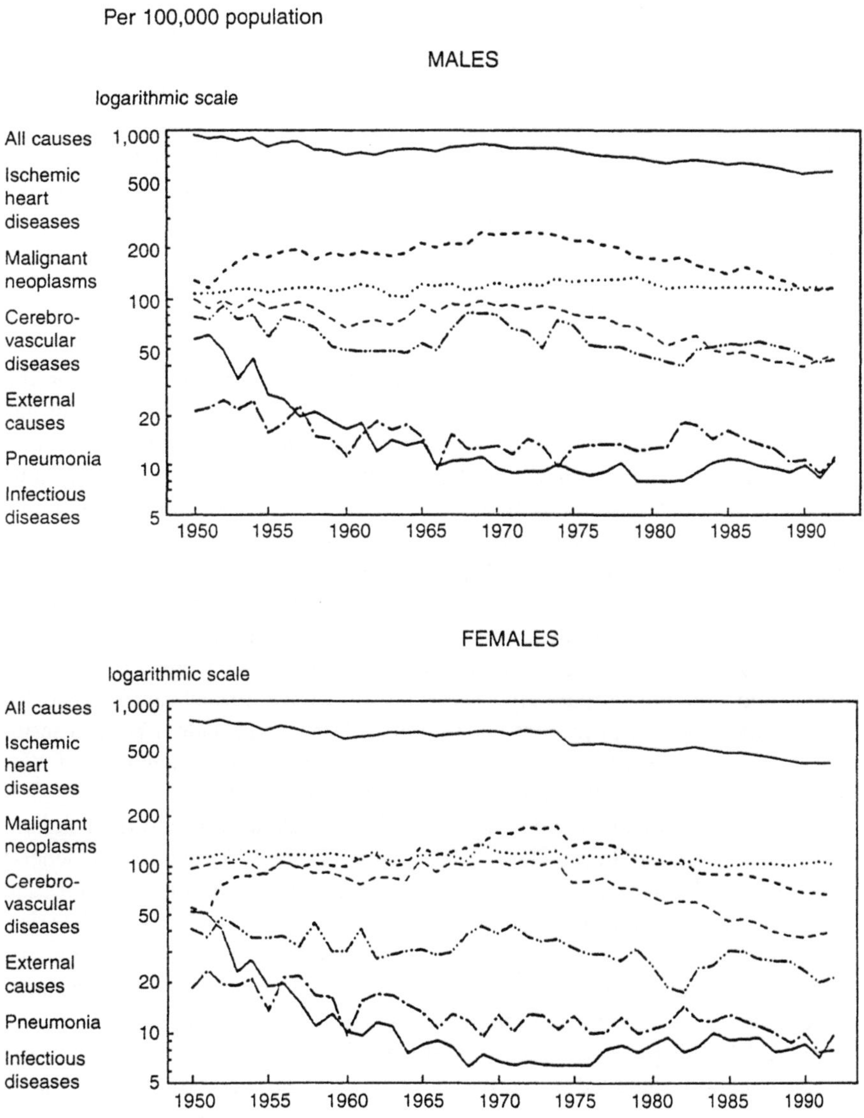

Source: Central Bureau of Statistics 1993.

by an exceptionally higher-than-usual proneness of Israeli women (especially those from North Africa) to die of diseases included in that large group of causes or by heart diseases. This finding should foster medical and epidemiological research in the field. However, it is likely that the phenomenon is linked to the migratory experience and adjustment of large parts of the Israeli population. Some sociologists claim that the group that underwent the largest strain was that from North Africa—because of, among other reasons, the negative selection of migration, the relative delay of the process, the lower adaptability of the human capital brought to Israel, and the largest disruption of communal life. As we already indicated, North Africans are exposed to death more than others (Jewish); North African women, in particular, might have been particularly sensitive to the large changes in life patterns (housing, food, military tension, etc.) they faced in Israel—with minimal family and communal support.

THE ISRAELI HEALTH SYSTEM: BASIC STRUCTURE AND CURRENT CHANGES

As a young but developed country Israel has made tremendous strides in the health status of its population. During the 47 years of its existence, Israel has established a health services network that is both extensive and complex. Despite a pluralistic structure of finance and delivery, Israel has achieved nearly universal access to health services, mainly through a system of voluntary sick funds. One of the most momentous policy changes in the history of the state went into effect on January 1, 1995, when National Health Insurance (NHI) became the law of the land. Passage of the law represents a trend to move from voluntary to obligatory health insurance and to reduce the pluralism in the system by having sick funds compete over bundles of services that were previously financed and delivered separately. These changes have special significance for public health and health promotion. In this section, we provide a brief description of the Israeli health system as it existed previous to implementation of NHI and the implications of the changes that have been introduced.

The main components of the Israeli health services network are the Ministry of Health, the Kupot Holim Clalit (KHC), which is the sick fund of the General Federation of Labor (GFL), three smaller sick funds (Leumit, Maccabi, and Meuhedet), local authorities, voluntary/nonprofit agencies, and private agencies. The sick funds supply, either directly or by purchase from other providers, ambulatory curative services and hospitalization services on a voluntary basis in exchange for insurance premiums. Psychiatric, geriatric, as well as public health and health promotion services are provided largely by government and are not generally included in the basket of services provided by the sick funds. Table 2 shows the shares of these sectors in provision of care.

In 1994, approximately 96 percent of the population of 5 million was insured through the sick funds, with KHC serving about 64 percent of the population; Maccabi, 18 percent, and Leumit and Meuhedet, about 9 percent each. An im-

Table 2
Institutional Shares of Provision of Care as a Percentage of National Health Expenditure

Institution	Percentage of Expenditure
Central government and local authorities	22
Sick funds	40
Non-profit Institutions	13
Others--private commercial providers	25

Source: Central Bureau of Statistics 1994.

portant aspect of the system, and a major focus of recent changes, relates to the political and organizational links of the sick funds. Kupot Holim Clalit and Leumit belong to labor unions. Until implementation of NHI, KHC members paid a tax to the GFL. Approximately 70 percent of these funds were transferred to the sick fund. A similar arrangement existed in Leumit. In part due to philosophical and political guidelines of their parent organizations, which limit selectivity in enrollment, both Clalit and Leumit insure an older and a financially less secure population. Older members (age 65+) make up 13 percent of Clalit's membership, 7.2 percent of Leumit's, and 4.8 percent and 4.1 percent, respectively, for Maccabi and Meuhedet (Central Bureau of Statistics 1994). Kupot Holim, Maccabi, and Meuhedet are not affiliated with any labor or trade union. They tend to accept members who are generally healthier and of higher economic status. These policy differences in population selection yield varying revenues and expenditure patterns among the funds, with consequences for their relative financial stability. KHC, in particular, has accumulated large financial debts in large part due to these disparities.

Although coverage in Israel is nearly universal, and health system resources appear adequate by international standards, physical access is constrained (Chernichovsky and Chinitz 1995; Ellencweig and Chinitz 1993). At times in the past, in many sick fund clinics the quality of primary care was low, and long waiting lists existed for elective procedures in the hospital. The health system as it exists does not always appear to be answering the needs of the population it serves—hence, the increasing market for private medical services (both ambulatory and hospital based) and the proliferation of extended and supplementary insurance (both through the sick funds and the private sector). These events have significantly increased the ''out-of-pocket'' expenses paid by the medical consumer.

Spending 7.7 percent of its gross national product (GNP) on health, Israel fares quite well compared with Organization for Economic Cooperation and

Table 3
National Expenditures on Health by Financing Sector, 1984 and 1992 (in percent)

Financing Sector		1992
General Taxation	30	21
Earmarked Employer Tax	22	25
Sick Fund Member Dues	12	23
Private out-of-pocket and insurance	19	29
Other	16	1

Source: Central Bureau of Statistics 1994.

Development (OECD) countries (Central Bureau of Statistics 1994). However, trends in the composition of health system finance sources raise other concerns. Research in OECD countries has suggested that higher proportions of public finance in the health sector are associated with lower overall health expenditures (Shirom 1994). Public financing is defined as deriving from either general government revenue or social insurance tax payments, which are usually income linked. Private finance is defined as direct out-of-pocket payments or private insurance. Until the end of the 1970s, public financing of the Israeli health care system was about 80 percent. As seen in Table 3, by 1992 this percentage stood at 70 percent. Direct government funding and the earmarked employer health tax together accounted for 47 percent of national health finance. Member dues to the sick funds, paid on an income-linked (though ultimately regressive) basis, accounted for 23 percent. Out-of-pocket expenses were 20 percent in 1985 and 29 percent in 1992 (Central Bureau of Statistics 1994). The reduction in public financing was mostly as a result of the government's decision to decrease the portion of the budget allocated to the Ministry of Health (Chernichovsky and Chinitz 1995; Shirom 1994).

Within this pluralistic system of finance and delivery, public health, preventive activities, and health promotion are provided primarily by central government and the local authorities. There are no clear data on the proportion of national health expenditures devoted to these fields. Within the Ministry of Health, about 5.5 percent of the budget is devoted to the public health services (Ministry of Health 1994). Out of overall national health expenditures, 34 percent are spent on public clinics and preventive medicine, but this includes the curative primary care clinics of the sick funds.

Personal preventive services are provided primarily by 460 family health stations of the Ministry of Health, by mother and child stations operated by the Jerusalem and Tel Aviv municipalities, as well as by KHC. The smaller sick funds have also begun to provide some preventive services in recent years. The main services provided under this rubric are prenatal preventive care; immunization, developmental monitoring, and early disease detection for infants; and health education. In the view of the State Judicial Commission of Inquiry into the Health System in Israel (1990) and subsequent assessments, these services are in need of improvement and should be integrated into the service baskets provided by the sick funds. The same sources cite deficiencies in school health programs, environmental health, health education, and occupational health (State of Israel 1990; Shirom 1994).

Passage of NHI and initiation of other reforms in the health system are aimed in large part at reducing the pluralism of the system by concentrating finance in the hands of central government and by bundling of health services previously provided by a multiplicity of providers into an expanded sick fund basket. Sick fund member dues have been replaced by a health tax. The government will pool the revenues from this tax with all other sources of finance and from this pool make capitation payments to the sick funds, ensuring that funds intended for the health system are not diverted to other uses. Sick funds will be prohibited from selective enrollment, in an attempt to streamline competition and reduce inequities in provision of care. The Ministry of Health will be removed from day-to-day operation of services thereby, allowing it to play the role of planner and regulator, seeking to ensure that citizens have adequate access to the services included in the basket.

MATERNAL AND CHILD HEALTH PREVENTIVE SERVICES

At the beginning of the twentieth century, Palestine was a province of the Ottoman empire. The population was poor, and malaria, trachoma, blindness, high infant mortality (144/1,000 in 1922), and lack of a basic sanitary system characterized the region (Grushka 1968). The initiative to establish Maternal and Child Health Stations to improve child health and reduce infant mortality and educate women on issues of personal hygiene came from the voluntary organization of Hadassah, the Women's Zionist Organization of America. From the modest initiatives of providing advice on personal hygiene and nutrition, and distributing supplementary feeding through the "Milk Stations," a network of Maternal and Child Health Stations has developed, and parallel with it in the early 1920s, the Department of School Hygiene. The latter provided services for schoolchildren who suffered mainly from skin diseases and eye problems. Health education was the foremost concern, with the public health nurse playing a most important role.

In the 1920s, a comprehensive health insurance scheme was established by the general Federation of Jewish Labor, with the aim of providing curative and preventive services in the cities and even in the smallest agricultural settlements.

The basic principle of the health services was, and still is today, accessibility and availability to all levels of society with more attention to the problems of the weaker classes and new immigrants.

These services formed the nucleus of the preventive health services of the State of Israel established in 1948. The first decade of existence of the State of Israel was dominated by the need of absorption of the large number of new immigrants from different countries. Infectious diseases, malnutrition, and high infant mortality were the main physical problems, in addition to mental problems arising from suffering during World War II and the difficulties of adjustment to a new society and environment.

The preventive services provided by Hadassah were handed over to the Ministry of Health during the 1950s, and the ministry became the main provider of preventive services. The Labor Union's Health insurance plan (Kupot Holim) and that of other agencies (Kupot Holim Ammamit, etc.) continued to provide mainly curative care for the population insured with them.

The network of Maternal and Child Health services (MCH) has developed throughout the years into an extensive preventive care system with 1,000 stations, in the 1990s, dispersed equally throughout the country. As of today, two thirds of the MCH Stations are run directly by the Ministry of Health, the others by the Labor Union's health insurance plan and in the large cities by the municipalities. The public health nurse carries the main load of the service. Pediatricians, gynecologists, and family physicians carry out routine checkups. In some centers, there is a psychological adviser.

The preventive services are free of charge; only a small fee is paid by the population attending these services, and exemption is provided for the poor. The service is utilized by 95 percent of mothers with their infants; the average number of visits is 10.2/child during the first year and 3/child during the second year. Attendance drops to 50 percent by the fourth year. The immunization rate of children up to the age of two years is high for all sections of the population: diphtheria, tetanus, pertussis—87 percent for the Jewish and 91 percent for the Arab population. Similarly, the combined OPV (poliovirus vaccine live oral) and IPV (poliovirus vaccine inactivated) immunization, and MMR (measles, mumps, rubella) was applied to 88 to 90 percent of the population (Table 4). The high rate of immunization eradicated the infectious disease morbidity and mortality of the child population. The infant mortality had declined to 7.8/1,000 in 1993, and the "under 5 mortality rate" to 11/1,000, placing Israel among the levels achieved by the developed countries (Central Bureau of Statistics 1993).

The focus in the preventive services is on prevention and early detection of chronic conditions, enhancing optimal psychosocial and cognitive development, provision of more intensive services for the high-risk groups, that is, low birth weight babies, and special support for new immigrants who came recently from the former USSR and Ethiopia. Children with health problems diagnosed during routine surveillance are referred for diagnosis and treatment to their primary

Table 4
Immunization of Children up to Age Two, Registered at Maternity and Child Health Centers, by Population Group, 1980–1990 (in percent)

	D.P.T. Vaccine			Poliomyelitis Vaccine			Measles Vaccine		
	Total	Jews	Non-Jews	Total	Jews	Non-Jews	Total	Jews	Non-Jews
All of Israel									
1980	84.0	85.0	81.0	85.0	86.0	80.0	81.0	81.0	79.0
1990	88.0	87.0	91.0	88.0	88.0	90.0	91.0	90.0	92.0

Source: Ellencweig and Chinitz 1993.

Table 5
Causes of Death of Youth Aged 10 to 19, by Population Group, 1981–1986 (in percent)

	Jews	Non-Jews	Total
Accidents	41.4	30.3	37.7
Suicides	3.5	2.5	3.2
Homicide	2.7	3.2	2.9
Other External Causes	7.6	4.9	6.8
Unknown	7.4	14.1	10.3
Congenital Anomalies	2.3	3.9	2.8
Heart and Vascular Diseases	2.6	3.7	3.0
Infections	4.6	7.2	5.4
Neoplasms	15.0	10.6	13.6
Other Diseases	12.8	17.6	14.3
Total	100.0	100.0	100.0

Source: Israel Central Bureau of Statistics 1993.

care physician at the various health insurance plans or to the 21 Child Development Centers of the Ministry of Health, where a multidisciplinary health team is carrying out assessment and treatment for chronic conditions such as hearing and vision impairment, developmental retardation, and cystic fibrosis.

The utilization of the curative health services in childhood is high: 12 visits/year/child for the zero to four years old. These visits to the primary care physician or pediatrician are in addition to the visits at the preventive services (Neumark et al. 1992).

School health services are provided by the team of the Maternal and Child Health Station in the region; they include surveillance of the health status of the students, immunization, health education, and attendance to acute problems. Budgetary constraints limit these activities. School-based and/or school-linked adolescent health services are being developed to address the specific health care needs for youth (e.g., accident, smoking and alcohol abuse prevention, and sex education). Interdisciplinary health promotive and preventive actions have been taken to reduce accident mortality, the main cause of death among youth (Table 5) (Grushka 1968).

All pregnant women receive prenatal care, either from the Maternal and Child Health Stations, health insurance plans, hospital clinics, or private physicians. Utilization for prenatal care of the public health services, the MCH Stations, is high in the rural regions and small townships (90 percent), whereas in the cities, it is less than 50 percent. Privatization characterizes prenatal care among the urban and better-off population. The average number of visits during pregnancy is ten; of them three to five are checkups by the physician. The maternal mortality rate is 6/100,000, comparable to that in most developed countries. The rate of low birth weight has increased during the 1980 and 1990s, from 6.6 to 7.8 percent. One of the determinants is probably the increased use of assisted reproduction technologies (Central Bureau of Statistics 1993).

Due to the increasing cost of health services, the enlarging percentage of the uninsured population in the 1990s, particularly among the new immigrants and the Arab population, and the overutilization of the preventive and curative services, National Health Insurance was implemented as of January 1995. Within this new framework, it is planned to integrate the preventive health service network (the Maternal and Child Health Stations) with the curative care services provided by the various health insurance plans. Public health professionals express anxiety about the planned integration of the curative with the preventive services and fear that the preventive aspects of care will receive less attention in the curative service setup.

The achievements of the preventive services, since its establishment 80 years ago, are remarkable. The ever-changing society of Israel with a high rate of immigrants, nuclear families, and an increasing percentage of one-parent families needs the preventive services for medical reasons and for social support of the high-risk groups.

THE CHALLENGES FACING THE ISRAEL HEALTH CARE SYSTEM

The major challenges facing the health service system of Israel as we near the end of the twentieth century are the result of a fascinating interaction between a number of factors. These include:

1. The changing demography of the population and especially the effects of continued mass immigration of diverse population groups.
2. The changes in the health status of the population and in the major risk factors for morbidity, disability, and mortality.
3. The recent National Health Bill and its potential implications (both positive and negative) for the health services and the health of the nation.
4. The Peace Process and its effect both on Israel and on the region.

While the past and future aging of the population is a product of the fall in infant mortality, continued high fertility, and migration, there has also been a recent observation of an increasing life expectancy at age 65 (Friedlander and Tamir 1994), which has important implications for the total health needs of the elderly population and for the resources required for their care. In this connection, it is of interest to note that the capitation formula (decided on in the framework of the recent health reform) that forms the basis for the resource allocation to the sick funds is calculated taking into account the size of the insured population and its age distribution—the latter because of the fact that the aged utilize a disproportionate amount of the resources available. The National Health Bill defined an extensive basket of services that have to be provided from the monies allocated to the sick funds. There is a tremendous challenge to these funds to, on the one hand, provide the defined services and, on the other, remain within their budgets while serving an aging population.

There is an obvious link between the above and the spiraling cost of health services, fueled by developing medical technology. The challenge will be to define the indications and priorities for the use of these diagnostic and treatment modalities based on their proven effectiveness. While there has, to date, been little success in limiting the utilization of expensive interventions where these are not clearly indicated, this will have to be done if available resources are to cover the costs.

The second change in the population structure has been the 47 years of immigration. While many thought that it had ended, or considerably lessened, the political changes in the former Soviet Union have brought a half a million immigrants to Israel since 1989. While numerically this was an increase of 10 percent in the population, a much smaller immigrant group is no less significant in health terms. The two waves of migration from Ethiopia since the early 1980s have confronted the health services with a markedly contrasting challenge. While the Soviet migrants bring with them the morbidity and risk of the major chronic diseases, the Ethiopians typify the meeting of the First and Third Worlds. The challenge is intriguing. Can the health services, for example, reduce the risk of cardiovascular disease in the former while preventing its occurrence in the latter? We failed with the immigration from North Africa in the 1960s (Epstein and Zaaroor 1982). Are we planning and organizing to succeed this time?

While the population structure has been altered, the change in the major health problems is no less dramatic. Mortality from coronary heart disease has fallen by more than 50 percent since the mid-1970s (Epstein 1979). In this way, we are no different from many other industrialized countries (Thom et al. 1985). However, the causes of this are not known. Whether this is a result of a reduction in incidence (change in risk factor status) or a fall in case fatality (possibly the effect of acute care), or both, is unknown. This lack of information precludes logical planning for the future, especially in relation to the future provision and need for sophisticated cardiological intervention. This is a challenge that is beginning to be met. The establishment of the Israel Centers for Disease Control has as its objective the systematic collection of epidemiological data that can form the basis for policy decision making in the future.

While individual diseases are a challenge, a wider issue is that of the health status of different population groups. The issue of the immigrant health differential has been referred to above. There are two other issues that should be cited. Sabatello has referred to the low male/female ratio in mortality and the reported different relative positions that men and women have in comparison with other countries (Thom et al. 1985). The excess of female cerebrovascular morbidity and mortality (Epstein and Zaaroor 1982), their relatively high coronary mortality, and the rise in breast cancer (Ministry of Health 1993) and its catapulting the malignancies to first place in the causes of female mortality have all been shown epidemiologically. There is a need to recognize that a problem exists and attempt to plan accordingly.

There are differences in various health indices in the Jewish and essentially Arab population in the country. As an example: While infant mortality has fallen dramatically in both, and the absolute differences in the rates become substantially smaller, the rate ratio between them has not changed.

The relative needs of different population groups are not reflected in the National Health Bill, and it will be a challenge to the planners to attempt to include this variance in their attempts at needs-based resource allocation.

One cannot omit an additional entity in this discussion of health status. This relates to the "epidemic" of accidents, especially involving motor vehicles. Until recently, Israel with an unenviably high MVA (motor vehicle accident) rate did not, at least, have this problem linked to alcohol. This has changed dramatically in recent years, especially in young people. While this is not a problem of the health services alone, it has a tremendous impact on morbidity, disability, and mortality. It highlights a question that has become central in health planning in recent years, that is, the need for intersectoral cooperation and collaboration in order to provide the necessary services related to health. The challenge has begun to be met by the developing Healthy Cities movement in Israel. This has as its basis the widened modern concept of health promotion and the attempt to achieve this by, amongst others, planned intersectoral activity. On the other hand, the new Health Bill does not highlight this need for a wider collaboration in trying to meet some of the major health problems that will take us into the next century.

The identification of persons at risk and the attempt to change this have been the basis for organized public health activity for generations. In the last few decades, this has become more and more focused on the subject of risk behavior as a major constituent of lifestyles. The above reference to alcohol is only one example of the problem. Modern society is typified by the health risks associated, amongst others, with cigarette smoking, drug usage, alcohol, and unprotected sex. A major focus is on youth who until now have not been a high-priority group for the health services. The role of health education at early ages and the critical requirement for cooperation between the different service agencies (health, education, welfare, police, judiciary) will provide a severe challenge if there is to be a successful war waged on the untoward effects of behavioral risk.

While the discussion above refers to the challenges that face the health services, the greatest test is probably in the recent changes in the health services structure and functioning. These have come about from a variety of factors that manifested over the years, including the subjects discussed above but also taking into account the professional and public dissatisfaction with the services even though there has been almost complete access over the years.

There are many questions that at this stage can only be asked:

- What will be the relevance of the fact that the Health Bill did not include defined health objectives (as was done in the recent reorganization of the British National Health Service? [Her Majesty's Stationery Office 1992]).
- Will the compulsory health insurance provide sufficient funding for the basic basket of service?
- Will the introduction of competition (laudable in itself) help to control costs or be responsible for them spiraling out of control?
- Will the planned introduction of private practice into the public hospitals relieve the congestion or result in a two-tier system where quality health care is the prerogative of the wealthy?
- Can one ensure that the payment for hospitalization on a diagnosis-related group (DRG) basis will not result in differential admission and discharge practices that are deleterious to the health of patients?
- Will primary health care and especially its promotive and preventive elements be preserved and expanded when the health insurers receive responsibility for them?
- Will the aged, the chronically ill—whether physically or mentally—and the disabled

receive the care they require in the competitive economically (almost entirely) oriented system?

- Will the admirable accent placed on the development of quality assessment and improvement and of quality management really occupy a central position in the activities and not only in the ideology of the health reform?
- Will the need to balance a budget result in the neglecting of education and research in the health care system?

The above questions, and many others, are reflected, up to a point, in the legislation, but the outcome is far from certain. The challenge is clear and will require a monitoring system that is planned for but not, as yet, in place. The change in the role of the District Health Authority from direct provision of preventive health services to being a mini-ministry responsible for the ongoing assessment of population needs, the degree to which they are met, and service evaluation is an integral component of the health reform. The success of this change in its function may well determine the outcome of the whole exercise.

No discussion of the challenges facing the health services would today be complete without reference to the greatest potential for change in this part of the world. There is little doubt that the Peace Process has changed the political and social thinking in a very short period of time. International cooperation in the health field was one of the defined articles in the Declaration of Alma Ata in 1978 and a stated constituent of the Health for All ideal (Alma-Ata WHO Conference 1978). The foundations are being laid for cooperation as the process moves ahead. Palestinian students have over the years studied in the Hebrew University–Hadassah School of Public Health and Community Medicine, and this has recently been extended. Joint training and research programs are being planned. Cooperation and collaboration in the health field could well represent the microcosm of the entire process. Its success could well have a profound effect on the health of all peoples in the region. It could well be the greatest challenge of all.

It is clear from the foregoing discussion that there is no single challenge that, if answered, will solve all the problems. The thesis presented in this chapter is that the challenge is in recognizing the conglomerate whole and the identification of the interface between the different elements. There is frequently the tendency to compartmentalize the subjects in an attempt to limit their complexity and allow for feasible and limited action. This strategy is problematic when considering the interrelating facets of the challenges facing the Israel health service system.

We have to identify the different trees in the wood, or we will not see the wood for the trees.

REFERENCES

The Alma-Ata WHO Conference on Primary Health Care. (1978). *WHO Chronicle*, 32, 409–430.

Bachi, R. (1976). The population of Israel. *CICRED Series. Paris.*

Central Bureau of Statistics (CBS). (1993). *Statistical Abstract of Israel.* Vol. 44. Jerusalem: Ueterpress Enterprises. 671–680.

Central Bureau of Statistics (CBS). (1994). *National Expenditure on Health 1991 and Preliminary Estimate for 1992.* Jerusalem: Central Bureau of Statistics.

Chernichovsky, D. & Chinitz, D. P. (1995). The political economy of health system reform in Israel. *Health Economics,* 4, 418–428.

Eizenbach, Z. & Sabatello, E. V. (Eds.). (1991). Demographic and socio-economic aspects of population aging in Israel. *CICRED/INIA Series.* Paris/Volletta.

Ellencweig, A. Y. & Chinitz, D. P. (1993). Israel's health system reform: The role of management in ensuring and improving health status. *European Journal of Public Health,* 3, 85–91.

Epstein, L. (1979). Ischemic heart disease in Israel: Patterns of morbidity and mortality over 30 years. *Israel Journal of Medical Science,* 15, 993–998.

Epstein, L. & Zaaroor, M. (1982). Mortality from ischemic heart disease and cerebrovascular disease in Israel. *Stroke,* 13, 570–573.

Friedlander, D. & Tamir, Y. (1994). *Socioeconomic Characteristics and Old Age Mortality in Israel.* Jerusalem: Institute of Gerontology and Human Development.

Grushka, T. H. (1968). *Health Services in Israel.* Jerusalem: Ministry of Health.

Her Majesty's Stationery Office. (1992). *The Health of the Nation. A Strategy for Health in England.* London.

Israel Central Bureau of Statistics. (1993). Socio-demographic characteristics of infant mortality (based on data for 1985–89). *Special Series no. 932.* Jerusalem.

Ministry of Health. (1994). *Proposed Budget for 1995.* Jerusalem: Ministry of Health.

Ministry of Health, Department of Epidemiology. (1993). *Cancer in Israel: Facts and Figures 1989.* Jerusalem: Israel Cancer Registry.

Neumark Y., Palti, H., Donchin, M. & Ellencweig, A. Y. (1992). Utilization of pediatric health service in Jerusalem. *Journal of Community Health,* 17, 271–282.

Shirom, A. (1994). Preventive health service. In: Kop, Y. (Ed.). *Allocating Resources to Social Services.* Jerusalem: Center for Research on Social Policy in Israel.

Sicron, M. Immigration to Israel 1948–1956. *Special Series no. 60.* Jerusalem: Central Bureau of Statistics.

State of Israel. (1990). *Report: The State Judicial Commission of Inquiry into the Health System in Israel.* Jerusalem: Government Printer.

Thom, T. J., Epstein, F. H., Feldman, J. J., et al. (1985). Trends in total mortality and mortality from heart disease in 26 countries from 1950 to 1978. *International Journal of Epidemiology,* 14, 510–520.

United Nations (UN). (1993). *Demographic Year Book 1992.* New York.

World Health Organization (WHO). (1994). *Health in Europe.* WHO Regional Publication. European Series no. 56. Copenhagen.

World Health Organization (WHO). (various years). WHO Year Books. Geneva: WHO.

ITALY

Franco Cavallo and Giovanni Renga

MAJOR HEALTH PROBLEMS FACING THE COUNTRY

Population Development

If we consider the development of the Italian population during the last 100 years, we can realize that the demographic trend, formerly steadily increasing, has been slowing down, remaining since the 1970s and 1980s substantially unchanged (Figure 1). The number of births has been drastically reduced, lowering the birthrate from 37.6 percent in 1861 to 9.9 percent in 1989 (Figure 2); the number of live births, which was over a million in 1921, is now around 500,000.

Since the beginning of the 1960s, in Italy as in most European countries, a demographic transformation has taken place, characterized by a decrease of the birthrate and fertility rate and by a parallel decrease of the probability of death in older ages (mainly for females). Therefore, by the end of the 1980s, a negative demographic balance was reached. As a consequence, a deep modification in the age structure of the population was determined, as one can see from the typical tower shape of the age pyramid and from the increasing difference between male and female population at the older ages, due to the different life expectancy in the two genders (Figure 3).

Besides these changes in age and gender structure, important modifications have also taken place in the mortality rates (Buiatti et al. 1993a).

The Modification of Mortality Rates and of Prevalent Diseases

The infant mortality rate has markedly decreased during the last 30 years, going from 227 per 1,000 live births in 1861 to 159 per 1,000 in 1905 and to

Figure 1
Demographic Trend of the Italian Population Since 1871

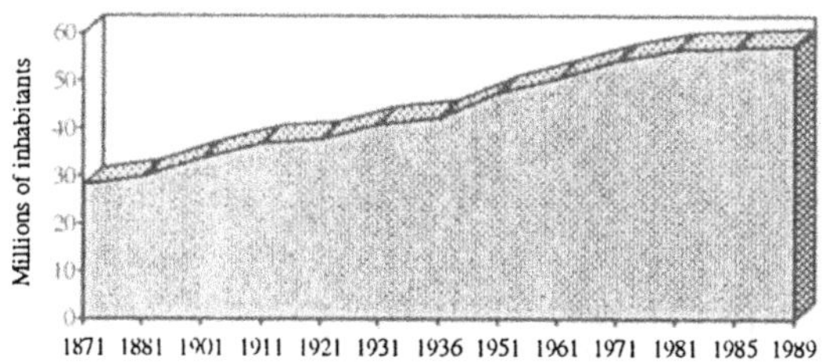

Source: Buiatti, Carnevale, Geddes, and Maciocco 1993a.

8.3 per 1,000 live births in 1989 (Figure 4). The different subrates of infant mortality have also changed. From 1960 to 1988 the percentage of the infant mortality taking place during the first week of life (early neonatal mortality) has gone from 40.6 percent to 65.3 percent; the mortality taking place from one week to one month of life (late neonatal mortality) has gone from 13.9 percent to 13.0 percent; the mortality taking place after one month of life until one year (postneonatal mortality) has decreased from 45.5 percent to 21.7 percent. The causes of death have also been sharply modified. Infectious and diarrheal diseases, which were the cause of 30 percent of deaths during the first half of the century, now have a negligible importance; the role of respiratory diseases has also decreased. Nowadays perinatal conditions are responsible for 60 percent of deaths before one year of age, and congenital malformations are attributed to another 25 percent.

Overall mortality has also decreased. Life expectancy has gone from 35.1 years for males and 35.6 for females in 1881 to 73.7 for males and 80.4 for females in 1990, with the more consistent gains for females, who have now an almost 7 years longer life expectancy with respect to males. Notwithstanding this general situation, important differences can be evidenced in the overall mortality in the different geographical areas of Italy, with, for example, a higher mortality for males in the northern regions and for females in the south (Buiatti et al. 1993a).

As for mortality rates for specific causes of death, or subgroups of causes, we can point out that during this last century in Italy, as in most other industrialized countries, the importance of infectious diseases has been reduced in favor of chronic diseases (tumors and cardiovascular diseases) (Figure 5) (Checcacci, Meloni, and Pelissero 1992). The only infectious disease following an opposite trend is AIDS (acquired immunodeficiency syndrome), whose annual incidence rate has been sharply increasing after 1985 (Figure 6) (COA 1994).

During the last 20 years, an annual increase for all types of tumors has been registered (0.7 percent), a greater one for lung tumors in men (2.9 percent) and

Figure 2
Birthrates in Italy Since 1905

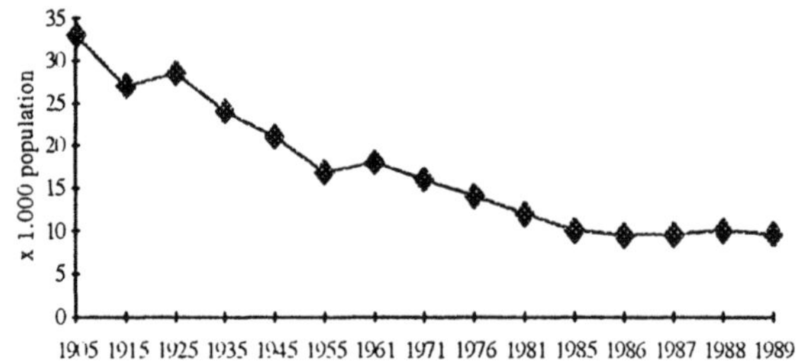

Source: Buiatti, Carnevale, Geddes, and Maciocco 1993a.

for breast cancer in women (Figure 7). Stomach cancer is decreasing in both genders at a constant rate of 2.2 percent yearly; colon cancer shows a slight increase in men, while rectal cancer is stable in both sexes (Checcacci, Meloni, and Pelissero 1992).

Cerebrovascular diseases are steadily decreasing in both sexes. Cardiovascular diseases are also decreasing in males and females; myocardial infarction and ischemic heart diseases show a reduction in men, starting from 1979, at an annual rate of 1.4 percent, while women have been steadily decreasing even before (Buiatti et al. 1993a).

Lifestyle, Nutrition, and Environmental Hazards

Alcohol. Alcohol consumption is very common and widespread all over Italy, but there are no reliable figures concerning its diffusion by gender, age, or geographic area. What we know with regard to wine consumption is that its diffusion is higher in the northeastern regions, while southern regions are below the national average.

Data coming from ISTAT give a rough idea of the per capita consumption in terms of liters/year of the different types of alcoholic beverages (wine, beer, superalcoholics). These data show that, after a reduction of wine consumption during World War II, there has been a sharp increase up to the beginning of the 1970s, followed by a steady decrease in wine consumption in the following decades, along with a considerable increase in beer consumption (Figure 8). Also superalcoholic beverages have been decreasing since the end of the 1980s.

Generally speaking, the total estimated per capita pure alcohol consumption, which was at its peak at the end of the 1960s (15 liters/year per capita), came down, 20 years later, to 9.6 liters/year per capita, with a 30 percent reduction, mainly due to the reduction in wine consumption (Buiatti et al. 1993b).

Figure 3
Age Pyramid of the Italian Population, 1951 and 1981

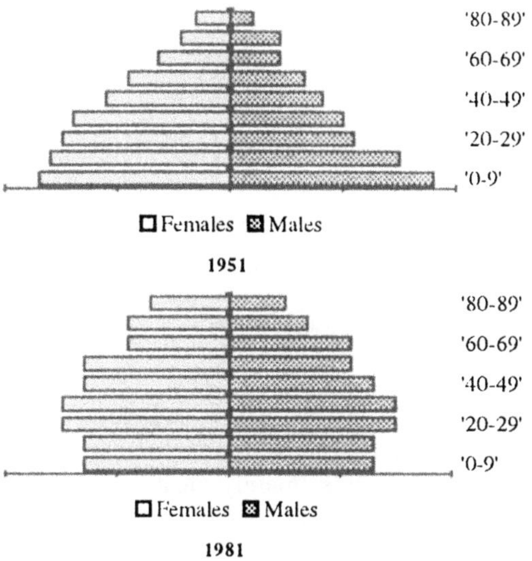

Source: Buiatti, Carnevale, Geddes, and Maciocco 1993a.

Tobacco. The smoking habit is showing a changing pattern during the last 15 years. While the previous trend was that of a rapid increase in men of all ages and of a similar, even if lower, one in females, since the beginning of the 1980s the trend has sharply reversed in men (Figure 9). The smokers' prevalence went down from more than 50 percent to less than 40 percent, and it still seems to be decreasing. The same phenomenon is not true for women, where—even if at much lower figures—the smokers' prevalence is still increasing (Geddes and Cellerini 1990).

As for the characteristics of the smoking population, this seems well described by school degree. In fact, in men, the previous situation was that of a prevalence in favor of higher-degrees people; now, prevalence is higher in lower class people, so that the decrease in smoking habits has been much higher in the highest school degrees. The opposite is true among women, where the more cultured ones are those with a higher increase in smoking.

Nutrition. Data from the National Institute of Nutrition show the modifications that have taken place in the Italian population from the beginning of the century. A sharp increase in the consumption of proteins (animal and vegetable), together with an overall increase in calorie intake, which has taken place since the end of World War II, is the main characterizing phenomenon. Animal fat consumption also shows a slight increase, while carbohydrate and vegetable fat consumption are quite stable (Figure 10) (Angelillo 1993).

Figure 4
Infant Mortality in Italy Since the Beginning of the Century

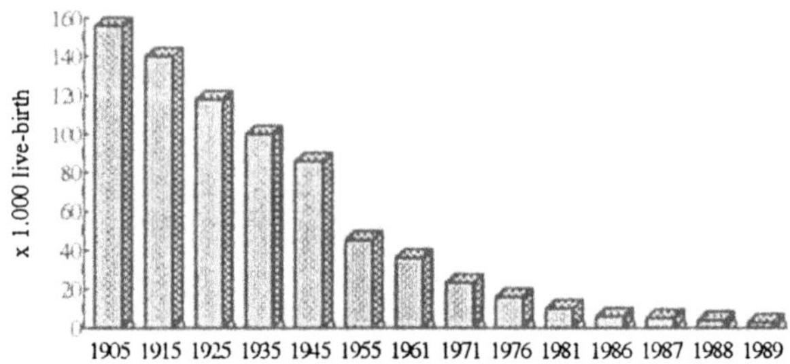

Source: Buiatti, Carnevale, Geddes, and Maciocco 1993a.

These data are paradigmatic of the Italian situation, where a considerable increase in population income has facilitated higher expenditures in foods that were previously almost inaccessible (mainly meat of any kind), but it has not changed the traditional structure of the Mediterranean diet, based on a good balance between fats and carbohydrates as calorie-intake foods (Buiatti et al. 1993d). The preliminary data on current eating habits seem to show a reverse tendency in overall calorie intake and protein consumption.

Environmental Hazards. A detailed network for monitoring environmental pollution has not yet been set up in Italy, with the exception of big cities, where specific law has set the obligation for continuous monitoring of environmental pollutants. The latest data given by the *Health Status of the Population Report* of 1992, edited by the Environment Ministry, show an overall decrease of some pollutants in the latest years (mainly SO_2 and CO), while others are stable (organic volatile substances [SOVs]) or increasing (dust and NO_2).

Health and Inequalities

Unequal distribution of health and of health services access throughout Italy has been investigated during the last decades as an important indicator of efficient and effective functioning of the National Health Service. Differential mortality for all causes of death, and for specific subgroups, with respect to social status (indexed by school degree of the head of the family and/or by house ownership), is normally used for these analyses. More recently, other indicators having to do with morbidity, perceived health status, and use of health services have been used. This has become possible since ISTAT, the Italian National Institute for Statistics, began carrying out a nationwide inquiry every three years (starting in 1980), based on a large representative sample of the population, concerning health status and use of health services by the population.

Social differences are even more striking if the different geographical areas

Figure 5
Number of Deaths from Infectious and Chronic Diseases in Italy, 1903–1985

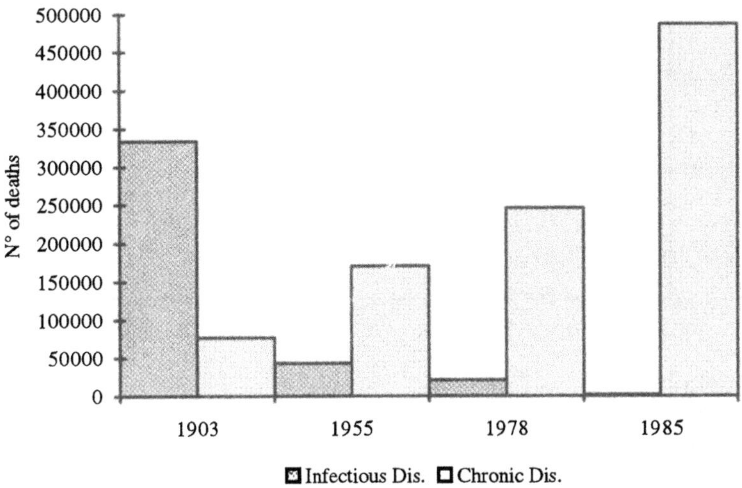

Source: Checcacci, Meloni, and Pelissero 1992.

of Italy are considered: Southern regions, for example, show higher mortality rates for some diseases that recent therapeutic progress has made less severe, like cervical cancer and respiratory diseases; moreover, perinatal mortality rates are still much higher than northern and central Italy (South: 10.2 percent; Center: 7.1 percent; North: 6.0 percent).

As for general mortality, the school degree index identifies remarkable differences among different categories: An illiterate person has a mortality risk almost twofold that of a university graduate (RR [Relative Risk] = 1.64 for males and 1.81 for females) (Faggiano et al. 1995), and a blue collar has a higher risk than a white collar (OR [Odds Ratio] = 1.4 for males in Torino) (Faggiano and Costa 1990). Unemployed people have a suicide rate higher than other persons, and the employment rate is three times lower in the South than in the North.

Also, disability is more frequent in the southern regions and in the islands: While 36 percent of the Italian population live in these areas, 46 percent of invalid people come from them; if we consider that disability is strongly linked with age, these data are even more striking, as southern regions have a mean age lower than the rest of Italy.

Studies on utilization of health services are still limited in our country. Nevertheless, it appears clear that citizens from higher social classes use health services in a more selective way, mainly for preventive and specialized services.

As for the distribution of health services, while differences in the distribution

Figure 6
AIDS Annual Incidence Rate per 100,000 Population in Italy, 1982–1993

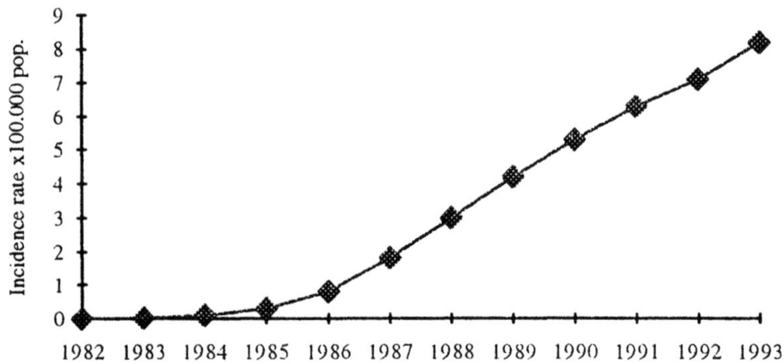

Source: COA 1994.

of health facilities (hospitals, for example) are evident in terms of beds per population, even if not striking for public hospitals, intensive and subintensive therapy wards are much more widely represented in the northern regions.

Health of the Immigrants. Immigration to Italy from abroad began to increase and exhibit some consistent patterns in the 1980s. By the end of 1992, foreigners with regular permissions to live in Italy numbered 1,230,000, plus an illegal quota estimated at around 500,000. Immigration from the European Community (EC) covers only a small percentage (15 percent) of this population, while the African component gets the higher share. From the health point of view, apart from some peculiar pathologies brought from the countries of origin, mainly of infectious origin (parasitic or other tropical diseases) or acquired "in loco," due to nonexposure to the local etiologic agents or to poor housing conditions (tuberculosis and other pulmonary diseases), this population is not much different from the indigenous one. This phenomenon is also due to the "healthy immigrant" effect.

The main problem of the immigrant population is in fact the physical and psychological distress of being in a foreign country in a precarious situation, which is itself an important health risk factor. Being an outcast, being able to work only as black labor, and the difficulty in accessing health and social services are the main elements affecting their health status. Specific high-risk categories are probably children and mothers; higher maternal and infant mortality, with respect to the local population, are in fact registered among this population (Lemma and Costa 1990). But, as a whole, the main problems faced by the health services in those areas where immigration has been heavy are those coming from the deep cultural differences between the immigrant person and the health professionals. The already difficult relationship between doctor and pa-

Figure 7
Cancer Incidence Rates per 100,000 Population in Males and Females, Age Standardized on the 1971 Italian Population

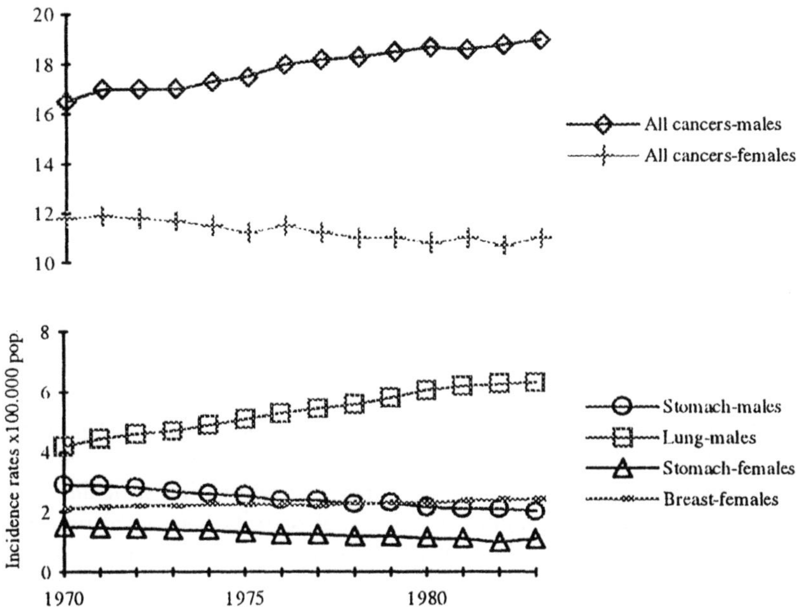

Source: Checcacci 1992.

tient is complicated by a miscomprehension gap that makes intervention often ineffective. It seems therefore that juridical and communication problems will be key issues in this situation. Providing regular access to health and social services and training health professionals who may act as intermediary actors between the services and the health needs of the immigrants is likely to be the most effective way to cope with this new and formerly unknown problem (Consiglio Sanitario Nazionale 1993).

PROVISION, UTILIZATION, AND IMPACT OF HEALTH SERVICES

The Organization of the Health System in Italy

The Crispi-Pagliani Act of 1888 has been the first attempt to give a rational structure to the health system in Italy. In this framework, the responsibility for public health matters (which were mainly represented by infectious diseases control and prevention, water and soil protection, guarantee of a minimum health

Figure 8
Trend of Alcoholic Beverages Consumption, 1950–1985

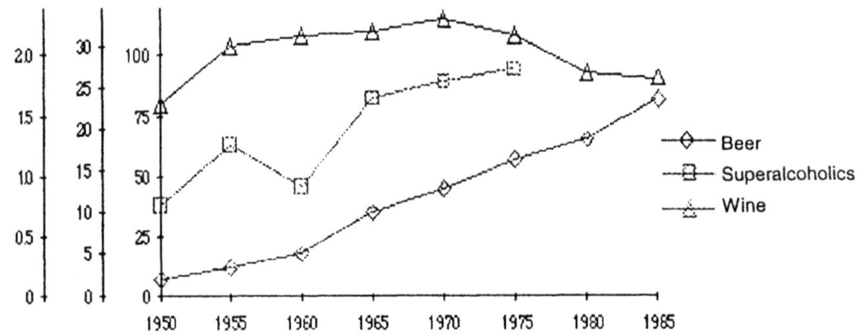

Source: Buiatti, Carnevale, Geddes, and Maciocco 1993c.

and social care for the more disadvantaged people) was taken up by the state, through the regional and municipal administrations. The curative side (essentially hospitals) was taken care of by charity institutions (most of them under the aegis of the Catholic Church), while social security was based on a social insurance fee, paid out of each worker's wage, partially by him and partially by the employer.

This model has remained substantially unchanged for around 90 years, being only marginally modified by the institution of the Health Ministry as an autonomous body from the Ministry of Internal Affairs in 1958 and by a law passing all hospitals of public interest under the control of the public administration (1968).

In 1978 a National Health Service (NHS) was finally set up, giving full accomplishment to what was required by Article 32 of the Italian Constitution: ''[H]ealth is a fundamental right of the individual and a main interest for the community.'' With this law, an NHS was planned, based on the principles of the individual's right to health, of a global approach to health (from prevention to diagnosis, therapy, and rehabilitation), of equity in access to health services for all, of community participation in the planning, managing, and monitoring of health services activities, and of a close coordination between health and social services.

The responsibility of running the whole system was distributed among three institutional and administrative levels: state, regions, and municipalities, through the local health unit (USL) (Giannico 1993) (Figure 11).

The State Level. The state level is mainly charged with the duty to give directives for health services management and development. The Parliament has to define the general legislative principles and the objectives to be reached; the government and the Health Ministry give concrete application to these objec-

Figure 9
Smoking Prevalence in Males and Females in Italy, 1975–1990

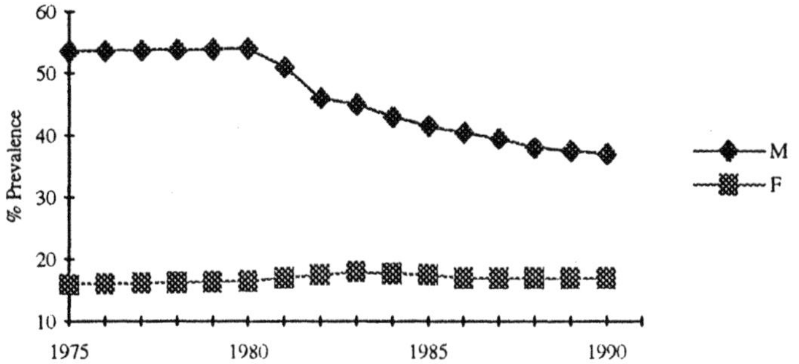

Source: Geddes and Cellerini 1990.

tives, allocating an annual budget to the regions, coordinating the regions' activity, and monitoring the way resources are utilized by the regions. Direct control is kept on a few activities of general interest, like dealing with the control of tropical diseases and negotiating international matters on health.

Along with these administrative bodies, some technical and consultative bodies help the ministry in taking its decisions:

- *Higher Council for Health (CSS).* It is the technical adviser to the ministry for all matters concerning public health and matters of public interest concerning health.
- *Higher Institute for Health (ISS).* It is a technical and scientific body giving information and consultancy to the ministry and other public administrations; it takes care of organizing short courses for continuing education of health professionals.
- *National Institute for Working Safety (ISPSL).* It deals with research, experimentation, and counseling on new methodologies for preventing work accidents and professional diseases.
- *Permanent State-Regions Conference (CSR).* It is composed of well-known experts, representatives of different national organizations dealing, or having to do, with health, representatives of unions and business organizations, and representatives of regional administrations; it is responsible for drawing the general health policy directives and setting up the objectives for the triennial National Health Plan.
- *Inter-Ministry Committee for Economic Planning (CIPE) at the Ministry of Health.* The CIPE gives rules for drawing up the national health plan and is charged with the subdivision of the national health budget among the regions.

The Regional Level. The regional administrations have similar competencies as the state, at the regional level; they have to draw up a regional health plan, and to make laws and other administrative acts in keeping with the state direc-

Figure 10
Evolution of Italian Dietary Habits

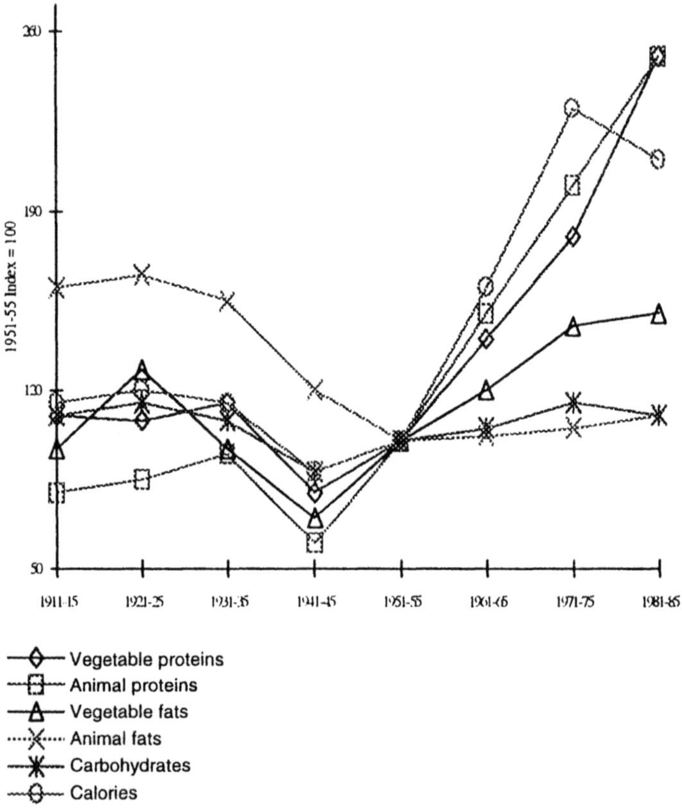

Source: Angelillo 1993.

tives; they have to allocate the regional health budget among the USLs of the region.

In addition, the regional administration has to define the territorial limits of the USLs and their organizational structure, up to the health district level, where the first approach of the citizen with the health service usually takes place. The region also sets rules for running hospitals and secondary care services, for organizing public health and veterinary services, and for organizing continuing education of health professionals.

The Municipal and Local Health Unit Level. The situation has changed very recently in this respect, as now the third level is directly that of the USL; in the original NHS law, the municipal administration(s) in charge of the USLs terri-

Figure 11
National Health Service Organization

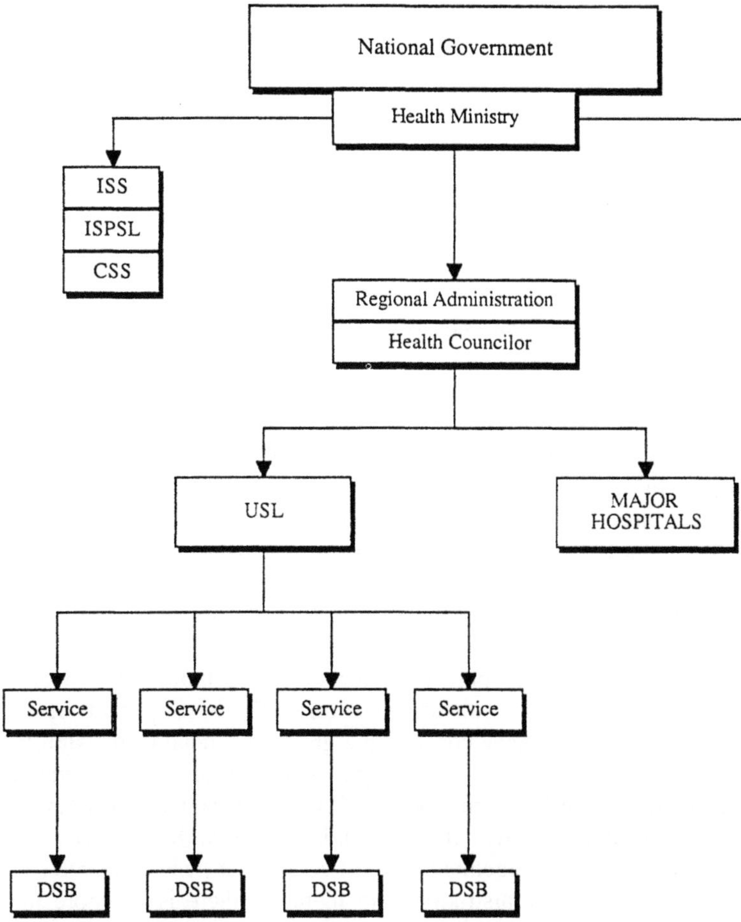

Source: Giannico 1993.

tory had the power to nominate the running body of the USL, whose members were appointed with a mix of technical-political criteria. A USL territory may coincide with that of a local municipality, be a part of it, or sum up a number of smaller municipalities. Its dimension was supposed to lie between 50,000 and 200,000 inhabitants.

To fulfill its preventive duties, the USL Prevention Department is generally organized in different services (the detail can be different for each region) covering the following matters:

- Public Health and Hygiene
- Health Education and Promotion
- Food and Water Control
- Wastes Control
- Environment Protection
- Work Safety
- Primary and Secondary Care
- Rehabilitation
- Legal Medicine
- Continuing Education of Health Professionals

To carry out all these tasks, the USL is organized in different services. The organizational model is somehow different for each region, but they are all based on a common set of services having to do with primary care, public health, secondary care (hospital care and specialist care), pharmaceutics, veterinary care (animals and food control), legal medicine, and social assistance. All first-level services, where the first contact of the citizen with the health system usually takes place, are organized at the district level (DSB), the most decentralized subunit of the USL.

In recent years, two laws were passed by the Italian Parliament (1992 and 1993), partially modifying the overall organization of the NHS (Buiatti et al. 1993b). The major innovations have concerned a greater financial responsibility given to the regional administrations, the average dimension of the USL (which was increased to allow for a lower number of USLs), and their transformation into quite autonomous administrative entities, run by a general director who has direct responsibility for the management of the budget. The general director is nominated by the regional administration, and therefore there is no more involvement of the local municipalities in running the USLs. As for the hospitals, the major ones (highly specialized, polyclinics, or a mix of the two) have acquired an administrative status similar to that of the USL, with a general director and an autonomous budget.

From the point of view of the citizen's right to health care, a set of essential interventions has been defined, which all USLs are obliged to give through the NHS to every citizen entitled to care.

Generally speaking, all these innovations are trying to push the system toward a kind of "internal markets" dynamics acting within the NHS, based on the distinction between health care producers and consumers; up to now, it is very difficult to foresee what the impact of these modifications will be on the overall organization of the health system (Montagnani and Zanetti 1993).

Figure 12
Health Expenditure and per Capita Income in Italy, 1984–1993

	1984	1988	1990	1993
Hlth expend. per-cap ($)	770	1070	1236	1450
% hlth expend. on GDP	6.8	7.6	7.7	8.3
% public hlth expend./ total hlth expend.	78	78	77	74

Source: Dirindin 1992.

Health Care Financing in Italy

Italy, as most Western developed countries, has faced a steady increase in health care expenditure in the last decades. Population aging, the increasing prevalence of chronic diseases, the introduction of new and expensive technologies, and the expanding demand for health care are only some of the causes of this phenomenon (Barbuti et al. 1993).

Main Components of Health Expenditures. Public health expenditure has reached 1,450 dollars in Italy in 1993. At the beginning of the 1970s, total health care expenditure was around 5 percent of the GDP (gross domestic product), while in 1984 it had reached 6.8 percent and in 1993 8.3 percent (Figure 12).

Data from 1991 show a further increase, reaching 8 percent of the GDP (Balma and Zanoni 1994). The Italian situation, however, is, from this point of view, quite in line with that of most well-developed countries. On the other side, our country has one of the highest percentages of health care expenditure financed from public money (around 74 percent). As for the services produced by the private sector, the share of the total expenditure is around 53 percent (Dirindin 1992).

If we analyze the structure of health care expenditure coming from the state budget, we realize that the greatest part goes for the personnel (40 percent), followed by goods and services (19 percent); drugs expenditure is around 13 percent.

As for the type of care for which the expenditure is done, 50 percent of the total health care expenditure is going for hospital care (supplied by public and private hospitals). Expenditure in public hospitals has been decreasing during the last decade, 1980 to 1990, due to the lower number of beds per inhabitant and to the shortening of the average length of stay.

Prevention, which was supposed to be the hinge of the new health system, has only 4.5 percent of the total budget.

The imbalance among different regions with respect to per capita health care expenditure is quite remarkable. Western and central regions show, in general, a higher level of per capita expenditure with respect to southern regions, even if the difference has been decreasing during the last years, due to a better distribution of the national health budget. Liguria and Emilia-Romagna are the regions with the highest per capita expenditure, while Calabria is the one with the lowest. From the point of view of the difference in health services use in the different parts of Italy, primary care expenditure is quite similar all over Italy, while northern Italy has a higher consumption of hospital and specialized services, and southern Italy a higher consumption of drugs.

Sources of Revenues for the NHS. The Reform of 1978 stated that health care is a right of each citizen and therefore has to be guaranteed by the state, which, if the revenues coming from the compulsory insurance contributions from public and private employers and employees are not sufficient, is bound to cover the remaining part from general taxation and borrowing. A small part also comes from local revenues going directly to the USLs for the payment of fees for services, or copayments, or for services given on direct payment by the citizen.

The central government is responsible for determining the share of public resources dedicated to health care (national health budget). More than 50 percent of this budget comes from the workers' contribution taken directly from employers and employees. The other part comes from general taxation. This same general mechanism has been confirmed by the more recent laws modifying the Reform of 1978; now, however, the contribution coming from workers' wages goes directly to the regions, and consequently the budget allocated by the state government is lower.

During the last years, there have been a number of measures concerning health costs sharing by the citizen; this has been quite important in the area of drugs expenditure, where 11 to 13 percent of the total costs have been paid by the citizens during 1985–1990 (highest percentage in 1986, with 15 percent; and lowest in 1987, with 8 percent). The latest directives from the state allow the regions to put even higher fees on drugs or other services. Quotas for health care expenditures coming from fees and copayments are difficult to estimate and vary widely from north to south, due to the very different criteria used by local administrations to identify people exempt from payment.

Allocation of the National Health Budget to the Regions. The national health budget is allocated to the different regions by CIPE, on proposal of the health ministry, advised by the National Health Council. The overall sum allocated to each region is divided into two parts:

- A share for capital expenditure, for expenses of renewal, maintenance, and transformation of existing structure; and

- A share for current expenditure, to finance all activities connected with actual supply of health services.

The overall allocation is made on the basis of the population and of the set of services to be guaranteed to everybody; it also takes into account interregional mobility of patients and the need to finance the existing structures, with an aim to ameliorate the imbalance between better-equipped and less-equipped regions.

Voluntary Help. Alongside of the NHS structures and activities, a wide and increasing area of voluntary work has shown up, which testifies to the increasing strength of social solidarity. The National Federation of Associations for Public Help and Support now has 425 associations all over the national territory, with about 670,000 members. They are active in all kinds of care services but especially in the field of drugs dependence services, AIDS, social deviance, elderlies, disability, and care for the chronically ill.

Preventive Health Care and Public Health Services

On the basis of the law introducing the NHS in 1978, each USL was charged to organize and develop its approach to prevention and environmental control in order to take care of all possible elements of danger/risk of biological, physical, chemical, or behavioral nature in the working and life environments. This situation determined a quite differentiated and dishomogeneous organization of preventive activities in different parts of the country. Due to a quite diffuse dissatisfaction with the effectiveness of the USL's interventions in matters of prevention, a popular referendum held in 1993 ruled out these norms, calling for a unified, and higher-level, organization of preventive activities, particularly those concerned with environmental protection.

The result was a new law, which has subdivided the competencies for environmental protection among the National Agency for Environmental Protection, Regional Agencies for Environmental Protection, and the Departments of Prevention of the USLs. USLs still have direct and full competence on the activities of rehabilitation, health education, and school medicine.

National Agency for Environmental Protection. The agency is charged to promote, countrywide, activities geared toward ensuring environmental protection, in connection with similar agencies based at the regional level. Its duties are the promotion of research on all elements of the ecosystem involved in causing, or preventing, pollution and environmental deterioration; the systematic collection, elaboration, and diffusion of data and information on environmental status; and the promotion of training programs in environmental protection. The agency is also charged to keep in touch with other national and international institutions involved in environmental protection, such as the European Agency for Environment and the Statistical Institute of the EC (EUROSTAT), in order to formulate guidelines for environmental activities, to be implemented by central and peripheral authorities.

USL: The Prevention Department. To fulfill its preventive duties, the USL Prevention Department is generally organized in different services (the detail can be different for each region) covering the following matters:

- Public health and hygiene
- Safety of the working environment
- Food and nutrition control
- Veterinary service (subdivided into three functional areas: animal health; production, trade, and preservation of food of animal origin; breeding and zootechnical production control)
- Epidemiology

Prevention activities stretch, therefore, from the identification and control of risk factors in working and life environment to data collection and diffusion to promotion of guidelines for risk factors removal. The department is also charged with the control and mapping of toxic substances used by industries and the compatibility between production activities and need to preserve workers' and population's health.

The Health Ministry, and its connected technical organizations, overlooks the departments' activities, pledging for a uniform implementation of national and international directives and supplying any information useful for a better knowledge of health risks.

Rehabilitation. Rehabilitation of physical and mental invalidity is one of the NHS objectives. This has become a priority need during the last decade, as population aging (the elderlies are now more than 15 percent of the general population) and the consequent increase of chronic diseases have widened the percentage of people needing rehabilitation. Following the most recent directives, rehabilitation is offered, to those who need it, in a global context, taking into account both health and social needs, through an integrated effort of health and social services.

Rehabilitation activities for persons with physical, mental, or sensorial handicaps are carried out directly by the USLs at the district level, sometimes in collaboration with similar services offered by the Social Departments of the local municipalities. If the USL does not have the ability to organize a rehabilitation service by itself, it can do so by buying such services from the private market, following a convention scheme approved by the Health Ministry.

School Medicine. School medicine is a long-standing institution in the Italian health and school organization. Since the beginning of the century, it has taken care of the hygiene of the school environment, of the control of the infectious diseases most common in the childhood communities, and of the diffusion and monitoring of vaccinations. After the reform law of 1978, school medicine activities are among the USL's duties.

School medicine's present concerns are:

- The periodic medical examination of children's health status, in connection, and without overlaps, with the functions of the general practitioner (GP).
- Carrying out the tuberculosis (TB) control tests during the first, third, and last year of the elementary cycle, along with a general activity of education concerning TB prevention.
- Organizing health education activities, together with the teachers, addressing students and parents.
- Taking care of specific health problems eventually involving the school (children with handicap; HIV [human immunodeficiency virus] positive students; children needing specific assistance, for example, in case of diabetes or thalassemia) where a close link with secondary care health structures and diffusion of information to the teachers and other students is highly needed.

School medicine activities are now playing a quite crucial role owing to the new situation brought about by the immigration of a consistent extra-EC population, with different habits and different needs from Italian ones and often without the possibility to access health facilities. In this context, the school doctor can play the important role of observer of the new needs emerging from this part of the population, of counselor on the right way to access the existing services, and of first resource in extreme situations.

Health Education. The need to achieve the capability for each citizen to autonomously deal with his own health is one of the cornerstones of the NHS; this goal has to be reached through adequate health education aimed at the individual and the community. Taking for granted that the health education function is part of the GP's duties in his relationship with the patient, the law assigns the formal duty to organize health education activities to the USL. In this context, the USLs have, as their first duty, to provide each citizen with full information on their rights, on the existing services and facilities, and on the easiest way to access them. In that frame, a specific aim is to increase citizen compliance with existing screening activities so that they can take full advantage of the existing programs.

In connection with the schools, and other educational agencies, the USL organizes specific health education programs for schoolchildren of any age on the subjects deemed relevant in that specific context. It also collaborates with national programs or campaigns addressing particular problems such as drugs, tobacco, alcohol, and HIV diffusion.

THE STRUCTURE OF PUBLIC HEALTH TRAINING IN ITALY

In Italy, university is responsible for professional training of all health professionals, medical and nonmedical.

Training in public health has developed coherently with the evolution of the health system, emphasizing the development of competencies for running activities of environmental and social prevention, control, and monitoring of health services activities, based on a purely bureaucratic approach. The evolution of the health system and, more recently, the introduction of competitive models in the national health system, have promoted the development of an epidemiologic culture and of managerial and assessment competencies.

Training in public health takes place in Italy at three levels: undergraduate, postgraduate, and continuing education.

Undergraduate training is carried out for medical and nursing students along their curriculum, where courses in biostatistics, epidemiologic methods, public health, and community medicine are offered. The impact of this kind of training is very limited, and the prevailing vocational choice of the average graduate is for clinical disciplines.

Postgraduate training may take place at the university or in other institutions and may end with formally recognized titles (diploma of ''Specialist in Hygiene and Preventive Medicine'') or with generally defined, not formally recognized ''Master'' titles. The curriculum is now undergoing a radical reform in order to adapt it to the new competencies needed for public health professionals (needs and risk analysis, technology assessment, management of health services) and is likely to change its name to ''Specialist in Public Health Medicine.''

University in Italy is the only legally recognized institution entitled to give professionally accepted diplomas in the different branches of specialist medicine, public health being one of them.

The postgraduate course in public health is run by the Schools of Specialty in each university; only medical doctors are admitted, and the number of admissions are limited (around ten students per year for the biggest schools) in relation to the size of the area that the university is supposed to serve. The student has to work full-time and is paid with a Health Ministry scholarship. The title of specialist in public health is specifically required for a number of positions in the NHS: public health services of the USLs, hospital direction, and primary care services direction.

As public health competencies different from those traditionally provided by the university schools of specialty are highly needed, together with the need to offer public health training to nonmedical professionals as well, a considerable—even if sometimes confused—offering of postgraduate courses has been growing.

Good-quality public health–related courses are run by a number of training agencies (public or private) and university institutions such as, for example, the ISS, the technical body of the Health Ministry; the Business School of the ''Bocconi'' University in Milan; the National Agency for Training Improvement in Southern Italy (FORMEZ); the Center for Health Economic Research of Torino (CRESA); and the Centre for Nursing Training (CESPI of Torino). Also, the Smith Kline Foundation, World Health Organization (WHO) Collaborating Center for Health Manpower Training, has developed, over the many years, a series of training initiatives (short seminars, conferences, university staff meetings) focused on public health.

All these institutions run courses from a few days to several weeks (exceptionally for one academic year), which can serve simultaneously as postgraduate training or as a continuing education opportunity for professionals already trained. Training usually focuses on health administration and management, health economics, planning and evaluation of health services, areas that normally are not sufficiently covered by the existing university schools of specialty.

The hope for this new season of the Italian NHS is that the different disciplinary cultures associated with public health will be able to structure a training system coherent with the country's needs.

MAJOR CHALLENGES FOR THE HEALTH SERVICES

Currently, the Italian NHS is facing a major transformation of its structure and organization with the aim to limit the costs of care and to rationalize a system that has many functioning distortions and diseconomies. The main innovation will try to achieve a system where the service suppliers will be financed according to a fee-for-service-supplied. A "service" may consist of a laboratory examination, a visit, a hospital admission, or the treatment of a disease (for example, in hospital); every administration will have to negotiate the price of the activity with the demanding consumer, eventually competing with other service suppliers of the same USL or of other USLs in order to cover its costs. This new system is likely to trigger competitive phenomena within the NHS, and between public and private services, which are so far not known to our system and whose consequences are difficult to predict. Moreover, service management will be given to a fully responsible general director of the USL (or of the autonomous hospital) who will have to report periodically to higher authorities and be judged on his ability to match costs with expenses.

For these reasons, it will be of the utmost importance in the coming years to monitor the effects of the new system, paying attention to the health of the population, to health services accessibility, and to consumers' and health workers' satisfaction. Particularly critical will be the activities for monitoring services quality and verifying health professionals' behavior. From the point of view of health manpower, the biggest challenge will be that of identifying as soon as possible a sufficient number of health and administrative services executives with the needed qualities of managers able to behave in a less centralized and bureaucratic system, allowing for greater professional autonomy. For this reason, a large effort is currently under way to train human resources, especially coming from the health field, to have a sound competence in administration and a high level of managerial skills. This involves of course, first of all, people and institutions being required to have postgraduate training in public health, which means, in Italy, attending the university schools of specialty in public health for medical doctors.

Other specific achievements are expected from the NHS in the coming years, having to do with a number of objectives to be reached in well-defined strata of the population or for the population as a whole.

Objectives for Specific Subgroups of the Population

Pregnancy and Childhood. The main expected achievements are:

- To provide more effective care of the pregnancy, through an adequate and well-disseminated network of district services for normal pregnancy monitoring and control, preparation to delivery, identification of at-risk pregnancies for referral to higher-level care, and postpartum home care;
- To achieve a complete vaccination coverage for measles, rubella, whooping cough, and mumps;
- To set up an efficient screening program for some preventable childhood disabilities such as ambliopia;
- To implement home care services for chronically ill and severely handicapped children; and
- To implement ad hoc services for women and children from extra-EC countries.

Adolescent People. Consultancy centers for adolescents should be established, where ad hoc trained personnel, with considerable availability in terms of their personal willingness and time schedule, gather young people to give them help and support and favor their healthy development.

Elderly People. The main objectives should be:

- To implement outpatient services for rehabilitation;
- To implement an integrated care system, home based, for over-sixties not self-sufficient, partially self-sufficient, or at high risk of not self-sufficiency; and
- To implement home hospitalization for elderlies with nonacute diseases.

Immigrated People. The main problem with this growing category of persons is that of implementing primary care services that, working in close connection with higher-level services, have the possibility:

- To filter/orient the demand for care, actively working on high-risk groups, in connection with other types and levels of services and groups of people of the same ethnic community;
- To utilize specific mother-language ''mediators'' coming from the same ethnic community, whose specific involvement should be given high value, to allow for a continuity of the relationship of the immigrant with the country of origin; and
- To give them access, if needed, to the different health services (for medical or laboratory examinations, drugs consumption, hospital admission) of the primary and secondary levels, to which they are not usually formally entitled.

Environmental Risks

Environmental monitoring and control constitutes a main task of the NHS. Important progress has been made with the implementation of stricter rules for atmospheric and water pollution control, despite legislative activity that moves forward or backward depending on the availability of resources to invest in environmental control and pressure coming from the industrial sector to lower production costs.

With respect to the working environment, great emphasis is put at present on the necessity to monitor and improve worker safety and worker health. Toward this end, a complete information system should be set up to censor all industrial activities, to list the existing risk profiles for each firm and each activity, to enumerate all substances used, and to file all data on work accidents and professional diseases. This information system should steer all consequent preventive activities, both at the individual level and in the working environment.

Planning, Assessment, and Quality Assurance

NHS planning activity, though greatly emphasized in the law, has been poorly implemented. Only once has a national health plan been defined (it should have been done every three years since 1978!), and few regions have coherently set out their triennial plan to define objectives and directives for the services. Consequently, assessment activity has been poor, even though many studies and suggestions for an indicator system aiming to evaluate NHS achievements have been carried out. The Health Ministry has given, on some occasions, different sets of indicators for specific services or activities, but it has never been able to set up a comprehensive system—nor to implement a monitoring or surveillance activity of the NHS outcomes.

Recently, great attention has been put on the quality issue, coming mainly from professional bodies reacting to a number of paradigmatic examples of bad-quality service underlined by the national press. The National Society for Quality Assurance has also given a strong push in this direction, and as a result, many activities have started. National and regional acts have also called for the implementation of Committees for Quality Assurance, which are now getting an organized set of activities under way. In the coming years, we expect stronger and stronger emphasis on these aspects, with consequent improvement of health activities and greater health assurance for Italian citizens.

REFERENCES

Angelillo, B. (1993). Epidemiologia sociale. In: *Manuale di igiene*. Milan: Masson: 276–279.

Balma, R. & Zanoni, M. (1994). Elementi di economia, di pianificazione e di programmazione sanitaria. In: *Guida all'esercizio professionale per i medici chirughi e gli odontoiatri*. Torino: C. G. Edizioni Medico Scientifiche S.r.l.

Barbuti, S., Bellelli, E., Fara, G. M. & Giammanco, G. (1993). *Igiene e medicina preventiva*. Rome: Monduzzi Edizioni.

Buiatti, E., Carnevale, F., Geddes, M. & Maciocco, G. (1993a). Demografia e statistiche sanitarie. In: *Trattato die sanità pubblica*. Rome: La Nuova Italia Scientifica.

Buiatti, E., Carnevale, F., Geddes, M. & Maciocco, G. (1993b). Evoluzione dell'assistenza e dell'ordinamento sanitario in Italia. In: *Trattato di sanità pubblica*. Rome: La Nuova Italia Scientifica. 31–72.

Buiatti, E., Carnevale, F., Geddes, M. & Maciocco, G. (1993c). L'ambiente sociale. In: *Trattato di sanità pubblica*. Rome: La Nuova Italia Scientifica. 455-457.

Buiatti, E., Carnevale, F., Geddes, M. & Maciocco, G. (1993d). La nutrizione. In: *Trattato di sanità pubblica*. Rome: La Nuova Italia Scientifica. 134–144.

Checcacci, L., Meloni, C. & Pelissero, G. (1992). Epidemiologia e prevenzione delle principali malattie non infettive. In: *Igiene*. Milan: Casa Editrice Ambrosiana.

COA (Centro Operativo AIDS). (1994). Aggiornamento dei dasi di AIDS conclamato notificati in Italia al 31 dicembre 1993. *Notiziario dell'Istituto Superiore di Sanità*, 7 (no. 5), 3–8.

Consiglio Sanitario Nazionale. (1993). Aspetti demografici e sociali. In: *Relazione sullo stato sanitario del paese 1990–1991*. Rome: Istituto Poligrafico e Zecca dello Stato. 50–60.

Dirindin, N. (1992). La sfida degli anni '90. Evoluzione e tendenze della spesa sanitaria in Italia. In: *Il cambiamento organizzativo in Ospedale* (Campana, A. & Olivero, G. Eds.). Torino: Rosemberg & Sellier.

Faggiano, F. & Costa, G. (1990). Classe sociale e mortalità a Torino negli anni '80. *Polis*, 4, 471–496.

Faggiano, F., Lemma, P., Costa, G., Gnavi, R. & Pagnanelli, F. (1995). Cancer mortality by educational level in Italy. In: *Cancer Causes and Control*. Torino: University Torino Research Report 2, 1–20.

Geddes, M. & Cellerini, A. (1990). I fattori di rischio: Il fumo. In: *La salute degli Italiani. Rapporto 1990*. Rome: La Nuova Italia Scientifica. 173–174.

Giannico, L. (1993). Cento anni di sanità pubblica in Italia. *Federazione Medica*, 42, 5.

Lemma, P. & Costa, G. (1990). Stranieri in Italia: Lo stato di salute e il sistema sanitario. In: *La salute degli Italiani. Rapporto 1990*. Rome: La Nuova Italia Scientifica. 225–235.

Montagnani, U. & Zanetti, M. (1993). Modelli socialisti e modelli liberali: Quali soluzioni per il sistema sanitario Italiano? *Epidemiologia e Prevenzione*, 34, 272–274.

JAPAN

Atsuaki Gunji

MAJOR HEALTH PROBLEMS FACING THE COUNTRY

Japan is the archipelago located in the east end of Asia. The four main islands are fairly mountainous and densely inhabited by approximately 120 million people. A warm current flows up to the north end of the islands along their northern side, and in winter, winds blow from the continent to the Pacific Ocean. The wet wind brings much snow to the north side of the islands and the mountains, creating a reservoir of water to grow rice in the spring. In summer, wind blows from the Pacific toward the continent, and it is very hot and humid. This climate facilitates the growth of rice and a variety of agricultural products. A cold current comes down along the southern coast and collides with the warm current around the middle of the main island. This produces good fishing areas, and the Japanese have traditionally depended on fish as their main source of protein.

The origin of the Japanese is still unknown in spite of extensive research, but at present, it is generally thought that Japanese people are a mixture of multiple races. The government of Japan was substantially unified about 400 years ago by the Tokugawa family, but they closed the door of the country during their about 300 years regime. In 1868, the Meiji Restoration occurred. The Meiji government opened the door of the country and modernization commenced.

Demographic Transition and the Population Structure

Japan's demographic transition had to wait until the early 1900s when the standard of living in Japan substantially improved. Following a salient peak death rate recorded in 1913, because of an influenza epidemic, the death rate started to decline. At that time, the infant mortality rate had been hovering around 150 per 1,000 live births. This rate is much higher than the present situation in some parts of the world where the economic and hygienic situation is worst. Since then, the death rate has continued to decrease consistently. The latest data on the infant mortality rate is 4.5 per 1,000 live births in 1992.

The fertility rate had long been sustained at a fairly high level. Before World War II, it was influenced by the policy of the military government that encouraged people to have more babies. After the war, a baby boom occurred, which resulted in periodical waves in the fertility rate. However, the pure reproduction rate went down below 1.00 in 1984, when ''oil shock'' ran through the world and Japan's economic growth lost speed. Therefore, Japan started its demographic transition in the early 1900s and completed the change at around the 1980s.

Epidemiological Transition

Along with the demographic transition, the pattern of prevalent diseases has also changed. In the early 1900s, the infant mortality rate had long been hovering around 150. At that time, major causes of infant mortality were acute infections such as penumonia and dysentery. In 1940, it went below 100, and after the war, it continued to decrease very rapidly down to 4.4 in 1991.

During wartime, tuberculosis (TB) was endemic and the top killer disease of this nation (Figure 1). Therefore, the salient TB hump is observable in the death rate trend in this period. This chronic infectious disease ebbed away and relinquished the position to brain stroke by 1951. Brain stroke also began to decrease and was taken over by cancers and next by heart diseases. Today, death rates are highest first from cancers, followed by heart diseases and then brain strokes. These three diseases constitute about 60 percent of total deaths.

The known human immunodeficiency virus (HIV)-positive population in Japan was 3,022 in 1994, with 713 patients being symptomatic. About 58.6 percent of the positive population are hemophiliacs; 7.5 percent are deemed to be infected by homosexual contact and 20.5 percent by heterosexual contact, which is recently increasing the most. The ratio of drug abusers is 0.3 percent (9 persons).

Pneumonia is again stepping up in the order of the causes of death, along with the graying of the population, and has now come up to the fourth position.

When the death rates are adjusted by age structure, some different features come up. The age-adjusted death rate due to cancers is not increasing but, rather, is decreasing in women because two major cancers, gastric and cervical, are decreasing. Among cancers of different organs, gastric cancer had long been most prevalent among the Japanese. However, the death rate by gastric cancer had consistently been decreasing, and in 1993, it was taken over by lung cancer. On the other hand, the death rate by colon cancers is increasing. If the trends are extrapolated up to the end of this century, the sequence of prevalent causes of death by cancers will become, by descending order, lung, colon, liver, and

Figure 1
Death Rate Trends, 1900–1990

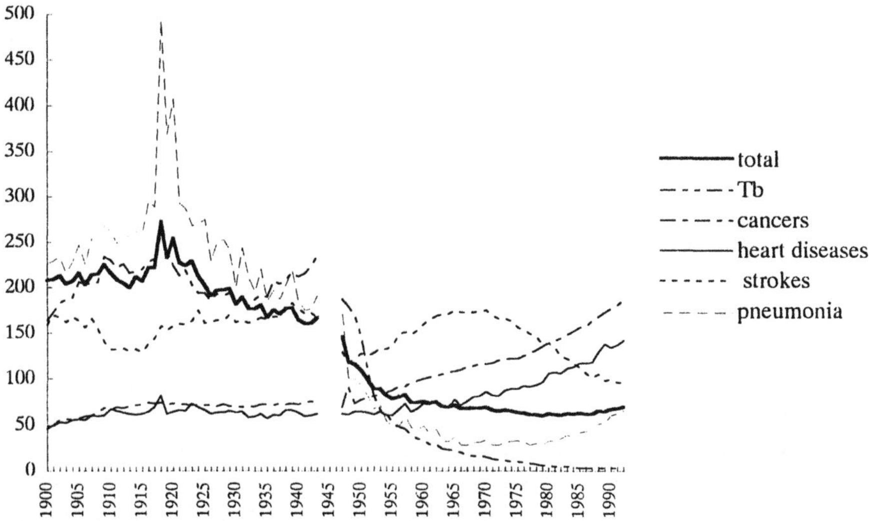

Note: The total death rate is the number per 10,000, and those by causes are per 100,000 population.
Source: *Annual Report on Health and Welfare*, various years.

gastric cancer. This sequence is quite similar to those of Western countries. However, the extrapolation of the trend of liver cancer is not certain because hepatitis B has already become controllable by diagnosis method and vaccination; moreover, hepatitis C has also become possible to diagnose, and it has become clear that interferon is effective to some extent.

Age-adjusted death rate for strokes is decreasing; especially the rate for brain hemorrhage is very rapidly decreasing compared with those of embolism and thrombosis. Ischemic heart disease is less prevalent in Japan than in Western countries, but the national data on the age-adjusted death rate for the disease are still decreasing, although there is a report that it is increasing among the urban sedentary workers in large cities.

Mental Health

According to the predictions of the Institute for Population Research, Japan is going to see peak aging of the population in the first quarter of the next century. In 1990, there were about 1 million people suffering from dementia. It is forecast that the dementia population will reach about 2.5 times that number at the peak.

Graying of the Population

One of the inevitable consequences of the demographic transition is the graying of the population. In 1992, the ratio of the population of 65 years old and older was 13.1 percent. It is expected to peak at 25.8 percent in 2025 when the generation of the baby boom reaches that age. The ratio of that population versus the working population will be 1: 2.3 at that time. After that, the ratio will go down a little and then toward a stable state, although the wave of fertility will continue.

Health Situation

The most comprehensive and standardized measure of the health status is the life expectancy at zero age. The latest directly measured life expectancy was 75.92 years for males and 81.90 years for females in 1990.

However, the morbidity of the elderly has been increasing since 1982. In light of this, it is questionable to say that the health status of Japanese is improving when the quality of life is taken into account. We have calculated an index that may mean "healthy life expectancy" while actually the index has been worsening since the early 1980s. We assume that this is the effect of a mass screening program started in the same year by the legislation of the Act for the Health of the Elderly. One supportive datum for this inference is the fact that the production of antihypertensive drugs suddenly started to soar, although the trend had long been stable up to 1982.

Nutrition

There is reason to think that nutritional status is the factor that is most conducive to the longevity of Japanese. The intake of nutrients remains well balanced. According to the annual *National Survey on Nutrition*, the average energy uptake per person per day at around 2,050 kilocalories has not changed for ten years, and the proportion of fat still remains at around 25 percent of the total energy uptake. Only the high intake of salt is problematic, especially in some areas in the northern part of the country, where the average salt intake per person a day is about 27 grams. The national figure had been in a decreasing trend until 1987 when it was 11.7 grams per person a day and again turned to an increasing trend.

Environmental Hazards

Japan has experienced many unfortunate events caused by environmental pollution in the course of its economic development, such as mercury poisoning ("Minamata disease"), cadmium poisoning ("Itai-Itai disease"), and massive air pollution. A series of measures to control pollution seems to be successful to solve these problems, but there are still problems left unsolved such as pollution by NO_2 and SPM (suspended particle matters), especially in the areas along busy roads in big cities. Land development is still going on and continues to endanger wildlife. Many species are still threatened with extinction.

PROVISION, UTILIZATION, AND IMPACT OF HEALTH SERVICES

Public Health

Health services are classified into preventive services and medical services. In Japan, preventive services and other public health services are provided by the government as one of the public services. However, medical services are in principle deemed to be the matter of the private sector with some exceptions. For example, the government commits psychiatric patients who threaten to hurt themselves and/or someone else. The government reserves the right to force them to be admitted to a hospital and covers the fees. A tuberculosis patient who is excreting bacteria can also be forced into a hospital.

The organization of the preventive services is a four-headed organism. The Ministry of Health and Welfare has the prime responsibility for public health services and engages in actual provision of the services for the people who are living in communities through the administrative machinery of the local government. The local government has one Health Center placed in an area of about 100,000 population, which is working as the front base of public health activities. The Ministry of Labor is responsible for worker health at the work site, and the Ministry of Education is responsible for school health. The Environmental Agency is responsible for nature preservation and control of pollutions. The infrastructure is important for the policies and programs to function as they are intended. Professional associations such as medical associations and nonprofit organizations are indispensable to implement them in local communities.

There are also many voluntary organizations cooperating with professionals in the communities in Japan. All the municipalities have voluntary organizations for TB control, and they contribute to propagation of knowledge and cooperate in mass screening programs by visiting homes and summoning people to the program. Along with ending the TB epidemic, they have changed their target to the preventive activities of chronic diseases. It is quite common that communities have volunteer organizations promoting maternal and child health. They also cooperate with the activities of the local Health Center. Among these are the so-called rearing schools (*Kosodate Kyoushitu*) that are now popular among those who have a newborn baby or who are pregnant for the first time.

About 170,000 volunteers are working for the improvement of nutrition in communities all over the country. These volunteers mentioned above are all women activists.

Medical Care

Medical care is in principle deemed to be the matter of the private sector. Although there are a variety of ownerships of medical facilities, there is theoretically no difference among institutions of different ownerships in terms of kinds of services provided, the population to be served, and fee schedules. The Medical Care Act, which regulates the medical facilities, classifies medical facilities into four kinds; the clinic, the hospital, the general hospital, and the long-term care ward, which is newly added by the amendment of the act in 1992.

The salient organizational characteristic of the Japanese medical care system is that for historical reasons the majority of hospitals are privately owned small hospitals. The origin of this characteristic resides in history, and this characteristic has profound influence on the administration of the system.

Welfare services are essentially public services for those who cannot support themselves. Therefore, it means that tact and discretion on the part of the government are necessary for a client to become the beneficiary of the services. However, along with the graying of the population has come the realization that welfare services are not only benefits for citizens suffering hardship but are rather services many people need to be the users of. The government forged the ten-year "Golden Plan" in 1988 to develop and improve the welfare system. It recently announced plans to commence an insurance program of the welfare services for the elderly.

Evaluation of Japanese Medical Care System

The medical care system is a multifaceted entity. Therefore, in order to comprehensively evaluate the system, a framework is necessary. Many frameworks have been proposed in the past, but it seems to be consensus in this field that the health care system has to be evaluated not only on its effectiveness but also on its efficiency and equity (Figure 2). These factors are not completely independent but are interrelated. Especially nowadays, when the utilization of the market mechanism has become the major concern in many countries, the trade-off relation between efficiency and equity has emerged as a confrontational problem in many countries.

Accessibility. The accessibility to medical care is determined by various factors such as (1) quantity of resources and (2) their distribution. More important, (3) economy seriously influences the accessibility, and sometimes (4) cultural differences become a barrier to access to medical care, for example, when people of a particular cultural background have a sex preference regarding the doctor to attend them.

The accessibility of the Japanese health care system is excellent. One of the reasons for this is that quantity of medical resources in Japan is abundant at present. The number of medical doctors is about 170 per 100,000 population in

Figure 2
Framework of the Health Care System

- effectiveness
  - accessibility
    - quantity
    - distribution
    - economy,culture, etc.
  - quality
  - integration
- efficiency
  - macrospective
  - microspective
- equality, equity

1992 and is estimated to be doubled in the middle of the next century if the present rate continues.

The number of beds has been increasing for several decades and reached the level of about one bed per 100 citizens. According to Organization for Economic Cooperation and Development (OECD) data, the number of hospitals and beds in Japan is an outlier among 24 member countries, and the number of beds is also more than two times that of the United States.

The average size of Japanese hospitals is smaller than any other country. Privately owned hospitals have about 80 beds, and they constitute about 14 percent of all the hospitals. Jurisdictional Persons have around 140 beds and constitute 41 percent. Therefore, about 70 percent of the hospitals and 55 percent of the hospital beds belong to the private sector.

Many small private hospitals are distributed throughout the small land. Furthermore, the economic barrier is very low because the universal health insurance scheme covers the whole population in Japan. Hence, the accessibility of the Japanese medical care system is excellent. The distribution of medical facilities is weighted toward city areas. The areas where people have serious problems of accessibility to medical facilities are restricted to some small islands and the remote villages when they are isolated by deep snow fall in winter.

After World War II, a mission from the United States came to Japan and recommended that Japan create universal health insurance. The Korean War allowed the Japanese economy to take off, and in 1961, universal health insurance schemes covered all citizens, although the depth of coverage was not as comprehensive as at present. The schemes are classified into two groups. One is the scheme that organizes the people at their work sites and is called the Social Health Insurance Scheme (SHIS). This scheme covers about two thirds of citizens, and half of them are the dependents of the workers. The other is the scheme that organizes people where they live and is called the National Health Insurance Scheme (NHIS). This covers another one third of citizens. Large organizations such as big companies and public organizations can organize insurance organizations of their own, but in the case of small organizations such as small companies, the government takes the role to organize an insurance organization and invites them to join together to share the risk more safely.

The latter insurance schemes are actually organized by the local governments. Japanese government is a three-storied building: the central government, prefectural governments, and municipalities; cities, towns, and villages are named according to their size of population. Each municipality is responsible for organizing a health insurance organization. Therefore, the name National Health Insurance Scheme is misleading. Instead, it should rather be called a Municipal Health Insurance Scheme.

Equity. There are some inequities among the schemes in terms of premium rates and benefits. The copayment of the insured at work sites is 10 percent of the bill, but the dependents of workers and the insured by the NHIS have to pay 30 percent of the bill. Workers are usually in the SHIS while they are working, but after retiring from their jobs, they come in to NHIS. Getting old, they naturally have to consume more medical services than in their young days. Along with graying of the population, this inequity between generations has become a more urgent problem to be solved. To solve this problem, the Insurance Scheme for the Elderly was separated from the NHIS, and 70 percent of the fund is shared by the SHISs and the rest is paid by the government.

Quality. Regarding quality, there are no official data on this aspect nor any mechanism to ensure the quality of medical care in this country. The real situation is unknown.

Integration of Institutions. Integration means how well the institutions and their different functions are coordinated. Integration is very poor in Japan because there is no explicit referral system. It is very rare for industrialized countries not to have an explicit referral system in their health care systems. Doctors who are practicing in their clinics have to make a personal effort to refer their patients or to establish such a system.

Efficiency. It is difficult to measure the macrospective efficiency of the medical care system because it is difficult to define an appropriate outcome of the system. Therefore, only spending for medical care is conventionally used as a denominator to compare the efficiency among countries.

The efficiency of the Japanese health care system is taken to be fairly good at least macrospectively, although it is well known that there are microspectively some extraordinary inefficiencies such as very long average length of stay in hospitals and overprescription of medicines.

The OECD publishes the data on provision and utilization of medical care according to the standardized rule. Looking at these data on medical spending per person a year, Japan is located at a little lower than the middle among the member countries (Table 1). The national expenditure for medical care in the countries is almost linearly proportionate to the gross domestic product (GDP). Only the United States is an outlier high above the regression line, and Japan is well below the line. According to our analysis, it seems that countries whose government has more commitment to finance medical care distribute more distantly below the regressed value.

In summary, the Japanese health care system is excellent in terms of accessibility but very lacking in terms of integration. Quality may be divergent, and it is dubious that the system is efficient. Regarding efficiency, further analysis will be done in the last part of the chapter. Next, history has to be reviewed to understand why these characteristics have been brought about.

History of the Medical Care System

The origin of these characteristics of the Japanese health care system resides in its history. The reason why, in Japan, accessibility has become so good and integration has lost is as follows: Japan has historically been swinging between two alternative ideas in terms of the sector to which medical services should have belonged; one is the idea that medical care should basically be delivered by the private sector, and the other is that it should be one of the public services. Soon after the Meiji Restoration, the pendulum swung toward the public sector. Many hospitals were constructed by local governments. However, this trend came up against the opposition of the medical profession. Gradually, they got a greater say, and public and nonprofit hospitals could not be dominant in the Japanese health care system. The Red Cross and the Benevolent Society, which is a nonprofit organization funded by the Meiji emperor, constructed hospitals but not in great numbers.

After World War II, the American mission for the reform of social security very strongly advised Japan to create a network of public hospitals and abolish private practice. The Ministry of Health and Welfare followed this advice and devised a plan to construct the network throughout the country. Actually, some hospitals were constructed following this plan, but the program was eventually only partially realized because of the lack of funds in both the central government and the local government.

When the Japanese economy took off after the Korean War and Japan succeeded in implementing a universal health insurance scheme, improved accessibility to medical care and accumulation of funds for medical facilities soon followed. Again, there emerged strong voices and pressures to swing back to the private sector, and they eventually got a greater say. In 1960, the Medical

Table 1
Per Capita Health Spending in OECD Member Countries

	1985	1986	1987	1988	1989	1990	1991	compound annual rate of growth
United States	1711	1824	1962	2146	2362	2601	2869	9
Canada	1244	1364	1461	1558	1666	1811	1915	7.5
Switzerland	1224	1267	1332	1435	1498	1640	1713	5.8
Germany	1175	1215	1287	1409	1412	1522	1659	5.9
France	1083	1135	1193	1295	1415	1528	1650	7.3
Luxembourg	930	978	1135	1219	1267	1392	1494	8.2
Austria	984	1046	4409	1191	1298	1383	1448	6.7
Iceland	889	1073	1220	1331	1373	1379	1447	8.5
Sweden	1150	1165	1240	1303	1390	455	1443	3.9
Finland	855	911	979	1044	1147	1391	1426	8.9
Italy	814	849	955	1058	1150	1296	1408	9.6
Australia	998	1072	1112	1171	1225	1310	1407	5.9

Belgium	879	931	992	1081	1153	1242	1377	7.8
Netherlands	931	990	1046	1101	1176	1286	1360	6.5
Japan	792	839	916	992	1092	1119	1307	8.7
Norway	846	1066	1043	1112	1128	1193	1305	7.5
Denmark	807	818	890	972	1013	1051	1151	6.1
New Zealand	747	806	871	900	954	995	1047	5.8
United Kingdom	685	739	795	858	912	985	1043	7.3
Spain	452	472	522	598	682	774	848	11.1
Ireland	572	580	596	620	651	748	845	6.7
Portugal	398	389	434	493	548	554	624	7.8
Greece	282	323	321	334	384	400	404	6.2
Turkey	66	89	100	110	118	133	142	13.6
OECD average	855	914	980	1055	1126	1212	1305	7.6

Sources: Schieber, Poullier, and Greenwald 1993; Letsch and Drummond 1992.

Financing Corporation was established to encourage and support the private sector in constructing medical facilities, and in 1962, amendment of the Medical Care Act passed the diet. The amendment prohibited only the construction of public beds when the area already had more beds than a certain limit defined by the act. Thereafter, the private facilities continued to construct beds, and especially while the country attained high economic growth, many clinics had grown up to small private hospitals. The government was so late to curb the investment that too many beds were constructed by the private sector. In such a way, Japan succeeded quickly to construct hospital beds not spending public funds. Therefore, the organizational characteristic was born that the system is composed of many small private hospitals. Hence, accessibility had become excellent.

As the facilities were competing with each other in the market, they were unwilling to refer their patients to their competitors and often caused feuds among them. Hence, integration of the Japanese health care system was lost.

THE INFRASTRUCTURE OF TRAINING AND RESEARCH IN PUBLIC HEALTH

There are four institutions specialized in training and research for public health. One is the Institute of Public Health, which belongs to the Ministry of Health and Welfare, and is engaging in research and training of public health workers who are mainly employees of the local government. This is the only public health school listed in WHO's (World Health Organization's) catalog of public health schools. The other three schools are under the administration of the Ministry of Education. However, they are not necessarily concerned with public health activities but are interested in more basic health sciences, social sciences, and nursing sciences.

The public health nurse had been educated mainly in a one-year course administered by nursing schools. However, these kinds of schools are rarely equipped for research work. Now, to meet the emerging needs for nursing, the Ministry of Education is proposing to transfer three-year colleges to four-year schools and to build new four-year schools and postgraduate schools in universities.

Medical schools mostly have two departments of social medicine, one of them focusing on individual patients' needs, the other on medical statistics. However, the area of public health is too wide for the few department staffs to cover, and external specialists are usually mobilized for education of public health for medical doctors. Nowadays, each department of specialty in medical schools is struggling with patient social problems because the more medical technology progresses, the more effort necessary to support them to rehabilitate the patient. In order to promote research and education to meet these needs, the new-concept public health school is wished for.

Table 2
Comparison of Health Spending per Capita Between the United States and Japan

	USA	Japan
Exchange rate	$2,600	$1,582
GDP-PPP	$2,600	$1,175
Medical-PPP	$2,600	$2,828

Source: Schieber, Poullier, and Greenwald 1993.

MAJOR CHALLENGES FOR THE HEALTH SERVICES

The most important challenge for administration of the country is to cope with the radical change in demography. The aging of the population in Japan is very serious not only because of the extremely high level of aging but also because of the high speed. Every structure of the society has to be adapted to this rapid change in demography. In particular, the construction and reconstruction of the social security systems have to be accomplished while the percentage of the working population is high enough to finance the reform. Therefore, it is a crucially important task to improve the efficiency of the security systems, to which of course the health care system belongs.

According to the OECD data, Japanese medical expenditure per capita adjusted by GDP-ppp (purchasing power parities) is rather less than the amount expected from GDP. The OECD prepares not only GDP-ppp but also medical-ppp. The medical-ppp may be considered as a kind of unit price, although it is an aggregated price of many items of services. Therefore, the total amount of spending divided by medical-ppp will yield the total volume of services purchased by the people. Table 2 shows the results of our calculation from OECD data. It shows that the volume of medical services consumed in Japan is exceptionally high and is more than that of the United States. The reason why total spending seems to be low in Japan is simply because prices of services are cheaper in Japan than in the United States. Further analysis shows that the volume of consumption of the inpatient services is rather lower than the average, but that of the outpatient and especially of medicines are exceptionally high in Japan.

Then, why is the volume of consumption so large in Japan? It is understandable through examining the macrostructure of the health economy in Japan.

All the medical institutions are competing for patients in the market, and the private ones have to be strictly self-supportive financially. They procure resources that are necessary for their practice such as nurses and other staff, medicines, devices, information, and monetary resources through each free market. On the other hand, their revenue side is substantially controlled by the government through the fee-for-service payment system. The prices of the Japanese fee-for-service system are itemized in detail; for instance, the ministry sets the price for each medicine. The ministry seems at least ostensibly successful at controlling the total health expenditure through the system—hence, the low health expenditure per capita of this country.

However, when the government tried to push down prices even more in order to control total health expenditure, it became clear that medical institutions have incentive to increase profit by increasing the volume of services to balance costs. So this system is not efficient and is threatening to endanger the quality of medical care. This threat will be aggravated by knowing that the Medical Care Act recommends that the owner responsible for financial management become the superintendent of the institution responsible for almost all aspects of patient care. It is obviously the easiest way to change care in a more profitable way when the institution may lose the balance and has to redress it. Therefore, some radical reform has to come in to change the incentive structure of the medical care system.

Japan puts heavy weight on secondary prevention through mass screening, among many other kinds of preventive activities. In spite of the fact that the epidemiological change has been accomplished and the major risks for lives have shifted from tuberculosis to cancers and chronic diseases, the Japanese government still clings to the preventive method used for TB control and is spending formidable financial resources for mass screening. About 30 percent of the citizens living in communities are screened and are given a chance to get further examinations for gastric, cervical, colon, and lung cancers, although the effect and efficiency of these programs are quite dubious.

If people are screened at large, the most common case to be screened out is hypertension. They are referred to medical facilities, where doctors readily prescribe antihypertensive drugs because economic incentive pushes them to do so. However, regarding mild hypertension, the concept of detecting early and treating early is quite controversial. Although some kinds of drugs are proved to be effective to prevent strokes, the effect of antihypertensive drugs for preventing coronary disease is quite dubious. On the other hand, the preventive effect of exercise is an established fact. It is also an established fact that smoking is the biggest risk factor, among others, for health in industrialized countries because it is a risk factor for both cancers and ischemic heart disease. However, commercials in mass media are still permitted in Japan, and smoking is increasing among young and especially female citizens. Radical changes are hoped for in the arena of public health.

REFERENCES

Annual Report on Health and Welfare. (Various years). Available from Japan International Corporation of Welfare Services, '1–2–9 Shinjuku, Shinjuku-ku, Tokyo, Japan 160'.

Ellencweig, A. Y. (1992). *Analysing Health Systems: A Modular Approach.* Oxford: Oxford Medical Publications.

Gunji, A. (1989). *Hospitals and the Medical Care System in Japan: Past, Present and Future.* History of Hospitals. Tokyo: Shiraishi Shoten, 161–176.

Health and Welfare Statistics Association. (1993a). *Health and Welfare Statistics in Japan.* Tokyo.

Health and Welfare Statistics Association. (1993b). *Kokumin eisei no doukou* (Trends of National Hygiene). Tokyo.

Jeong, H.-S. & Gunji, A. (1994). The influence of system factors upon the macroeconomic efficiency of health care: Implications for the health policies of developing and developed countries. *Health Policy*, 27, 113–140.

Letsch, S. & Drummond, M. (1992). National health expenditures, 1991. *Health Care Financing Review*, 14, 148–181.

Schieber, G. J., Poullier, J. P. & Greenwald, L. M. (1993). Health spending, delivery and outcomes in OECD countries. *Health Affairs*, 12, 120–129.

KOREA

Yong-Wook Lee and Jong-Gyu Kim

MAJOR HEALTH PROBLEMS FACING THE COUNTRY

The health status of Koreans has improved greatly in the past decades. The life expectancy has increased for males from 53.0 in 1960 to 67.7 in 1992 and from 57.8 to 75.7 for females, in the same period. Changes in socioeconomic structure, lifestyles, and improvement of health and medical care have drastically modified the causes of death in Korea. In the past, the main causes of death were acute and communicable diseases, but now they have been replaced by chronic and noncommunicable diseases.

Infectious Diseases

Acute Communicable Diseases. The incidence rate of acute communicable disease in the Republic of Korea has been markedly reduced by improvement of sanitation, successful operation of disease prevention programs, and promotion of public health. However, some imported cholera cases and increase of human immunodeficiency virus (HIV)–infected persons make it necessary to establish control programs for newly imported diseases. Measles incidence had been over 3,000 per year but has decreased below 500 due to the strength of the measles vaccination policy. Few cases of diphtheria and tetanus have been reported in this decade, and no poliomyelitis has occurred since 1984. The incidence rate of major communicable diseases is 3.2 per 100,000 in 1991, 2.4 in 1992, and 4.5 in 1993, respectively. Annual change in cases of acute communicable diseases is shown in Tables 1 and 2.

Chronic Communicable Diseases. The incidence or prevalence rate of tuberculosis, leprosy, and sexually transmitted diseases—so-called chronic commu-

Table 1
Class 1 Communicable Disease—Number of Cases by Year

Disease	Year					
	'70	'89	'90	'91	'92	'93
Total	5,841	156	262	350	481	452
Cholera	206	-	-	113	-	-
Typhoid fever	4,221	133	232	187	221	307
Diphtheria	567	-	-	-	-	-
Bacterial dysentery	814	11	13	34	240	113
Paratyphoid fever	33	12	17	16	20	32

Source: Ministry of Health and Social Affairs (MOHSA) 1994a.

nicable diseases—has rapidly decreased owing to the successful operation of prevention programs, the advancement of chemotherapy, the promotion of public health, and the improvement of standards of living. However, due to the change of sexual activity, acquired immunodeficiency syndrome (AIDS) is emerging as a new problem. Appropriate measures should be taken for the prevention of these new diseases.

The nationwide tuberculosis surveillance survey was launched in 1965 by the government, and it has been performed since then every five years. According to the sixth nationwide tuberculosis prevalence survey performed in 1990, the radiological and bacteriological prevalence rates were estimated to be 1.8 percent and 0.24 percent. These show over 60 percent decreases compared with those in 1965, 5.1 percent and 0.94 percent, respectively.

In order to improve sexually transmitted disease (STD) control, the Ministry of Health and Social Affairs (MOHSA) registered prostitutes, service girls, waitresses, dancers, and so on, at public health centers and forced them to receive regular STD checkups. The total number of registered women was 120,000 in 1992, and they have been regularly checked for STD infection. Under the government STD control scheme in 1991, free treatment and medication at government expense were given to 47,000 patients who were STD infected.

Since the first identification of HIV seropositives in December 1985, 255 persons have been reported infected with HIV by the end of February 1993. Among them, 12 persons developed AIDS as reported to the World Health Organization (WHO). The epidemiologic pattern of HIV transmission in Korea is in transition from an imported case–dominant pattern three to a homosexual-dominant pattern one.

The number of registered leprosy patients was 22,310 in 1993. Among the total registered patients, 1,103 cases (4.9 percent) are bacillus positive. The

Table 2
Class 2 Communicable Disease—Number of Cases by Year

Disease	*Year* '70	'80	'90	'91	'92	'93
Total	**24,426**	**7,729**	**5,973**	**996**	**552**	**1,496**
Poliomyelitis	176	14	—	—	—	—
Pertussis	3,818	1,554	174	118	41	39
Measles	3,625	5,097	3,415	258	38	765
Mumps	813	866	2,092	382	253	474
Japanese encephalitis	27	107	1	3	3	4
Rabies	24	—	—	—	—	—
Malaria	15,926	—	*6	*2	—	*3
Murine typhus	—	1	20	6	1	11
Scarlet fever	—	26	139	119	110	76
Amoebic dysentery	—	40	18	22	29	8
Meningococcal meningitis	17	3	2	1	1	7
Hemorrhagic fever with renal syndrome	—	20	106	85	76	109
Tetanus	—	1	—	—	—	—

*Imported cases.

Source: MOHSA 1994.

average age of registered cases rose from 46 in 1976 to 58 in 1993. The young age group under 20 years among newly detected cases had decreased from 138 to 8 cases during the 1973–1990 period.

Parasitic Disease. In the past, the parasite prevalence rate in Korea was high due to the deep rooted habit of eating raw foodstuffs. Recently, owing to the general improvement in environmental sanitation and the promotion of people's awareness of individual health, the parasite prevalence rate has decreased from 84.3 percent in 1971 to 3.8 percent in 1992. The liver fluke was an intractable disease until curative medicines were discovered, and this has marked a turning point in the eradication of the disease.

Chronic Diseases

The main causes of death are now chronic and noncommunicable diseases. Mortality rates of adult diseases (or noncommunicable diseases) are increasing in Korea. It is anticipated that this tendency will become more pronounced because of the aging of the population structure, change in dietary habits, an increase in the smoking population, and a decrease in physical activities. The crude mortality rates (per 100,000 population) of major adult diseases in 1992

Table 3
Crude Mortality Rates of Major Adult Diseases (per 100,000 population)

Classification	*'85*	*'86*	*'87*	*'88*	*'89*	*'90*	*'91*	*'92*
Malignant neoplasm (cancer)	85.9	92.1	94.5	99.5	105.2	110.4	105.3	110.9
Cerebrovascular disease	76.6	77.0	73.5	73.3	74.1	75.1	72.6	80.4
Hypertension	48.2	47.2	45.2	39.9	37.3	35.6	29.9	27.5
Chronic liver disease	28.4	29.0	29.2	28.4	30.0	29.6	28.8	28.6
Infectious and parasitic disease	23.2	21.4	19.9	17.4	16.0	15.7	14.4	13.8
Diabetes mellitus	6.8	7.6	7.7	7.4	9.4	11.8	12.4	13.5

Source: National Office of Statistics 1993.

in Korea were: malignant neoplasm, 110.9 and cerebrovascular disease 80.4 (Table 3).

Cancer is the first among the causes of death in recent years in Korea. The cancer patients who were diagnosed in general hospitals are registered and controlled at the National Medical Center (NMC), and there were 55,029 patients registered in 1992.

Mental Health

The number of mental patients was estimated to be approximately 960,000—that was 2.16 percent of the total population—in 1993. About 111,000 patients, or 11.6 percent of total patients, needed hospitalization. At the end of 1993, there were 18,694 psychiatric beds in 463 mental hospitals and clinics, and there were 74 other approved mental care institutions.

Age, Gender, and Social Class Effects

The Republic of Korea had a population of 43 million in 1990, registering a density of 437 persons per square kilometer. The composition of population by age group and sex is shown in Figure 1. When we observe the demographic characteristics of the total population in Korea, it is anticipated that persons aged 0 to 14 years will decrease because of a continuing low fertility rate and persons aged 65 years and older will increase. The population of people aged 65 or more is 2,450,000, or 5.5 percent of the total population in 1994. Compared with other developed countries, the number of aged is not yet a serious problem in Korea. Nevertheless, the population of the aged is expected to increase rapidly in the near future owing to better medical care and living envi-

Figure 1
Composition of Population by Age Group and Sex

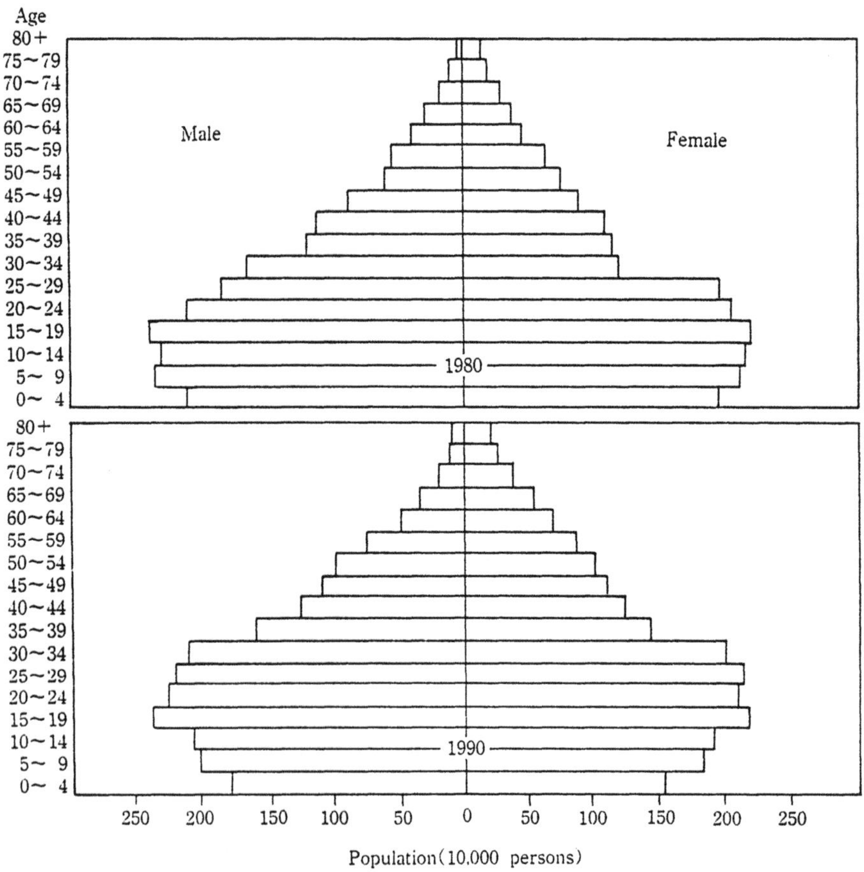

Source: MOHSA 1994b.

ronment. The total dependency ratio will drop to 38.8 percent in 2000 but again increase to 40.6 percent in 2021 (Table 4).

At the end of 1993, there were 21,879,000 women in Korea, which was 49.7 percent of the total population. The number of females between 15 and 64 years was 16,551,000. The sex ratios (number of men per 100 women) were 100.7 in 1960, 102.4 in 1970, 101.8 in 1980, and 101.3 in 1990. The ratio will increase according to the National Statistical Office. Rapid economic growth and industrialization have accelerated urbanization and concentration of population in the urban areas. Currently, 1 out of every 4 lives in Seoul. The urban population was 75.6 percent in 1992 and is predicted to increase to 77 percent by the year of 2000.

Table 4
Demographic Characteristics of Korea

Classification	'80	'85	'90	'94	'95	2000	2021
Total population (thousand pers.)	38,124	40,806	42,869	44,453	44,851	46,789	50,586
Age composition(%)							
0 - 14 years	34.0	30.1	25.8	23.8	23.2	21.2	15.8
15 - 64 years	62.2	65.6	69.2	70.7	71.1	72.0	71.1
over 65 years	3.8	4.3	5.0	5.5	5.7	6.8	13.1
Dependency ratio(%)	60.7	52.5	44.5	41.5	40.6	38.8	40.6

Source: National Statistical Office 1992.

Population Development

Fast development growth was once a serious social problem in Korea, but it dropped to an average of 0.93 in 1990. Korea has attained comparative success in controlling its population growth by means of family planning. According to the population census conducted in 1990, Korea had a population of 43 million in 1990. And the natural population increase rate dropped from 1.67 percent in 1980 to 1.02 percent in 1985, again to 0.98 percent in 1990, and finally will drop to zero in 2021 with the population at 50,586,000. The total fertility rate (TFR) dropped to 1.6—less than 2.1, which is the replacement level of TFR. The government expects this low fertility trend to stabilize at between 1.5 and 2.0.

Crude birthrate and crude death rate in 1992 were 15.4 and 5.8 per 1,000 persons, respectively. The infant mortality rate was 12.8 per 1,000 births in 1992, and maternal mortality rate was 3.0 per 10,000 births in the same year. Life expectancy was 71.3 years—67.4 for males and 75.4 for females in 1990. It is anticipated that life expectancy will be 77.0 in 2021.

Environmental Hazards

While Korea has achieved considerable success in areas such as improvement of income level through continuing economic growth, industrialization and urbanization have caused several negative side effects such as environmental pollution and food hazards.

Imported Food. Food imports to Korea are expected to increase very rapidly in volume, varieties, and countries of origin as the national economy grows and with the liberalization of the Korean market to foreign business. Various foods and raw or processed materials from developed or developing countries are imported. As a result, hazardous factors are imported as well.

Air Pollution. From the late 1970s, the Korean Environmental Protection Agency (KEPA), which is now the Ministry of Environment, has issued air quality standards for air pollutants. In August 1983, KEPA identified six pollutants as requiring some National Ambient Air Quality Standard (NAAQS). These six were sulfur dioxide (SO_2), carbon monoxide (CO), nitrogen dioxide, photochemical oxidants, particulate matter, and hydrocarbon. In February 1991, KEPA added lead to the list. Hydrocarbon has been deleted, and the standards for SO_2 and CO became more stringent in December 1993. The major contributors of air pollution, in decreasing order, are carbon monoxide, sulfur dioxide, nitrogen dioxide, hydrocarbons, and total suspended particulates. The trends in SO_2 level in Seoul are depicted in Figure 2. According to KEPA, ambient sulfur dioxide levels decreased from 1980 and dropped to 0.023 ppm (parts per million) in 1993, though several times the 24-hour maximum is exceeded in winter. So KEPA amended the standard from 0.05 ppm to 0.03 ppm in December 1993.

PROVISION, UTILIZATION, AND IMPACT OF HEALTH SERVICES

Organization of Health Services

MOHSA is responsible for the maintenance and promotion of national health and social welfare in Korea. In order to carry out these functions, MOHSA is divided into two main areas of work, with assistant ministers responsible for each. One assistant minister is responsible for social welfare policies; the other for planning, management, and general health services.

The other organizations in central government connected with the health services are the Ministry of Finance and Economy, the Ministry of Home Affairs (MOHA), the Ministry of National Defense (MOND), the Ministry of Education (MOE), the Ministry of Labor (MOL), the Patriots and Veterans Affairs Agency (PVAA), the Ministry of Government Administration (MOGA), and the Ministry of Environment (MOE). Local government implements the health services and develops community health services independently. The local offices in charge of health services are as follows: Bureau of Health and Social Affairs in Seoul; Bureau of Family Welfare in smaller cities and provinces; and Bureau of Health and Social Affairs in cities of more than 300,000 people.

Public and Private Insurance

The medical insurance introduced in 1977 expanded its coverage to the self-employed in rural areas in January 1988, the employee employed in a private company with more than five employees in July 1988, and the urban self-employed in July 1989. It only took 12 years to provide medical insurance coverage for everyone (Table 5).

In the 1980s, the government—with the cooperation of the nongovernment

Figure 2
Trends in Sulfur Dioxide Concentration in Seoul in Relation to the NAAQS

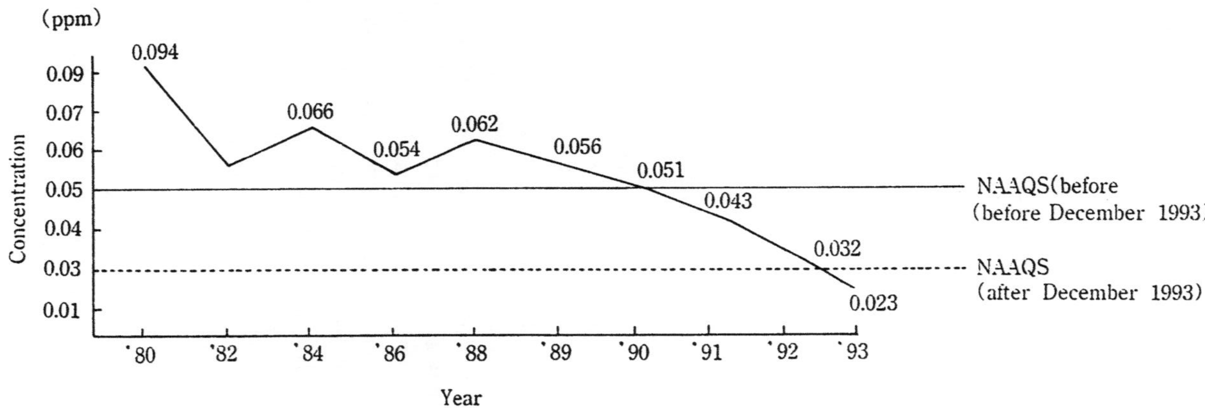

Note: The concentrations are calculated as annual averages.

Source: Ministry of Environment 1994.

Table 5
Current Status of Coverage by Medical Security, December 1993 (1,000 persons)

	Classification	*Coverage*	
		Persons	*Ratio*
Total (whole population)		44,575	100.0%
Medical insurance	Subtotal	42,209	94.7
	Employees of industrial establishment	16,158	36.3
	Government employees, private school employees, etc.	4,729	10.6
	Self-employed persons in rural areas	5,586	12.5
	Self-employed persons in urban areas	15,736	35.3
Medical aid, assistance		2,366	5.3

Source: MOHSA 1994a.

institutions and experts on medical insurance—designed a model of self-employed medical insurance (SMI) suitable to Korea. In addition, the government made nationwide efforts to improve the quality and availability of medical care in the rural areas, which lacked adequate medical facilities.

The medical insurance system has been developed as a social insurance scheme that is mandatory for all individuals. The scheme is managed by the medical insurance societies, which are nonprofit organizations established on the basis of either the workplace for wage earners or residence area for the self-employed. However, a Medical Insurance Corporation for the government/private school employees administers a medical insurance program for these employees throughout the country. Also, to assist and support each society and the corporation, one national federation—National Federation of Medical Insurance (NFMI)—exists in Korea. All medical insurance societies and corporations are members of the federation. The federation plays a very important role in the implementation of medical insurance policies.

The main source of finance for medical insurance is contributions. Employees and employers pay half of the contributions for the employees' medical insurance program. The government pays half of the contributions for its own employees and 20 percent of the contributions for private school employees. In addition, the government subsidizes self-employed medical insurance societies for the societies' administrative costs from general revenue.

The other prominent characteristic of the Korean medical insurance scheme is the partial sharing system of the medical care costs borne by the patients. The Korean medical insurance scheme has a "third-party" payment system in which medical services for the beneficiaries are provided by the medical practitioner or medical facilities not owned by the insurer, and those medical service providers are reimbursed by the insurer, on the basis of fee-for-service. Each year, a committee in MOHSA evaluates all the items of medical services and medicine available for the beneficiaries and sets the fee schedule. Medical service providers bill for their services according to the fee schedule, and each insurer (society or corporation) pays the fees to them after deducting the amount borne by the patient.

To secure medical care for those who cannot afford to pay the contributions, the government administers noncontributory programs, the Medical Aid and the Medical Assistance Programs, that are financed from general revenue. This kind of scheme was introduced in 1977 when the medical insurance program was first launched and at present covers 5.3 percent of the whole population.

Health Care Financing

General taxes, specific taxes, premiums, user charges, and charitable contributions support the health care system in Korea. Among them, premiums and user charges are the two main financial sources for health care. In the case of medical insurance in Korea, it is financed on the basis of the principle of social insurance in which contributions are levied and collected in proportion to the income level of the insured.

The gross national product (GNP) in 1992 was U.S.$325 billion, growing at 5.0 percent, and the average per capita income was $6,740. Health and social welfare expenditure was 0.66 percent of the GNP in that year. The proportion allocated to health and welfare out of the total government budget has been growing rapidly over recent years. The increase has resulted in the strengthening of various social security programs, such as medical insurance and national pension. The social welfare budget in 1994 amounted to 1,772 billion won (U.S.$2.16 billion, approximately), 4.7 percent of the total Korean budget, which increased by 7.1 percent compared to 1993.

Relation Between Ambulatory and Hospital Health care

The referral system for patients that had been partially implemented in January 1988 as part of the self-employed medical insurance program, was expanded to all programs on July 1, 1989. The self-employed medical insurance program that was launched in January 1988 required the use of the primary and secondary insurance medical care institutions locally available. The aim of this policy was to achieve sound financial stability and to maximize the utilization of local institutions. The tertiary medical care institutions were to be designated by the NFMI.

The primary insurance medical care institutions are all hospitals, clinics, health centers, and midwifery centers located in each *gun* area (county) and equivalent institutions within the radius of daily living community boundaries. The secondary insurance care institutions are all medical care institutions excluding the primary and tertiary insurance medical care institutions located within the provincial boundary and country towns and special hospitals for mental patients and tuberculosis patients. The tertiary insurance medical care institutions are general hospital–level and university (teaching) hospitals.

So the covered person should visit the primary insurance medical institutions first and, if necessary, may be referred to the secondary institutions. However, patients can visit the secondary insurance institutions directly in case of emergency. The three-tiers referral system was modified on the basis of two types of medical zone: the small-scale medical care zone (city or county level) and the large-scale medical care zone (provincial level).

According to the new, referral system, patients can freely visit primary insurance medical care institutions from health centers to hospitals with less than 500 beds within their small medical zone. However, where patients want to visit insurance medical care institutions outside the small-scale medical care zone (in the large-scale medical care zone) or to visit hospitals with 500 or more beds, they must take a referral letter from the doctor who offered them medical service first. When patients want to visit insurance medical care institutions in a large-scale medical care zone, they must have a doctor's referral letter.

Preventive Health Care

In creating national public health programs, the Korean government has laid great emphasis on preventive services rather than curative and on education for people to acquire basic knowledge of health to maintain and promote their health. The MOHSA has developed various materials for health education and distributed them to the local governments and other government authorities concerned. It has also arranged training courses for health personnel to cope with the rapidly evolving health environment. To enhance the effectiveness and efficiency of the health education system, the MOHSA established a health education material development center that collects and publishes available information and will develop revised education materials.

Production of Health Education Materials. The MOHSA produced and distributed various education materials for the local health workers' activities. Five thousand copies of "Weekly Health Information" were distributed weekly to the local governments, other ministries, health societies, and so on. Many kinds of materials for health education, such as slides, videotapes, and pamphlets, were distributed to the health centers, health subcenters, social education institutions, health workers, and military personnel for the purpose of improving the level of public health consciousness.

National Dietary Guidelines. The government has been encouraging people to be well acquainted with and practice the national healthy life guidelines and the national dietary guidelines established for disease prevention and health promotion and has been publicizing in every health-related publication and distributing posters in public places, hospitals, restaurants, and so forth.

Antismoking Program. In order to make the public aware of the dangers of smoking, the government reinforced the warning phrase printed on cigarette packs after conferring with the agencies concerned in 1989. For protecting nonsmokers, the government has gradually enlarged nonsmoking areas at public facilities. The tobacco retailers have been prohibited from selling tobacco to minors since it was proclaimed to be detrimental to minors' health by law in 1992. The Tobacco Business Act was revised in 1993 so that part of the income of tobacco companies is contributed to health or medical programs.

Immunization Program. The Expanded Program on Immunization (EPI) in Korea was launched in 1953 by giving BCG (tuberculosis vaccine) to part of the target population. In the following year, BCG immunization was expanded nationwide and since 1960, BCG has been produced domestically. In 1960, DPT (diphtheria, pertussis, tetanus) was included in the national EPI, and in 1965, poliomyelitis immunization started. In 1971, immunization for Japanese encephalitis was added. In 1980, MMR (measles, mumps, rubella) was included, and in 1985, hepatitis B vaccination started. Due to the increase in national demand, immunization for leptospirosis (1988) and hemorrhagic fever with renal syndrome (1992) began. Each immunization program was extended nationwide within a couple of years from its start. At present, vaccinations against diphtheria, pertussis, tetanus, poliomyelitis, measles, mumps, rubella, Japanese encephalitis, typhoid fever, and hepatitis B are being administered as a regular part of the EPI prescribed by law. The immunization coverage rates achieved in infants by 1991 were as follows: BCG, 93.7 percent; DPT, 96 percent; polio vaccine live oral (OPV), 96 percent; and measles, 92.4 percent. The estimated coverage rate of basic immunization for infants is 95 percent.

Tuberculosis Control Program. In order to improve tuberculosis control through prevention, earlier case finding, and treatment services, the ministry has been performing the following activities. First, to improve the effectiveness of therapeutic services for about 64,641 registered patients, the ministry plans to reduce the defaulter rate by strengthening the program as stipulated in the manuals of the national tuberculosis control programs. Second, to expand the immunized population against tuberculosis, the ministry gives BCG vaccination to eligible infants and preschool children. In addition, BCG vaccination is given to primary school students through health centers, hospitals, or nursing rooms in schools. Third, for the purposes of earlier case finding and prevention of transmission, persons and their families showing symptoms of tuberculosis are checked by sputum and X-ray examination. Fourth, to decrease the patient's discontinuity rate of receiving treatment, the ministry introduced a successful nine-month short-course chemotherapy. However, the ministry plans to introduce a six-month therapy nationwide if the result of the pilot treatment project under study is successful.

Leprosy Control Program. To enhance people's awareness and to provide accurate information on leprosy, the ministry has been developing publicity campaigns using audiovisual materials and magazines.

AIDS Control Program. The ministry is implementing an education program for prostitutes, seafarers, and international travelers and providing education materials especially for homosexuals and youth. Specific counseling services with voluntary HIV testing for homosexuals are provided. HIV screening for blood has been made mandatory for every blood unit since July 1987, and now efforts are being made to strengthen quality control of laboratory work. Case management is focusing on counseling and education, health monitoring, financial support, and AZT (azidothymidine) treatment.

Mental Health Program. The ministry is preparing for the enactment of the Mental Health Law to ensure human rights of mental patients, to promote preventive activities against mental diseases, and to establish a medical care system through the participation of central and local government, communities, and all people.

Early Diagnosis of Adult Diseases. The 13 adult disease screening centers of the Korea Health Control Association (KHCA), where screening is performed at low price, are carrying out early diagnosis of adult diseases utilizing mobile screening teams. In 1992, the ministry carried out 3,868,382 examinations for detecting adult diseases through KHCA.

Cancer Registry. The NMC implemented the hospital cancer registry in 1980. Each hospital has to document cancer cases in a standardized form and send the files to the NMC.

Prevention of Disabilities. The incidence of disability can be reduced by strengthening the maternal and child health care systems and by early detection and treatment of disability producing sickness and injuries. A management system for maternal and child health care has been implemented. Infants and adolescents are vaccinated on a periodic basic. The Korea government initiated the pilot programs for the medical examination of inborn metabolic disorders. (Under these programs, over 35,000 babies were examined within three days following birth. Among them, eight cases of hypothyroidism and three cases of phenylketonuria [PKU] were identified.)

Public Relations and Education for Drugs Misuse Campaign. The ministry has carried out preventive activities for eradication of drug demand. Preventive programs toward the reduction of drug abuse are: first, wide showing of propaganda films and videotapes at cinema theaters and through cable television networks to raise awareness of the consequences of drug abuse by illustrating victims of the evil effects of drug abuse; second, production and distribution of antidrug posters, comic books, slogans, leaflets, booklets, and slides; third, education for students by counselors and school inspectors who are directly trained by the government; and finally, promotion of the continuous preventive activities of the Korean Anti-drug Campaign Center, which is a nongovernmental organization.

Training of Health Workers. The government employees engaged in the sector of public health have been trained at the National Institute of Health (NIH), an umbrella agency of MOHSA. The objective of these training courses is to provide them with proper skills and updated techniques in the field of public health. Various training courses have been arranged for senior and junior officers, the newly employed, health center directors, and public health doctors.

Rehabilitation Services

According to the sample survey conducted by the Korea Institute of Health and Social Affairs in 1990, the total number of persons with disabilities in Korea was estimated at 956,000 with an appearance rate of 22.1 per 1,000 persons. The Korean government tries to lay a foundation for comprehensive welfare programs for the disabled by amending related laws. By amending laws that have excessively high qualification standards for some certificates, the government has expanded opportunities for persons with disabilities to participate in society.

Public Health Services

Medical Services. The demands for quality medical service have been greatly increased with the improvement of living standards, the enhancement of health awareness, and the expansion of life expectancy. Moreover, the implementation of the medical insurance program nationwide disclosed potential demands for medical care, which resulted in the need for more medical manpower and facilities. The annual trends in the number of medical-related persons who graduated from medical education institutes and received licenses after passing the pertinent government examinations are shown in Table 6.

The number of doctors, medical colleges, and hospitals and clinics were 48,390, 32, and 25,691 in 1992, respectively. The number of doctors, including Oriental medical doctors, per 10,000 persons was 12 in 1993. There were 23 specialties and 27,631 specialists in that year.

Medical institutions in Korea are classified into general hospital, hospital, dental hospital, Oriental medical hospital, medical clinic, dental clinic, Oriental medical clinic, and maternity clinic. The population per hospital bed was 347.9 per 100,000 persons in 1992.

Maternal and Child Health Services. The maternal and child health (MCH) program aims at improving the level of national health by means of perinatal care for pregnant women as well as health care services for preschool children. Population coverage of the MCH program in 1993 was 1,277,000 persons, which is equivalent to 8.2 percent of the target population, composed of 1,206,000 preschool children and 71,000 pregnant women. Some 71,000 pregnant women and 293,000 infants who are considered indigent are registered in health centers for regular medical examination. Pregnant women receive perinatal services at least nine times, including examination for anemia, urine, and blood pressure,

Table 6
Medical Manpower by Year (unit: person)

Year	Doctor	O Doc	Dentist	RN
1985	29,596	3,786	5,436	59,104
1986	31,616	4,041	5,995	64,270
1987	34,185	4,426	6,761	69,829
1988	36,845	4,932	7,657	76,143
1989	39,769	5,435	8,630	82,657
1990	42,554	5,792	9,619	89,032
1991	45,496	6,120	10,137	95,335
1992	48,390	6,839	11,285	101,140
1993	51,425	7,479	12,167	107,883

Year	N Aide	M/W	M Tech	M Rec
1985	106,340	6,247	21,681	396
1986	107,672	6,513	26,318	767
1987	116,348	6,849	31,463	953
1988	123,115	7,167	36,501	1,388
1989	128,867	7,397	40,705	1,808
1990	135,714	7,643	44,841	2,123
1991	143,760	7,862	49,482	2,486
1992	152,966	8,012	53,980	3,061
1993	162,047	8,150	56,680	3,564

O Doc = Oriental doctor.
RN = Registered nurse.
N Aide = Nursing aide.
M/W = Midwife.
M Tech = Medical technician.
M Rec = Medical recorder.

Source: MOHSA 1994a.

while infants receive nutrition, tooth and sight examinations, a congenital metabolic abnormality test, and medical examinations at the age of 6 months and 1.5 years. Those who are found to be abnormal receive follow-up examinations and then treatment if necessary. The government also provides free vaccinations such as polio, MMR, and DPT to 1,206,000 infants and babies among 3,966,000 under school age. As a result, the infant mortality rate has been reduced to 12.8 per 1,000 persons in 1991 from 17.3 in 1980. All MCH centers, private clinics, or hospitals that confirm pregnancies issue MCH handbooks to the patients.

Family Planning Program. The natural population increase rate has fallen to 0.95 percent in 1993 from 3.0 percent in 1960, while the total fertility rate dropped to 1.6 from 6.0 in the same period. In response to these changes, the government has been adjusting its direction from increasing the contraceptive supply for birth control to quality-oriented programs such as sex education for youth, prevention of induced abortion, and other MCH programs. The government has supplied contraceptive services to 19,970,000 people, including 4,209,000 sterilization operations.

Parasitic Disease Control. The ministry provides mebendazole and praziquantel, wide-ranging vermicides, to needy people and gives stool examinations and treatments to students, workers, and community people every year.

Pharmaceutical and Drug Abuse Control. The pharmaceutical administration policies of the Ministry of Health and Social Affairs aim at fostering the domestic pharmaceutical industry and enhancing its international competitive power. It has made great progress by adjusting dual aspects of competition and liberalization.

The ministry, which sets the basic program for liberalizing the import of all pharmaceuticals in the 1990s, laid the administrative foundation for the KGMP (Korea Good Manufacturing Practice) in July 1984 to create an atmosphere to produce qualified pharmaceuticals in the domestic pharmaceutical field. The ministry also actively secures the safety and efficacy of domestically manufactured pharmaceuticals through the Safety Research Center, who studies and surveys the safety and efficacy of all kinds of pharmaceuticals distributed in Korea. For improvement in public health, the government exerts pressure on manufacturers to supply customers with high-quality medicines and prevent manufacture and selling of low-quality medicines.

The pattern of drug abuse in the Republic of Korea has varied according to changes in the environment. Narcotics like opium and heroin were the most popular drugs at the beginning of the 1960s, cannabises in the 1970s; and methamphetamine arose as a serious social problem from the late 1970s to the late 1980s. Sniffers of volatiles—such as adhesives, organic solvents, and gas—and abusers of general drugs that are not under the control of drug regulations have frequently been reported since 1990. The purpose of drug control by the Korean government is to stop illicit drug trafficking and to eradicate drug abuse in the community. With a view to accomplishing these aims, the Korean government enacted the Narcotics Control Act on April 23, 1957, the Cannabis Control Act on April 7, 1976, and the Psychotropic Substances Control Act on December 28, 1979. These regulations have been the legislative base to actively participate in the international cooperation systems in line with the United Nations (UN) Conventions for drug control and to reinforce the capability of drug law enforcement in pursuit of eradication of illegal drugs from human society. The ministry amended the Narcotics Control Act and Psychotropic Substances Control Act on December 27, 1993, in order to prepare for ratification of the 1988 United Nations Convention Against Illicit Trafficking in Narcotic Drugs and Psychotropic Substances. According to the amended laws, the chemicals to be specified as raw materials in manufacturing narcotics and psychotropic substances by the presidential decree will be controlled and inspected by government by means of keeping transactions on record and preserved for two years.

Twenty-two national or public mental hospitals are designated as drug addiction treatment and rehabilitation centers by the ministry, which is responsible for the payment of the cost and for the supply of equipments. The Special Expertise Treatment and Rehabilitation Center, with 200 sickbeds and a planned opening in 1996, is under construction. With a view to protecting human rights, the ministry proclaimed the Presidential Decree on Protection for Drug Addicts in Treatment and Rehabilitation. The committee, consisting of psychiatrists, lawyers, and public officials, examines addicted inpatients so as to guarantee and further improve the human rights of drug addicts.

Food Sanitation and Control of Contaminants in Foods. To ensure food safety, standards and specifications for food and food additives are established and controlled under the Food Sanitation Act. If foods and food additives do not meet standards, they may not be produced, marketed, or imported. Standards are frequently updated as results become available from the National Institute of Health's research and information from other countries. Specifications for 117 general foods, 367 food additives, and 13 containers and packages have been published.

At the national level, residual contaminants in foods are monitored and evaluated every year by the National Institute of Health; in addition, each regional government's public health institute and local government environmental research institutes monitor as well. Gradually, target foods and the number of samples will be increased. In revising and supplementing the standards for contamination, the utmost efforts will be made to reduce any harmful effects.

MOHSA is in charge of control of imported food, and the duty of inspection is delegated to the 13 quarantine offices at ports. To make the inspection procedure for imported food more effective, a computer system was established in 1992. The system processes the information related to food safety and checks the history of the imported food to control hazardous factors and increase work efficiency. Major quarantine offices are connected with the computer network.

Drinking Water Supply and Management. At the end of 1993, the population with piped water supplies numbered 35,639,000, which was 80 percent of the total population. There are 37 drinking water–quality standards in Korea at present. The Ministry of Environment periodically checks the quality and monitors.

Social Welfare Services. The current social welfare system in Korea consists of three components: (1) social insurance (medical insurance, national pension, workers' compensation), (2) public assistance (livelihood protection, medical aid, veterans relief, disaster relief, disaster relief), and (3) social welfare services (for the disabled, the elderly, children, women, and the mentally handicapped).

Accessibility and Equity of Services

Sectoral and Regional Distribution of Health Resources. The Korean health care system mainly depends upon the private sector. Private clinics and hospitals have more than 99.7 percent of all medical facilities in number, employ 83 percent of physicians, and include 85.4 percent of total beds. Most facilities of the private sector are concentrated in urban areas. In Korea, while about 69.9 percent of the population reside in urban areas, 92 percent of the physicians and 85.9 percent of hospital beds are concentrated in the cities. This makes it difficult for the rural population to access medical care. The skewed distribution of medical resources is the result of the laissez-faire policy for the private medical care sector. The private sector tends to concentrate more in the cities where the demand for medical services is higher than in rural areas.

Regionalization of Medical Services and Patient Referral System. From July 1, 1989, the medical insurance program was extended to the whole population so that all people could have medical benefits. With overall coverage of medical insurance, the government has developed various measures to provide people with qualitative and effective medical services. One of them is to establish the nationwide regionalization system for medical services. Regionalization consists of two basic elements: the delimitation of a region and the development of graded services and patient referral system.

THE INFRASTRUCTURE OF TRAINING AND RESEARCH IN PUBLIC HEALTH

In order to carry out the functions of maintenance and promotion of the national health level, MOHSA has its own several umbrella agencies for training of health workers and supporting research. The major institutes are the NIH, the National Institute of Safety Research (NISR), and Korea Institute of Health and Social Affairs (KIHASA).

The NIH was established to conduct research, experiments, and training on public health. It has a long history and has contributed to national health promotion. The NISR was established in 1988 to conduct research and experiments on toxicology and pharmacology in order to ensure safety of drugs, food additives, and other chemical substances and experiments on the safety of new drugs produced by domestic pharmaceutical firms. KIHASA was founded as the Korea

Institute for Population and Health (KIPH). It carries out many research projects on public health and social welfare, such as migration studies and socioeconomic development.

There are government institutes of health and environment in every province and health centers at every district. Though the institutes and health centers are under the control of MOHA, they intensively perform health- and environment-related research, education, and services.

MAJOR CHALLENGES FOR THE HEALTH SERVICES

The Korean government has made continuous efforts in the fields of public health and social welfare in order to meet people's expectations and desires and to establish and promote social welfare policy, harmonized with income and economic level. To improve the level of health care, the government implements the following: (1) improvement of national nutrition and advancement of maternal and child health; (2) prevention of disease and effective management of acute and chronic diseases through strengthening of health education; (3) increase of quantity and enhancement of quality of medical services through expansion of supply; and (4) concentration of efforts on strengthening hygienic and safety control for food and medicine.

In addition, to improve social welfare services, the government has been carrying out the following: (1) stabilization of the medical insurance system, which was extended to everyone in July 1989; (2) establishment of a system for income security in case of sickness and death, with the extension of coverage of the national pension system to enterprises with five employees or more in 1992; and (3) expansion of social welfare services for vulnerable people such as the poor, the elderly, the disabled, and children.

Specific challenges for health and welfare services are as follows.

Strengthening Education for Adult Disease Prevention

The government will strengthen preventive education against various diet-related diseases such as hypertension, diabetes, and obesity and publicize national dietary guidelines through public advertisement and electric news boards.

Encouraging Breast-feeding

The Ministry of Health and Social Affairs has placed great attention on the nutrition policy, especially on infant nutrition, encouraging breast-feeding. The trend in breast-feeding practice around the world is that a growing number of educated mothers are now breast-feeding their babies because of increasing concerns about the physiological and psychological needs of their infants. With sufficient health information as well as increasing concerns about child raising,

Korea is witnessing transitions in its breast-feeding practice pattern—from the "transformation phase" to the "resurgence phase."

Antismoking Campaigns

The government will continue the antismoking campaigns cooperation with health, medical, and pharmaceutical associations and consumer groups.

Family Planning Program Prospects

The basic direction of the family planning policy is to maintain the present low fertility trend. In order to keep the present low fertility trend, government will enforce services for enhancing contraceptive practice attitudes, while supplying free contraceptive services to the limited indigent segment of the population, thus preventing unwanted pregnancies and induced abortions. As free government provision of contraceptives has been conspicuously reduced, IE&C services are becoming more important than ever before. Previously, family planning programs mainly concentrated on married people. But in the future, through sex education, the government hopes to reduce sex-related crimes, induced abortion, and parenthood of unmarried youth. Korea has successfully controlled population increase and attained demographic transition. With the accumulated experience of family planning programs, the government will strengthen cooperation with developing countries to help them attain their population targets. Since 1987, the Planned Parenthood Federation of Korea (PPFK) and KIHASA have been conducting international training for family planning staffs and women leaders. PPFK will continue such training programs with the assistance of the Korean government.

Strengthening Mental Health Care

At least one public mental care institution will be constructed in each province, and six national mental hospitals (four established and two planned) will be operated in cooperation with them.

Medical Management

The ministry established the medical management division in 1992 to improve medical management. Major contents of medical management are establishment and improvement of social intervention schemes against medical malpractice, control and guidance on medical services, safety management for diagnostic X-ray equipment, management of reduction for medical personnel and medical engineers, and control and management of medical wastes with suitable measures.

Supply of Good-Quality Pharmaceuticals and Development of New Pharmaceuticals

Major domestic pharmaceutical firms have come to greatly increase their investment in research and development (R&D) projects. In order to foster the systematic institutionalization of new drugs, the Korea Good Laboratory Practice (KGLP) system has come into force. The ministry plans to continue its new drug R&D assistance project in accordance with the Eleven-Year Plan for the Development of Science and Industry formulated by the government's High-Tech Industry Development Committee. The plan includes the establishment of R&D assistance organizations such as the Disease Model Research Center, the Clinical Trial Center, and the Medical and Pharmaceutical Literature and Information Center to actively support new drug development. It calls for a total investment of 317.2 billion won over an 11-year period that began in 1991.

Hazard Analysis Critical Control Point (HACCP) for Foods

In order to control food contamination, the ministry introduced HACCP analysis in 1994. HACCP will be implemented stepwise: for meat and milk products, in 1995; fish and fish products, in 1996; milk and milk products, in 1997; frozen foods, in 1998; and health foods, in 1999.

Environmental Pollution and Food Safety Monitoring System

The government will continuously monitor air and water pollution and contamination of foods to gather information systematically. Data will be analyzed and the collected information accessed to make decisions concerning appropriate corrective measures.

Health and Welfare Services for the Aged

The government will strengthen the services for the population aged 65 or more, enhance the spirit of respect for the aged, expand and diversify the welfare institutions and medical care, establish income maintenance for the aged. The government enacted the Old-Age Welfare Act on June 5, 1981, and promulgated the Charta of Respect for the Aged on May 8, 1982. In 1991, the government established the Old-Age Welfare Policy Committee, whose many experts from private and public institutions have been developing policies to improve the welfare of the elderly.

Recently, the number of aged who need to be admitted to institutions has been increasing because of the prevalence of nuclear families and larger numbers of aged. The government will categorize welfare institutions for the aged into eight classes: free nursing home, free sanitarium, cheap nursing home, cheap sanitarium, charged nursing home, charged sanitarium, elderly welfare center, and elderly welfare house. In addition, 415 regional elderly classes for leisure and hobby activities and 22,600 regional halls for the aged are in operation. Relaxation facilities for the elderly will be established in the near future.

Health and Welfare Services for the Child

Child welfare services are provided for children aged below 18 according to the Child Welfare Act amended in 1981. The government is endeavoring to prevent the occurrence of needy children by providing those in need with proper accommodation at child welfare facilities and by training social workers specialized in children's problems. The government will continue these programs; support for deprived children accommodated at welfare facilities; technical and vocational training for grown-up orphans; and support for child-headed families.

Women's Health and Welfare Projects

There are several projects for underprivileged women. On April 1, 1989, the Mother-Child Welfare Act was promulgated to support mother-headed families (projects for mother-headed families). In 1993, 3,695 million won was appropriated for families not only having middle–high school students but also bringing up infants under three years old. The government has offered rental apartment opportunities to low-income mother-headed households living in poor dwelling conditions. Mother-headed families with no shelter can be admitted to mother-child welfare facilities, where they may remain for as long as three years.

The Committee on Mother-Child Welfare and women's counseling centers have been established to provide underprivileged women and families with various social welfare services. The women's counseling centers help unmarried mothers, women separated from their husbands, and low-income women to reintegrate into society. There are 29 women's counseling centers and 98 women's counseling offices in the needed areas.

Education for the prevention of pregnancies in unmarried mothers and abandoned children is provided for people in the entertainment business and industrial workers at the central and provincial levels.

REFERENCES

Korea Institute of Population and Health (Institute of Health and Social Affairs). (1991). *National Fertility and Family Health Survey.*

Ministry of Education. (1992). *Statistical Yearbook of Education.*

Ministry of Environment. (1994). *Korea Environmental Yearbook.*

Ministry of Health and Social Affairs (MOHSA). (1992). *National Nutrition Survey Report.*

MOHSA. (1992). *Yearbook of Acute Communicable Disease Statistics.*

MOHSA. (1993). *Yearbook of Health and Social Statistics.*

MOHSA. (1994a). *Annual Report on Health and Welfare.*
MOHSA. (1994b). *Yearbook of Health and Social Statistics.*
National Office of Statistics. (1993). *Annual Report on the Cause of Death Statistics.*
National Statistical Office. (1991). *Report of Population and Housing Census.*
National Statistical Office. (1992). *Trends of Population Projection.*

MALAYSIA

Siti Norazah Zulkifli, Wah-Yun Low, and Khairuddin Yusof

INTRODUCTION

Malaysia comprises 13 states and two federal territories—Kuala Lumpur, the federal capital, in Peninsula Malaysia, and Labuan in East Malaysia. Peninsula Malaysia has an area of about 132,000 square kilometers, while East Malaysia (Sabah and Sarawak) covers about 200,000 square kilometers.

Out of the 18.6 million people in the country, 15.3 million reside in Peninsula Malaysia (GOM 1991). The population of Peninsula Malaysia is composed primarily of three ethnic groups, the Malays (55 percent), Chinese (34 percent), Indians (10 percent), and 1 percent other races. East Malaysia is distinct from the Peninsula in terms of the ethnic composition of its people, hence, adding to the rich cultural diversity of the country. In Sabah the majority (86 percent) of the population are classified as indigenous, termed Bumiputera, while about 11.4 percent are ethnically Chinese. The largest indigenous group in Sabah is the Kadazan or Dusun ethnic group who are about a third of the population, followed by the Bajau and Murut. In Sarawak, 70 percent of the population are classified as native, with Ibans followed closely by Malays and Bidayuhs as the major ethnic groups. Ethnic Chinese compose 28.9 percent of the population. As in Sabah, the remaining minority belongs to a variety of indigenous groups.

The per capita income (gross national product [GNP]) is estimated at U.S.$2,520, which places Malaysia as a middle-income economy (World Bank 1993). Measured in terms of ratio to the national average, the per capita gross domestic product (GDP) (1978 prices) in 1990 ranged from 0.40 for Kelantan to 1.73 for the federal capital (GOM 1991).

MAJOR HEALTH PROBLEMS FACING THE COUNTRY

The health profile of Malaysia resembles that of a country in transition from developing to developed economic status. Thus, health problems typical of both situations are evident, that is, infectious diseases and malnutrition, as well as chronic diseases associated with longevity and lifestyle changes, such as hypertension and heart disease.

Demographically, Malaysia has a relatively young population with about 38 percent under 15 years of age (1990). On the other hand, the elderly population, defined as above 60 years, is under 5.8 percent. Compared with developed countries—for example, Japan, which has about 18 percent above 60 years (1992)—the elderly population in this country is very small. Nonetheless, health problems associated with increased life expectancy will emerge.

Infectious Diseases

Malaysia has been successful in controlling infectious diseases through child immunization programs, provision of safe water supply, proper sanitation and waste disposal, and food quality control. For example, immunization coverage of infants for 1993 was 95.5 percent for BCG (tuberculosis vaccine), 88.5 percent for DPT (diphtheria, pertussis, tetanus), 88.1 percent for polio, and 77.8 percent for measles (Wan Othman 1995). The 1990 figures show that 96 percent and 66 percent of the urban and rural populations, respectively, have access to piped water supply (GOM 1991). Also, 93 percent have access to sanitary toilet facilities (GOM 1991). Improved literacy (78 percent) (World Bank 1993) and educational attainment among its people have also helped in disease prevention.

Information on certified cause of death for 1992 shows that septicemia, pneumonia, and tuberculosis were the most common fatal infections, accounting for 4.5 percent, 2.9 percent, and 1.3 percent of total deaths (35,612), respectively (Table 1) (Vital Statistics Malaysia 1992). Smallpox has been successfully eradicated—there were no cases over the past five years—and the number of deaths due to measles has progressively decreased from 62 in 1988 to 4 cases in 1992. Polio and neonatal tetanus have also been effectively reduced through widespread child immunization practices.

Among admissions to government hospitals in 1992, normal birth deliveries, complications of pregnancy, and accidents were the leading causes (Table 2). For the socioeconomically more advanced Peninsula, diseases of the circulatory system are the fourth most common cause. In East Malaysia, diseases of the respiratory system, that is, including infections such as pneumonia and tuberculosis, are prominent. In these two states, intestinal infections continue to be among the ten most common cause of admission to hospitals.

With regard to communicable diseases, Malaysia has not been spared the threat of the human immunodeficiency virus (HIV) and acquired immunodeficiency syndrome (AIDS). The number of HIV infections detected has increased

Table 1
Most Common Medically Certified and Inspected Deaths by Cause in Malaysia, 1988–1992

Cause of Death	*Percentage of Total Deaths by Year*				
	1988	*1989*	*1990*	*1991*	*1992*
TUBERCULOSIS	1.69	0.66	1.20	1.29	1.30
INTESTINAL INFECTIOUS DISEASES (cholera, typhoid, and paratyphoid infection and other intestinal diseases)	0.64	0.46	0.40	0.39	0.31
VIRAL INFECTIOUS DISEASE (whooping cough, smallpox, measles)	0.20	0.16	0.05	0.03	0.01
SEPTICEMIA	4.09	3.45	3.36	4.07	4.50
NEUROINFECTIOUS DISEASES (tetanus, meningitis and meningococcal infection)	0.83	0.69	0.67	0.59	0.63
MALARIA AND ALL OTHER INFECTIOUS PARASITIC DISEASES	0.70	8.84	0.77	0.88	0.74
NEOPLASM (malignant neoplasm of stomach, colon, rectum, rectosigmoid junction, and anus, trachea, bronchus and lung, female breast, uterus, cervix, leukemia, and other unspecified neoplasm)	10.59	10.93	10.84	11.16	11.50
HEART DISEASE AND OTHER DISEASES OF CVS (acute rheumatic fever, rheumatic heart diseases, hypertensive diseases, acute myocardial infarction, other ischemic heart diseases, atherosclerosis and other diseases of circulatory system)	21.12	20.27	19.46	20.45	19.85
CEREBROVASCULAR DISEASES	7.95	8.65	8.63	8.34	8.43
PNEUMONIA	3.28	2.92	3.05	2.65	2.92
RENAL PARENCHYMA DISEASE AND OTHER RELATED DISORDERS	2.87	3.06	3.41	3.08	2.46
CONGENITAL ABNORMALITIES	3.05	3.12	3.24	3.09	3.11
CONDITIONS ARISING FROM PERINATAL PERIODS (direct obstetric causes, indirect obstetric causes, birth trauma, and other conditions originating from perinatal period)	9.85	8.82	8.99	7.81	7.70
ACCIDENTS (motor vehicle traffic accidents, accidental falls, all other accidents and adverse effects)	9.42	8.16	8.04	8.46	8.67
SUICIDE AND SELF-INFLICTED INJURY	0.16	0.11	0.10	0.19	0.12
TOTAL	31,705	32,521	34,278	34,938	35,612

CVS=Cardiovascular system.
Source: Vital Statistics Malaysia 1992.

Table 2
Ten Principal Causes of Hospitalization in Government Hospitals in Peninsular Malaysia, 1992

PENINSULAR MALAYSIA			
No.	*Causes*	*No. of Discharges*	*% to Total Discharges*
1	Normal Delivery (ICD 650)	209,963	19.90
2	Complication of Pregnancy (ICD 630-648; 651-676)	130,604	12.38
3	Accidents (ICD E800-E848; E850-E929)	116,883	11.08
4	Diseases of the Circulatory System (ICD 390-398; 401-405; 410-438; 440-459)	69,284	6.57
5	Diseases of the Respiratory System (ICD 460-466; 470-478; 480-519)	63,231	5.99
6	Certain Condition Originating in the Perinatal Period (ICD 760-779)	59,850	5.67
7	Diseases of the Digestive System (ICD 520-579)	52,793	5.00
8	Symptoms, Signs, and Ill-defined Conditions (ICD 780-799)	49,640	4.71
9	Mental Disorders (ICD 580-599)	28,769	2.73
10	Diseases of the Urinary System (ICD 580-599)	28,691	2.72
	ALL CAUSES	1,054,976	100.00

Source: Vital Statistics Malaysia 1992.

from 206 in 1989 to 10,034 by the end of 1994. The Ministry of Health (MOH) has mounted an active campaign within its Healthy Lifestyle program to control HIV transmission via information, education, and communication strategies through the mass media, public exhibitions and talks, and dissemination of informational materials. A National Council of Non-Government Organizations on AIDS has been established to coordinate funds and activities in support of the government program.

Vector-borne diseases such as malaria and dengue still occur in parts of Malaysia. Malaria is common in Sabah, Sarawak, and some rural areas in Peninsula Malaysia, and outbreaks of dengue hemorrhagic fever occur periodically, more so in urban areas. The numbers involved, and the number of deaths, from a recent outbreak of dengue were enough for the government to launch a preventative campaign through the mass media.

Chronic Diseases

Chronic diseases have become more prominent in this country with time. A comparison of the ten most common causes of death in the country between 1970, 1980, and 1990 show the increasing prominence of noncommunicable illnesses, such as heart disease and cerebrovascular disease, compared to infectious diseases such as pneumonia (Table 1). Worthy of note, deaths due to diabetes mellitus, for example, have increased from 475 cases (1.49 percent of all deaths) in 1988 to 825 cases (2.32 percent) in 1992 (Vital Statistics Malaysia 1992). Diabetes is associated with obesity and dietary changes attributable to increasing affluence.

As mentioned earlier, accidents and diseases of the circulatory system are the most prominent cause of admission into government hospitals (1992) in Peninsula Malaysia. Again, this illustrates the prominence of noncommunicable diseases. In less-developed Sarawak and Sabah, diseases of the circulatory system constitute the seventh and ninth most common cause.

Currently, the most common certified cause of death continues to be cardiovascular, particularly acute myocardial infarction, and cerebrovascular disease (Table 1). As a group (hypertensive disease, myocardial infarction, ischemic heart disease, cerebrovascular disease, atherosclerosis, and other diseases of the circulatory system), these conditions constitute about 28 percent of total deaths.

Malignant neoplasms have increased as a contributor to total deaths in this country. Malignant neoplasms of the trachea, bronchus, and lung have progressively risen as a cause of death, from 2.02 percent in 1988 to 2.29 percent in 1992 (Vital Statistics Malaysia 1992). The magnitude of this problem has prompted the Ministry of Health to initiate an antismoking campaign, including legislation on no-smoking areas in government buildings and hospitals. The common cancers in this country are breast, lung, colorectum, cervix, oral cavity, nasopharynx, and liver (Lim 1991). With regard to nasopharyngeal cancer and liver cancer, Malaysia is regarded as being in the hyperendemic zone (Lim 1991). Steps to reduce the incidence of liver cancer have been taken with the implementation of a hepatitis B vaccination program for newborns and infants.

Mental Health

Relatively little attention has been paid to mental health issues in this country. Mental health problems tend to bear the stigma of shame and embarassment for family members and, hence, are kept concealed.

Malaysia has a plural health care system incorporating both modern medicine and traditional healers. Most ethnic groups in the country have their traditional healers, for example, the *bomohs* among the Malays, the *sinsehs* among the Chinese, the ayurvedics among the Indians, and the *bomohizan* among the Kadazan. Based on faith and spirituality, these healers are often called upon to exorcise and hence "cure" mental illnesses that are linked to supernatural forces.

As an indicator of mental health, the number of suicides over the past five years has been low at between 33 and 67 deaths per year. Data on attempted suicides admitted to a major public hospital in the capital city showed that the majority were women of lower income, low education, Indian ethnicity, and younger age (less than 39 years) (Mohd Hussain, Ganesvaran, and Agnes 1992–1993). Depression caused by maladjustment to psychosocial stressors, particularly financial problems and interpersonal conflicts with spouses, friends, and family members, was the main predisposing factor involved in the suicide attempt.

Health of Immigrants and Refugees

Historically, migration has played an important role in shaping Malaysia's population. The country has a sizable migrant population due to its high manpower needs and proximity to labor-exporting countries such as Indonesia and the Philippines. Besides its neighboring countries, Malaysia also has migrant workers from Bangladesh and Myanmar. The legal rights, protection, health care, and social needs of migrant workers in their host country deserve attention, and exploitative relations should be prevented. In addition, negative attitudes and prejudices among the host countrymen toward migrants may arise as their numbers increase. This should be monitored to attenuate potential problems and undesirable effects that may occur.

Migrants have access to public hospitals and clinics at nominal fees, as do Malaysian citizens. However, there may be barriers to utilization due to ignorance, lack of confidence, problems with language, cost, transport, time off from work, or negative interactions with health care providers. Thus, treatment may be sought late, when problems have become more severe, or not at all.

Limited data on migrants' health are available from a household-based survey on maternal and child health covering 1,515 married women in eight urban areas in Sabah (Zulkifli et al. 1994). Respondents in the survey were categorized as citizens or migrants. The latter had a significantly lower education level and household income than the citizens. A higher proportion of migrant respondents were also living without treated domestic water supply and sanitary toilet facilities. In terms of reproductive health, the findings showed that a significantly higher proportion of migrants had never attended antenatal care, had never used contraceptives, and had deliveries assisted by traditional birth attendants. Infant mortality was significantly higher among migrants (16 per 1,000 live births) than citizens (10 per 1,000 live births). This finding suggests that the poorer environment in which the migrants live may have a negative impact on infant health.

In terms of refugees, Malaysia has provided temporary asylum to Indochinese refugees before repatriation to other permanent host countries. According to a United Nations source, there were 10,077 Indochinese refugees in this country by the end of 1983 (United Nations 1985). During 1982–1983, almost 26,000 refugees arrived in Malaysia, while a comparable number left for resettlement elsewhere. A fenced-in refugee camp housing Vietnamese refugees is still operating in Kuala Lumpur. This provides basic shelter and amenities but without freedom of movement. At present, the policy is to persuade the refugees to return to their country.

Population Development

After independence in 1957, Malaysia adopted an antinatalist population policy. Couples were encouraged to have fewer children in order to reduce the population growth rate from 3 percent to 2 percent within 20 years (GOM 1965). A National Family Planning Board was established in 1966 under the Family Planning Act to coordinate and provide services throughout the country. Prior to this, family planning services were provided by private sources in urban areas, in particular, by Family Planning Associations. In 1958, the Federation of Family Planning Associations of Malaysia was formed, and by 1978, affiliates had been set up in each state.

In the late 1970s, the emphasis on controlling population had started to show signs of change, and in 1984, the policy was shifted toward a more pronatalist stance in order to achieve a larger population size. The National Family Planning Board was thus renamed the National Population and Family Development Board to reflect the New Population Policy's focus on birth spacing and family welfare rather than birth limitation. Some incentives were promulgated to encourage childbearing, for example, tax breaks for up to five children rather than the previous three. Maternity leave for civil servants was also increased to 60 days.

At present, natural increase is the main factor supporting population growth in the country. In this regard, fertility patterns vary by ethnicity and location largely based on social and economic differences among the people. In Peninsula Malaysia, fertility is highest among the Malays and lowest among the Chinese. Generally, the Chinese community in Malaysia is more urbanized, and have a higher educational attainment and income level and later age at first marriage. These are some of the factors related to lower total fertility in this group.

Nutritional Problems

The prevalence of undernutrition, particularly severe malnutrition, is relatively low. Death from protein-calorie malnutrition has declined from 36 cases in 1988 to 20 cases in 1992 (Vital Statistics Malaysia 1992). Although there is a less than 1 percent prevalence of severe malnutrition, about a quarter of children are moderately malnourished according to reference growth charts (Wan Othman 1995). The main nutritional problems among children are underweight and stunting due to protein-calorie deficiency, iron-deficiency anemia, and worm infestation. In general, malnutrition in children is more prevalent in rural than urban areas and increases with older age as nutritional requirements and deficits increase. For the higher-risk group, that is, rural children, breast feeding is still commonly practiced and for a longer period compared with urban infants. This confers some protection against malnutrition for infants.

As might be expected, malnutrition is a more common problem in the socioeconomically disadvantaged areas of the country, notably Sabah and Sarawak in East Malaysia. The nutritional surveillance program for children under seven years within the Department of Health and Medical Services in Sarawak documents the prevalence of moderate to severe malnutrition in 1991 as 9.8 percent among infants, 25.7 percent among toddlers aged one to four years, and 43.5 percent among preschoolers aged five to six years. Average and subgroup rates have all decreased compared with figures for 1982, particularly among the preschoolers. Similarly, based on a nutrition survey in Sabah in 1991 among children aged five years and below, malnutrition was reported to be higher than 40 percent in several districts, including two interior districts where the rates were 78 percent and 81 percent.

In certain parts of Malaysia, notably Sabah and Sarawak, iodine deficiency is relatively endemic. The extent of iodine deficiency in Sarawak, for example, exceeds 60 percent among populations above 15 years of age in interior regions (Kiyu and Tambi 1992). These nutritional problems are generally associated with children from lower-income and/or rural households in iodine-deficient areas. Since this deficiency may have protracted effects on child intellectual and physical development, several programs have been initiated in Sarawak, namely: (1) distribution of iodized salt to problem areas since 1957, (2) free distribution of iodized salt to pregnant mothers through maternal and child health clinics since 1979, and (3) steps to legislate mandatory import of iodized salt in 1982. Despite these efforts, iodine-deficiency disease is still prevalent in selected areas in this state. Most recently, the state government is experimenting with iodized piped water supply with the colloboration of the Institute of Medical Research in Kuala Lumpur.

With regard to nutritional problems among adults, anemia remains the most common in Malaysia, especially among women. The majority of cases are due to iron deficiency contributed by inadequate dietary intake and iron losses through menstruation and childbearing. As such, iron supplementation is routine practice in antenatal care. Steps need to be taken to increase intake among women from an earlier age to avoid further stresses during childbearing.

With rising affluence, problems related to overnutrition are becoming apparent. As mentioned earlier, diabetes—particularly non-insulin-dependent diabetes mellitus (NIDDM)—has increased in proportion as a cause of total deaths in the country over the past five years. There is also a cause for concern for rising occurrence of obesity in the population. Among schoolchildren, about 15 percent are above 100 percent of standard weight-for-age (Wan Othman 1995).

Environmental Hazards

The government's present thrust toward industrialized status by 2020 has made environmental concerns imperative in light of sustainable development. At the same time, population growth and agricultural activities have also contributed to land and water pollution. The extensive use of pesticides has already become an issue of concern as reported by a public interest nongovernment organization called Sahabat Alam Malaysia (Friends of the Earth). The government has expressed a commitment to environmental preservation as expressed in the Sixth Malaysia Plan 1990–1995 (GOM 1991).

In Malaysia, among 2,292 industries identified as major sources of water pollution in 1991, 40.5 percent were food and beverage industries, 14.1 percent were rubber-producing industries, and 11.8 percent were chemical-producing industries (Low 1993). In terms of organic water pollution, human and animal wastes and the manufacturing and agro-based industries are the primary sources.

PROVISION, UTILIZATION, AND IMPACT OF HEALTH SERVICES

Organization of Health Services

The Ministry of Health is the major government agency responsible for the delivery of health care. Health is a federal matter controlled by the Ministry of Health headed by a minister who is assisted by a deputy minister and chief secretary and the general director of Health. The general director is responsible to the minister for the overall administration. In carrying out the various functions, he is assisted by the deputy general director, the director of Medical Services, the director of Health Services, the director of Dental Services, the director of Planning and Development, the director of Pharmaceutical Services, and other directors of various institutions at the federal level. The staff officials at the Federal level are responsible for formulating policies, programs, and standards of procedures and techniques for various specialties.

At the state level, the director of Medical and Health Services, assisted by the deputies, the deputy director of Medical and Health Services (Medical), the deputy director of Medical and Health Services (Health), senior administrative officer, senior pharmaceutical chemist, and other officers, is directly responsible to the director general. The state director, consistent with the policies and objectives of the central government, through the Ministry of Health, plans, organizes, coordinates, directs, and estimates the expenditures and executes the medical and health program for the state. All state plans and programs are submitted to the ministry for review, processing, and consolidating in consultation with the respective state director before the overall plans are submitted to the government for approval. At the district level, the administration of the health services is under the medical officer of health or senior officer of health. He/she is directly responsible to the deputy director of Medical and Health Services (Health) for all health programs and matters related to health in the district. The medical officer of health at the district level is assisted by the medical and health officer at the main health center, the Malaysia Center of Health (MCH) Clinic at the health office, the senior health inspector, and a health sister and senior clerk and other staff. At the state level, the deputy director of Medical and Health Services (Health) is assisted by the MCH officer, health matron, an education officer, an entomologist, a senior public health inspector grade 1, and other staff. The medical service at the district level, on the other hand, is delegated by the state director to the medical superintendent of the district hospital or the medical officer in charge of the smaller district hospital. He/she is directly responsible to the state deputy director of Medical and Health Services (Medical).

Preventive Health Service

The government has played a dominant role in the provision of preventive and promotive health programs such as immunization and vaccination, control of communicable diseases, rural environmental sanitation, applied food and nutrition, occupational health and safety, health education, family development, and antidrug and road safety programs. The rural environmental and sanitation program provides a clean water supply and sanitation facilities for rural households. Up to the end of 1992, the total number of beneficiaries from water supply projects, gravity feed systems, sanitary wells, sanitary wells with house connection, and rain water storage systems totaled 1,378,895 houses with 7,174,254 people, constituting 79.3 percent of total rural houses or 79.5 percent of the total rural population. A total of 1,562,117 sanitary latrines have already been provided, benefiting 8,035,213 rural people. Nearly 90 percent of all rural houses now have this facility.

Efficient preventive health programs continue to be undertaken to reduce future expenditure on curative care. Much emphasis has also been placed on occupational health and safety as an important component of the preventive health care program. The same is true for the environmental and sanitation program, particularly in the rural and squatter areas, with a high prevalence of communicable diseases, where a potable water supply system is not available or affordable by the population groups concerned. The government is stepping up surveillance and enforcement on food quality control to ensure compliance with set standards.

Under the preventive dental services program, the fluoridation of water supplies, dental health education, and clinical procedures have been implemented. In 1992, there were 144 treatment plants with "fluoride feeders" out of a total of 418 treatment plants. The government has also introduced programs to improve the quality and increase the utilization of facilities at health centers and district hospitals to ensure effective delivery of health services to the public. In this regard, refresher courses for personnel in the management of curative health services have been organized.

The government has improved its referral system, making it more efficient and effective, to ensure that patients receive appropriate care based on need. Measures such as decentralized urban polyclinics and day care services continue in order to maximize the utilization of facilities and services at various levels and to ease congestion, especially at general hospitals. In consonance with the aim of more equitable distribution of services, district health systems have been strengthened with the provision of X-ray facilities and the upgrading of laboratory services in health centers and polyclinics (GOM 1991).

Health Care Financing

The commitment of government to health in general is evident from its budgetary allocation, which has steadily increased over the years. However, it constitutes less than 6 percent of the overall national budget (Wan Othman 1995).

For assessing public health commitment, an appropriate indicator is the percentage allocated to the program from the total MOH allocation. Data are available from 1990 onward, as follows:

Year	Total MOH Budget	Public Health Allocation	(%)
1990	1,756,410,770	573,165,920	(32.63)
1991	2,041,162,400	539,787,970	(26.45)
1992	2,352,678,600	550,939,300	(23.42)
1993	2,482,391,710	527,446,600	(21.50)
1994	2,390,504,900	723,839,900	(30.28)
1995	2,593,231,000	785,704,100	(30.3)

It is evident that 1994 was a significant year when the percentage allocation increased from 21.50 to 30.28 percent, which was to be maintained in 1995 (Wan Othman 1995).

Public health programs have greatly benefited from international funds—especially from UN-affiliated bodies such as WHO (World Health Organization), UNICEF (United Nations Children's Fund), and FAO (Food and Agriculture Organization). Other world bodies that have significantly contributed are the World Bank and Asia Development Bank, although most of these assistances are in the form of loans. Several agencies from Japan and the British Council have also given financial aid, usually indirectly in the form of fellowship attachments, consultancies, and donations of equipment.

Public and Private Health Insurance

The various types of health insurance available are (MMA 1987):

Fee-for-Service. This is a traditional form of insurance where for the payment of a premium an individual is protected against costs of any major illness that may befall him/her. The extent or limit of coverage is dependent on the premium paid.

Hospitalization and Surgical Insurance. This scheme provides hospitalization and surgical benefits such as:

- Room and board (per confinement/disability/day)
- Surgeon's fees, anesthetist's fees, and theater fees
- Drugs, dressings, hospital supplies, appliances, treatment fees, therapy fees, laboratory fees, X rays and diagnostic procedures (per confinement and per disability)
- In-hospital physician's visits to patient's bedside
- Specialist consultation fees when in connection with a disability requiring confinement in a hospital
- Emergency outpatient treatment for injuries arising out of an accident (per accident)
- Ambulance fees (per disability)

Outpatient "Private Doctor" Benefits. This plan is available for an additional premium. However, these schemes have not been widely utilized because (1) general practitioner visits are at present based on a fee-for-service; the average cost is RM15.00, inclusive of medicine, which is considered affordable even without insurance; (2) premiums are expensive; and (3) there is a possibility of abuse, as health insurance for general practitioner visits may be overused as a result of unnecessary visits.

Prepaid Health Plans. Here health care is paid for in advance at a predetermined rate.

Private Health Insurance

There are at least eight companies in Malaysia that offer health insurance (MMA 1987). It is estimated that over 250,000 individuals are presently covered under the various schemes offered, mainly through their employers. Health insurance companies only pay out 40 percent as returns on the payment of the premiums paid by the consumers, compared to the normal payout figure of 70 to 80 percent by health insurance companies worldwide (MMA 1987).

Health Insurance for the Poor, Aged, Indigent, and Disabled

A section of the population that is unable to afford any premiums for health insurance coverage include contract laborers, smallholders, farmers, estate workers, fishermen and some self-employed groups, the aged, and disabled. The government continues to take the main responsibility of providing health care to this section of the population either by paying for the health insurance premiums of these individuals or by bearing their health costs in government hospitals. Other sources of funding include: (1) cooperatives or estates—contributions for estate employees, padi farmers, mine workers, and fishermen made through their cooperatives or estates; (2) funds collected from estates that could be used to subsidize the payment of premiums of estate employees; and (3) Ministry of Social Welfare.

Self-Help Organizations

The voluntary agencies operating are the Malaysian Red Crescent Society, St. John's Ambulance Service, Leprosy Relief Association, National Cancer Society, Association for the Prevention of Tuberculosis, Association for Mentally Retarded Children, Association for the Blind, the Federation of Family Planning Associations, Cleft Lip and Palate Association of Malaysia, Anti-Dadah Organization (PEMADAM), Malaysian Aids Council, Diabetic Organization, National Autistic Society, and Malaysian Mental Health Association, as well as the professional bodies like the Malaysian Medical Association (MMA). Other self-help groups also include Alcoholics Anonymous, ALANON (association for those affected by someone else's drinking), Narcotics Anonymous, and Women's Aid Organization. Many, though not all, of the bodies are subsidized by the government as they complement and support public health care activities.

Rehabilitation Services

Drug addiction is spreading alarmingly and rapidly, particularly among the youths today. Due to the nature and severity of the problem, it is now considered a security problem, and as such, concerted measures in terms of prevention, curative, and rehabilitative actions have been undertaken.

In 1992, the number of drug dependents detected was 20,236, that is, an increase of 6 percent from the cases detected in 1991. The percentage of repeated cases showed an increment of up to 61.7 percent in 1992, as compared with 59.2 percent in 1991. The number of new cases detected in 1992 was 7,750 compared with 7,790 in 1991. This accounted for 38.3 percent in comparison to the repeated cases. At the moment, there are about 19 governmental drug rehabilitation centers in the country (Anti-Drug Task Force 1993).

From 1975 to 1992, 82,483 registered drug dependents went through the treatment and rehabilitation program. In 1992, 33,454 drug dependents underwent the treatment and rehabilitation program in governmental or private institutions: 6,433 in the governmental program, 8,117 in prisons, 372 in private centers, 11,618 in the supervision program, and 6,914 in the after-care program (Anti-Drug Task Force 1992).

Phasing out the leprosaria has resulted in the decreasing number of inmates at the National Leprosy Control Center in Sungei Buloh, Selangor, and in Sarawak. Those remaining were unable to be rehabilitated into the community. There are no new inmates being admitted to the leprosaria. In 1992, there were 890 institutionalized leprosy patients, compared to 1,770 in 1980, 1,378 in 1985, and 1,035 in 1990. At the end of 1992, there were 2,989 registered cases of leprosy in Malaysia.

Community-based and clinical-based rehabilitation for physically handicapped are also carried out. The nongovernmental organizations providing these services include the Kiwanis Down's Syndrome; Malaysian Care; Wisma Harapan for the mentally retarded; Rehabilitation for the Physically Disabled Center in Cheras, mainly for vocational training; Rumah Insan; and the Muscular Dystrophy Association. The Yayasan Sultan Idris Shah in Ipoh mainly provides community-based rehabilitation for the physically disabled.

Public Health Services

The provision and utilization of these public health services have a considerable impact on the health of the people. As shown in Figure 1, infant mortality rates have declined in Malaysia to fairly low levels for a developing country. In comparison, the average for middle-income countries is about 38 per 1,000 live births and for high-income countries is about 8 per 1,000 live births (1991 data—World Bank 1993). It should be noted that the infant mortality rates for Sabah and Sarawak are not comparable to that of the Peninsula because of underreporting. These states are less developed socioeconomically and have a higher proportion of births delivered by untrained birth attendants. Similarly, neonatal and perinatal mortality rates have also declined in Malaysia commensurate with indicators of social and economic progress (Figures 2 and 3, respectively).

As one indicator of women's health status, the maternal mortality rate in Malaysia has also declined to rather low levels. With the high relative proportion

Figure 1
Infant Mortality Rate in Malaysia, 1988–1992

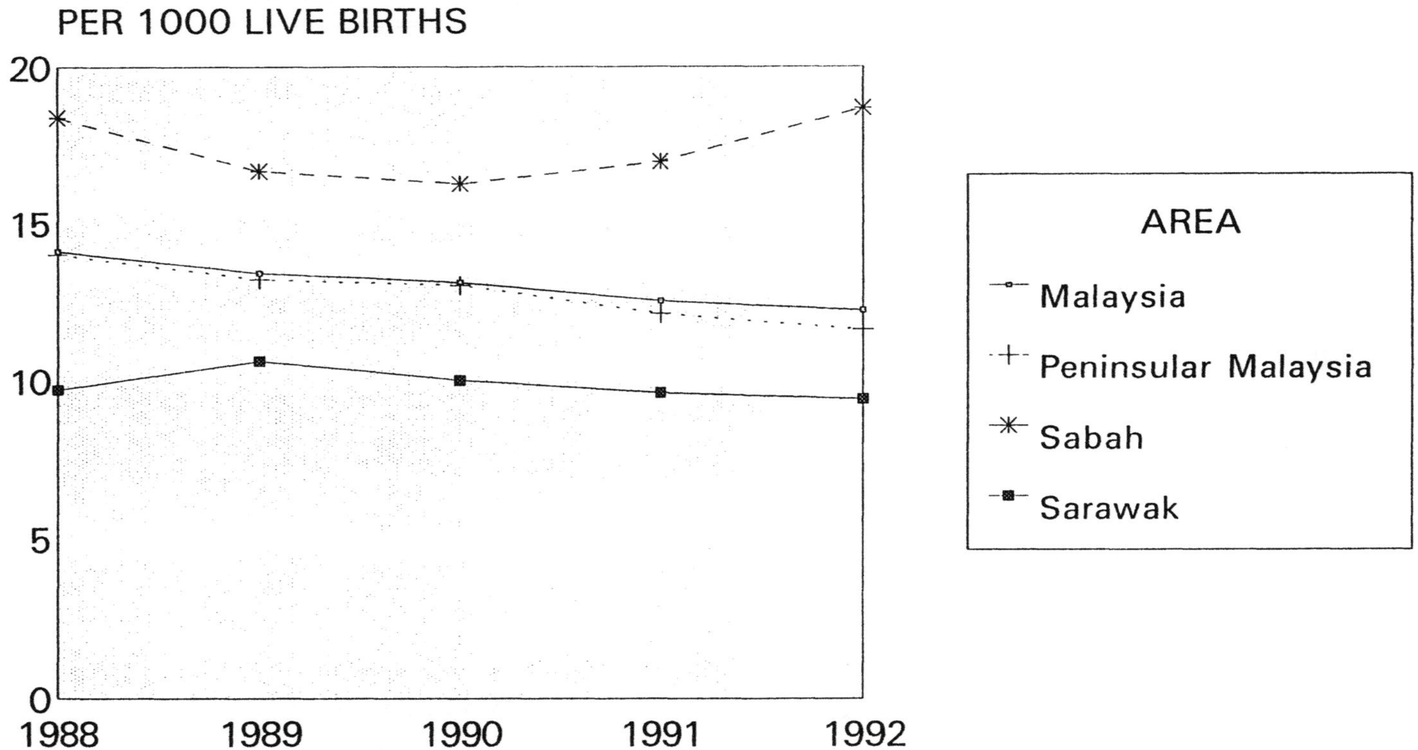

Source: Vital Statistics Malaysia 1992.

Figure 2
Neonatal Mortality Rate in Malaysia, 1988–1992

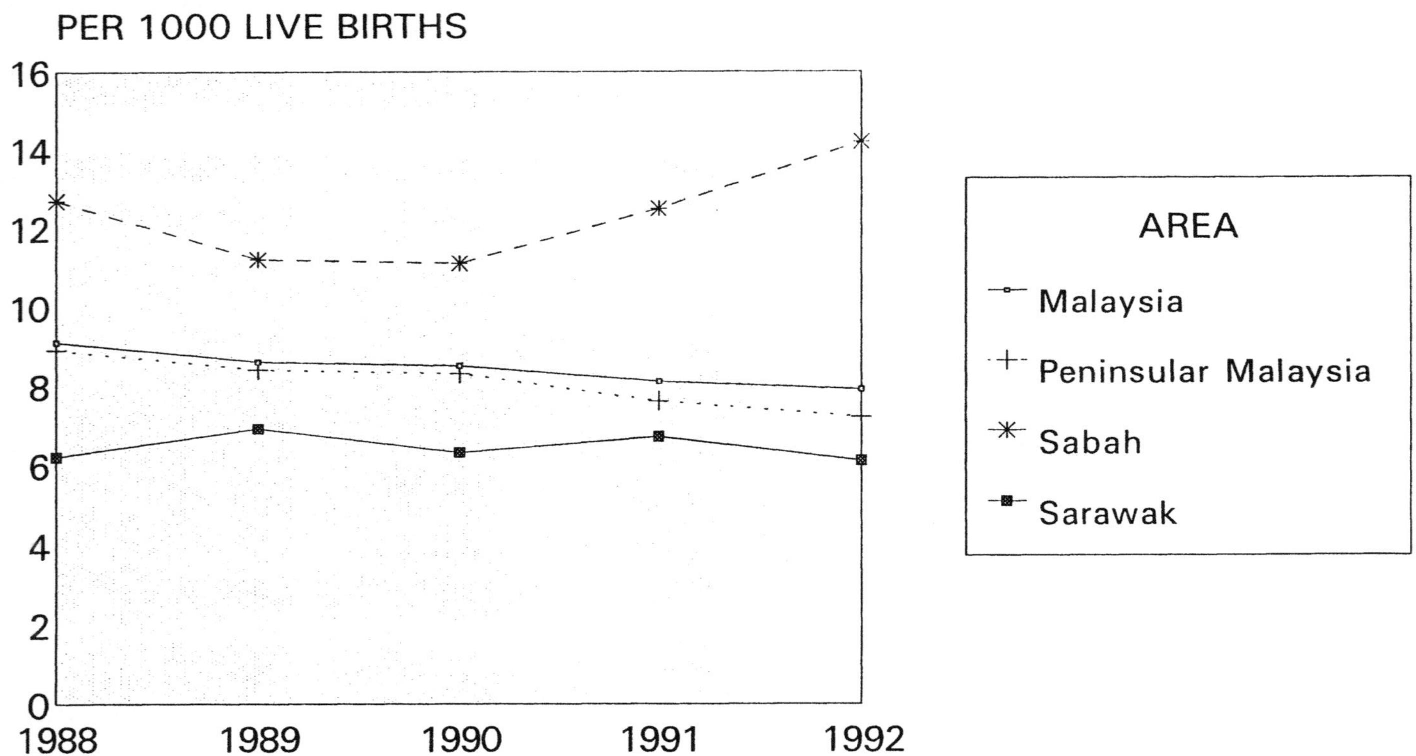

Source: Vital Statistics Malaysia 1992.

Figure 3
Perinatal Mortality Rate in Malaysia, 1988–1992

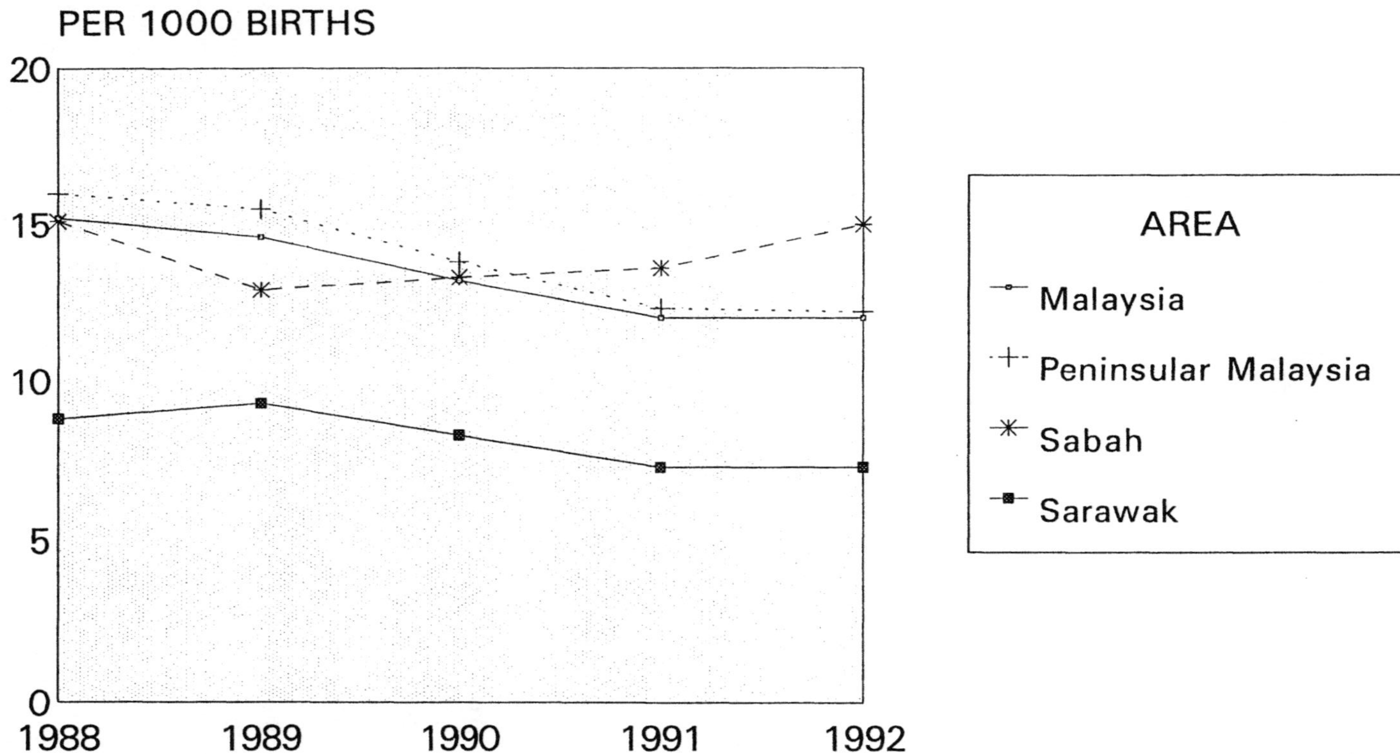

Source: Vital Statistics Malaysia 1992.

of children in the population and childbearing women and high fertility, due emphasis has been given to maternal and child health in this country. The current two-tier system of health care service delivery ensures a well-distributed provision of basic care, including maternal and child health through the *klinik desa* or community health clinic serviced by nurses with special training as rural health nurses. These nurses are trained to provide antenatal care and assist safe deliveries. Traditional birth attendants have been encouraged to enlist for proper basic training and become incorporated as trained midwives.

Accessibility and Equity of Services

The Ministry of Health is the primary government organization through which health care is financed and provided. The health care delivery system is financed by taxation, and this health care system is relatively accessible to all sectors of the population. The *World Development Report 1993* (World Bank 1993) named Malaysia as one of the few countries in which "public spending on health is biased toward the poor," which helps to "reduce inequities in access and health status."

The government aims to ensure access and equity of public health facilities and for this, one health center is designed to serve 15,000 to 20,000 population, while one *klinik desa* (community health clinic) should serve 2,000 to 4,000 population. In 1975, there was one health center for every 23,784 population, and this ratio improved to 1:23,000 in 1980 and 1:15,653 in 1993. In 1993 the *klinik desa* to population ratio was 1:3,899 (Wan Othman 1995).

The doctor to population ratios for selected years are shown below:

Year	**Ratio**
1975	1 : 4,650
1980	1 : 3,000
1990	1 : 2,533
1993	1 : 2,301

Besides the ratio itself, of equal, if not greater, importance is the distribution of doctors by regions and states in the country, which shows a very wide variance. In 1993, out of over 900 doctors working in Public Health, only 188 have postgraduate qualification in public health (Wan Othman 1995).

Current statistics of the Ministry of Health (MOH) document the change in policy of the MOH to move away from the 3-tier to the 2-tier system. It also shows a commitment to provide better coverage at community levels, as evident from the dramatic increase in *klinik desa* in the Fifth Malaysian Plan 1990 (773) from the Fourth Malaysian Plan 1985 (30) and the subsequent increase to 1,992 *klinik desa* in 1993 (Ministry of Health 1993).

TRAINING AND RESEARCH IN PUBLIC HEALTH

The Division of Training and Manpower Development under the Ministry of Health is responsible for planning, implementation, and evaluation of the Training and Manpower Development Program for doctors and paramedical personnel. Training is done at the national, state/institutional, and district/operational levels. Some training includes postgraduate training of public health engineers and biomedical engineers in the United States or the United Kingdom, and training of community nurses, midwives, and public health assistants.

The Public Health Institute, set up in 1966, is an important national institution under the Ministry of Health. The Institute covers the fields of training, research, dissemination of health information, and consultancy in health. It is currently one of the premier health institutions in Malaysia. The institute plays a major role in the training and education of health personnel from the Ministry of Health and other agencies in related fields such as health management for professional staff, quality assurance, health systems research, epidemiology and diseases control, environmental and occupational health, family health and nutrition, and community and patient health education. Training can be divided into three categories: preservice training; postbasic and postgraduate training; and short courses, workshops, and seminars. The institute conducts courses mainly for paramedical personnel, namely, public health nurses, public health inspectors, health education officers, and education technologists.

The institute actively carries out research, particularly in health systems research. In recognition of its research capability, the Public Health Institute has been designated as a WHO Collaborating Center for Health Systems Research.

Postgraduate degree courses—Master of Public Health (M.P.H)—are run by the University of Malaya and the National University of Malaysia specifically for doctors. Currently, both run a 12-month and 18-month course, respectively.

As far as research is concerned, the focus is on new emerging problems such as mental health, drug addiction, hepatitis, and AIDS. Another changing demographic is the increasing proportion of foreign population, and the larger proportion of aging population also warrants attention. Both problems bring new challenges and new demands on public health care services, thus opening up new areas of research.

The environment is a great concern for many and is of utmost importance in development planning because environmental degradation will undermine the sustainability of social and economic development. Three areas pertinent in environmental consideration and public health are water pollution, air pollution, and the management of solid waste (Mahbob 1995). Apart from these, other areas of research include child abuse, apathy in young people, and the increasingly observable incidence of HIV-positive cases in the country.

MAJOR CHALLENGES FOR THE HEALTH SERVICES

In 1995, the Ministry of Health organized the first national conference on public health. This conference covered the following future challenges of public health in Malaysia:

- Socioeconomic, political, and organizational aspects of public health
- Technology advancement and information technology in public health
- Research and human resource development
- Health promotion, behavior change, and healthy lifestyle

Subsumed under these four major themes are the current and emerging issues of the country, that is, the health impact of:

Social and demographic changes, in particular, related to:
- Industrialization
- Urbanization
- Migration
- Aging population
- Changing lifestyles and traditions

Economic development and environmental change

Innovation in public health to ensure acceptance and sustained health promotion through:
- Information communication to decision makers for priority setting, and appropriate and timely actions
- Effective health information, education, and communication to public through the mass media
- Increasing capabilities and skills among health administrators to persuade, negotiate, plan, and implement intersectoral action in health promotion

Health services organization, management, and financing, including privatization

Quality of life—concept of well-being

To prepare for these challenges, some actions that can be taken are suggested below:

Networking

Establish linkages with government institutions as well as nongovernment organizations for support and action implementation.

Build cooperation and participation with international health and health-related agencies, for example, World Health Organization, United Nations Fund for Population Activities, and International Labor Organization.

Set up information-sharing networks to prepare for a rapidly changing world.

Communication

Develop communication skills in report writing that is comprehensive and easily understood and interpreted by policymakers.

Develop some form of communication network between researchers, government, and the community.

Disseminate results and ideas to the community as an obligation and for accountability.

Develop abilities and skills in understanding cultures and political issues of other nations that affect this country.

Develop skills in advocacy.

Research and Training

Increase skills in forecasting and solving problems of the twenty-first century.

Emphasize research and manpower development that cater to policymakers' needs as well as community needs.

Identify and develop appropriate interdisciplinary academic and education programs to increase awareness and local capability in solving health-related problems.

Develop the structural organization for implementing intraregional programs in research, education, and training.

A very important resource will be manpower development and adaptability. In terms of clinical services, Malaysia has placed emphasis on maternal and child health services. As such, community-based maternal and child health clinics are most widely distributed, especially in the rural areas. As the country progresses, these clinics may incorporate services to cater to emerging needs, that is, reproductive health care to all women and geriatric care.

REFERENCES

Ali O., Khalid, B. A. K., Tan, T. T., Wu, L. L, Sakinah, O. & Ng, M. L. (1993). Prevalence of NIDDM and impaired glucose tolerance in Aborigines and Malays in Malaysia and their relationship to sociodemographic, health and nutritional factors. *Diabetes Care*, 16 (no. 1), 68–75.

Anti-Drug Task Force. (1993). *1992 Annual Report*. Malaysia: National Security Council, Prime Minister's Department.

GOM. (1965). *First Malaysia Plan 1965–1979*. Kuala Lumpur: National Printing Office.

GOM. (1991). *Sixth Malaysia Plan 1991–1995*. Kuala Lumpur: National Printing Office.

Kiyu, A. & Tambi, Z. (1992). *Iodine Deficiency Disorders in Sarawak, East Malaysia*. Paper presented at the WHO/UNICEF/ICCIDD Workshop on Iodine Deficiency Disorders, Manila, Philippines, 5–19 June 1992.

Lim, A. K. H. (1991). Cancer—a major health problem in Malaysia. Editorial. *Medical Journal of Malaysia*, 46 (no. 2), 114–115.

Low, K. S. (1993). A manual on river water quality management for Malaysia. *UNEP/*

JSWE Project: Assessment and Promotion of Human Resources for River Water Quality Management. Kuala Lumpur: Department of Geography, University of Malaya.

Mahbob, S. (1995). *Socioeconomic and Organisation Changes and Public Health Policy.* Paper presented at the Public Health Conference organized by the Ministry of Health, Genting Highlands, 24–26 January 1995.

Malaysian Medical Association (MMA). (1987). *Report on Health Assurance and Health Insurance for all Malaysians.* 15 March 1987. Kuala Lumpur: Malaysian Medical Association.

Ministry of Health (MOH). (1993). Annual report. Kuala Lumpur: National Printing Office.

Mohd Hussain, H., Ganesvaran, T. & Agnes, L. S. (1992–1993). Attempted suicide in Kuala Lumpur. *Asia Pacific Journal of Public Health,* 6, 5–7.

United Nations. (1985). *Asian Population Studies: Expert Group Meeting on International Migration in Asia and Pacific. Levels and Trends of International Migration in the Countries of the ESCAP Region.* United Nations Economic and Social Commission for Asia and the Pacific, Bangkok, Thailand, and Population Center Foundation, Manila, Philippines.

Vital Statistics Malaysia. (1992). *Preliminary Release.* Kuala Lumpur: Department of Statistics Malaysia.

Wan Othman, W. M. (1995). *Achievements in Public Health.* Special paper presented at the Public Health Conference organized by the Ministry of Health, Genting Highlands, 24–26 January 1995.

World Bank. (1991). *Asia Region Population Projections, 1990–1991 Edition.* Working paper WP599. Washington, D.C.: Department of Population and Human Resources, World Bank.

World Bank. (1993). *Investing in Health. World Development Report.* Washington, D.C.: World Bank.

Zulkifli, S. N., Khin, M. U., Yusof, K. & Wong, Y. L. (1994). Maternal and child health in urban Sabah, Malaysia: A comparison of citizens and migrants. *Asia Pacific Journal of Public Health,* 7 (no. 3), 334–351.

MEXICO

Gracīela Freyermuth Encīso and
Jaime Page Pliego

Mexico is located in a geographically strategic position, bordering the United States to its north and Latin America to its south. Its vast, diverse territory contains mountainous areas, jungles, desert, and large cities, one of them being the largest in the world. Among its various geographic regions exist diverse levels of socioeconomic development, only a few of which are highly industrialized. Other areas contain minor industrial infrastructures but do have commercial agriculture and cattle industries that employ high levels of technology. A major portion of Mexico, however, depends on subsistence agriculture and cattle raising.

The United States of Mexico (the official name of the country) has a population of more than 87 million inhabitants. Approximately 5.5 million are indigenous people distributed among 56 ethnic groups and live throughout the country (1,958,201 square kilometers), consistently in its poorest regions.

The socioeconomic status of Mexico's population ranges from a small, excessively rich elite to a majority that lives in extreme poverty. The standards of living vary throughout the country, depending upon the geographic region, employment opportunities, and the historic-cultural development of the region. A high percentage of the population lives in isolated, rural communities of less than 2,500 inhabitants who barely receive basic services such as running water, sewage systems, sanitation services, or electricity. Those who live in large cities, however, must contend with violence, overpopulation, and high levels of pollution.

The gross national product (GNP) for 1990 was $1,700 per capita. This statistical average does not reflect the income earned by the majority of the population. The devaluation in 1995 has reduced this figure to approximately $800 a year. This is due to the wide gap that separates them from the small group of excessively rich.

The coexistence of an impoverished majority, a small wealthy elite who benefit from the country's economic development, and an ample middle class who daily witness a decrease in their purchasing power contributes to the causes and characteristics of illness and death in the various socioeconomic regions of the country. Many of the principal causes of death are associated with poverty, including complications of pregnancy and birth and infectious diseases such as diarrheal disease, respiratory infections, measles, and tuberculosis. However, health risks associated with highly industrialized societies are also prevalent, including cancer, cardio- and cerebrovascular disease, diabetes, accidents, and the consequences of violence.

MAJOR HEALTH ISSUES IN MEXICO

The deterioration of the standard of living caused by the economic crisis and the consequent implementation of neoliberal policies are reflected in the diminishing quality of health services provided by the state, both in its public agencies open to the general population and in its health organizations that specifically benefit workers, called Social Security institutions. In addition, there has been an increase in morbidity and mortality rates and a resurgence of infectious diseases that had been previously eradicated, such as cholera, malaria, and dengue.

Infectious Disease

Although at the national level infectious diseases are last on the list of the leading causes of death, it is necessary to note that there exist serious inaccuracies in official public health records. The majority of deaths caused by infectious disease are not documented. These cases are not captured by the existing morbidity and mortality documentation mechanisms due to the fundamental lack of health services available to the poor. Although mortality indexes do indicate that timely prevention and intervention strategies have decreased the death rate due to infectious disease, they do not reflect the high level of infectious disease morbidity.

Although infectious diseases are not among the principal causes of death at the national level, they are still among the leading killers in the poorest regions of the country. For example, gastrointestinal illness lies tenth in the leading causes of death at the national level, with a mortality rate of 16.4 per 100,000 inhabitants. In the states of Oaxaca and Chiapas, it is the leading cause of death, with a mortality rate of 52.4 and 54.4 per 100,000 inhabitants respectively. Pulmonary tuberculosis, which occupies fifteenth place among the leading causes of death at the national level with a mortality rate of 5.2 per 100,000 inhabitants, has a mortality rate of 10.5 in Oaxaca and 12.5 in Chiapas. Acute respiratory infections do not appear among the 20 principal causes of death at the national level. However, they are the seventeenth leading cause of death in Chiapas, with a rate of 3.7, and the eighteenth leading cause of death in Oaxaca, with a rate of 5.5.

Human immunodeficiency virus (HIV) disease could become a serious public health problem for Mexico, as well. In 1992 there were 2,554 deaths attributed to acquired immunodeficiency syndrome (AIDS), indicating a rate of 2.9 deaths per 100,000 inhabitants and making it the nineteenth leading cause of death in Mexico. It is particularly prevalent in the more industrialized regions of the country, such as along the U.S. border.

Chronic Illness in Mexico

Chronic degenerative diseases are also among the primary causes of death at both the national level and the majority of regional levels. The primary cause of death in Mexico is heart disease, with a figure of 64.1 deaths per 100,000 inhabitants, primarily due to ischemic heart disease, which has a mortality rate of 37.1 per 100,000 inhabitants. Cancer is the second leading cause of death, with a rate of 50.4 deaths per 100,000 inhabitants. The most prevalent forms of cancer are tracheal, bronchial, and lung cancer, followed by stomach cancer and uterine cervical carcinoma. Diabetes mellitus occupies fourth place among the leading causes of death, with a mortality rate of 32.6 per 100,000 inhabitants, while cerebrovascular disease occupies sixth place, with an estimated rate of 24.7.

Mental Health

Mexico's resources for mental health care are limited. They consist only of hospitals concentrated in the large cities and serve only patients with serious illness, in acute crisis, and the chronically ill. In addition, there exist few qualified personnel trained to provide mental health care. As a consequence, there exist high numbers of homicides, the fourteenth principal cause of death in Mexico, with a mortality rate of 4.4 per 100,000 inhabitants. Suicide, although not among the principal causes of death at the national level, is the seventeenth leading cause of death in Mexico City, with a rate of 3.8 deaths per 100,000 inhabitants. Alcohol dependence, which in 1992 claimed 2,629 victims, holds eighteenth place among the leading causes of death in Mexico, with a rate of 3.0. These figures indicate the urgent need for prevention and treatment programs for mental health problems.

The Effects of Age and Gender in Mexico

The infant mortality rate was 18.8 per 1,000 live births in 1992. Prenatal complications are the leading cause of these deaths, although infectious diseases are also among the major killers. Pneumonia and influenza are the second leading causes of infant mortality, with a rate reaching 249.5 deaths per 100,000 live registered births. The fourth leading cause of infant mortality is intestinal infections, with a rate of 184.2. Mortality due to respiratory infections is in seventh place among the causes of infant death, with a rate of 41.0.

In 1994, 175,428 of 409,814 deaths in Mexico were females, constituting 42.8 percent of the total death rate. The principal causes of death among women was endocrine, metabolic, and immune system disease causing 19,062 deaths. Diabetes mellitus was the second leading cause of death, with 15,730 mortalities. Ischemic heart disease caused 14,114 deaths; 11,416 deaths were attributed to cerebrovascular disease; pulmonary, circulatory, and other heart diseases caused 11,054 deaths; and myocardial infarctions resulted in 10,678 deaths. These diseases hold third, fourth, fifth, and sixth place, respectively, in the principal causes of death among women. The tenth leading cause of death among women is cancer of the genitourinary organs, causing 6,454 deaths; 4,340 of these were due to cervical carcinoma.

Population Issues

Mexico has a young population. In 1992, 73.85 percent of the Mexican population was under the age of 34 years; 59.8 percent of the population were between 15 and 64 years of age and, it is assumed, able to participate in the workforce; 15.3 percent of the population were over 65 years of age. For the same year, the birthrate was 32.2 and the mortality rate was 4.7, both per 1,000 inhabitants. The life expectancy was 70.3 years of age, 73.7 years for women and 67.0 for men.

According to the same sources, 12.4 percent of the population over 15 years of age were illiterate (7.7 percent for women and 4.6 percent for men). Of those older than 16 years of age, only 25 percent had an education above that of elementary school. Of those over 18 years of age, only 11 percent had received an education at the professional training level. Of this group, only 0.5 percent finished professional training, and 0.8 percent finished the university level or higher.

Health Conditions for Immigrants and Refugees

Immigrants do not pose a serious problem for Mexico. The majority are South Americans, principally from Chile and Argentina, and Europeans. The former immigrated to Mexico primarily during the 1970s in search of political asylum. In 1981, as a consequence of the repressive political policies in Guatemala, thousands of peasants and entire communities sought refuge in Mexico, creating one of the greatest refugee influxes in Mexico's history. The Guatemalan immigrants were primarily indigenous people and peasants, with a small percentage of nonindigenous people (mestizos). These peasants settled along the Mexican-Guatemalan border in four areas of Chiapas.

The refugees suffered serious illnesses upon arriving in Mexico, particularly those who settled in the jungle. Their health and nutrition status had been precarious even while living in Guatemala and during their tiring, stressful escape. It then worsened upon being forced to live in overpopulated camps, in improvised housing without running water or sanitary facilities, and with many agents of disease transmission, particularly mosquitoes. These living conditions brought malaria, tuberculosis, severe anemia, dysentery, dengue, hepatitis, measles, and whooping cough. Mortality rates skyrocketed.

International refugee support agencies and national health institutions worked to create primary care resources in the form of networks of Guatemalan community health workers. They were trained by both government and nongovernment organizations. Secondary care was provided by a hospital created by the secretary of health. Among the principal programs that were implemented were health interventions and nutritional support for children under five years of age, health education, immunization programs, prevention and treatment of infectious diseases, prenatal care, and family planning programs.

In 1991, the leading causes of illness and death among the Guatemalan refugees continued to be infectious diseases, including acute respiratory infection, enteritis, and other diarrheal diseases, skin diseases, malaria, salmonella, and pulmonary tuberculosis. Perinatal complications were also among the primary causes of morbidity and mortality. The Guatemalans remained in these settlements for an entire decade. Then in 1992, with the help of international agencies, the refugee population began its return to Guatemala. Although large numbers of refugees have been repatriated, there still remain 33,800 of the original, officially recognized 40,150 refugees.

Nutrition Issues

Malnutrition is widespread in Mexico. Despite the fact that official statistics do not include the large number of undocumented cases, malnutrition was still reported to have reached eleventh place among the leading causes of death in Mexico, with a rate of 11.8 per 100,000 inhabitants. It is the fifth leading cause of death among infants and children under five years of age, with rates of 61.3 and 7.9, respectively. The magnitude of the problem is evident in the data acquired by a 1988 national study on malnutrition in which it was found that 41.9 percent of Mexican children suffered some level of malnutrition.

Environmental Concerns

Pollution is one of the primary environmental concerns of Mexico's large cities. The presence of industrial plants located in the inner cities, antiquated and obsolete city infrastructures, and the great number of cars and buses with poor emissions controls are the primary contributing factors to this problem. Severe ecological damage caused by the state petrochemical industry's (PE-

MEX) gases and toxic residues is also a major concern. It has affected air, earth, and water quality, as well as the agriculture, livestock, and fishing trades.

In addition, there has been unlimited destruction of the forests and trees in order to increase agriculture and livestock production. This has destroyed diverse ecological environments and created large erosion problems and consequent climatic changes.

MEDICAL ATTENTION IN MEXICO

In Mexico, before 1917, public health was the responsibility of the states and counties rather than the federal government. Because a public health service system did not exist, health care was provided by private foundations that provided hospital care on a charity basis. The state took responsibility solely for the sanitation control of ports, borders, and customs check posts.

The Constitution of 1917 offered a different perspective about the way in which the public health system would be managed from then on. Article 73 of the constitution declares that the federal government will be responsible for the public health needs of the country. As a result, the Health Department and General Health Council were created. Article 123 established the fundamental basis for federal social assistance benefits for workers, called Social Security. During the first 50 years of this century, new laws were created and institutions founded that would form the basis of the current health care system.

In 1937, the institution that today is the Secretary of Health (SSA), head of the health sector and coordinator of the National Health Care System, was established. In 1943, the Social Security Law was issued. This spawned the Mexican Institute of Social Security (IMSS), a decentralized public agency that initially provided health services for blue-collar workers and today also offers health care services to employees of private companies, merchants, artisans, independent businesspersons, and students. The system is financed by means of payments charged to the employees, employers, and the state.

In 1959, the foundations for health and comprehensive social benefits for state employees were established, which later were reorganized as the Social Security System for Public Employees. This system benefits all state employees and nonfederal institutions such as hospitals, universities, and banks. It is also financed by payments charged to the employee and employer, who in this case is the state. The current name of the institution is the Social Security Institute for State Employees (ISSSTE).

In 1973, a new federal assistance law was created that benefits marginalized groups through the program called Social Solidarity Program in Support of Marginalized Groups. Toward the end of the 1970s during a new presidential administration, the program was expanded and given a new name, IMSS-COPLAMAR. Its acronym stands for the Program of Social Solidarity Through Community Cooperation and was aimed primarily at rural marginalized communities. IMSS has been the institution responsible for implementing its programs. It is currently called IMSS-SOLIDARIDAD.

During the presidential term 1982–1988, the Mexican president proposed the creation of a National Health Care System. In 1982, Article 4 of the constitution was reformed to include a paragraph guaranteeing health care to the entire population. The creation of a National Health Care System has been a difficult task for the Mexican government due to the great diversity of health institutions, each with its own legal status, administration, and financial resources. Among the state institutions that provide services to the entire population are the SSA, the National System for the Integral Development of the Family (DIF), the IMSS-SOLIDARIDAD program, and local, state, and county hospitals. There also exist institutions that provide benefits specifically to workers, including the previously mentioned IMSS and ISSSTE, as well as the medical services for Mexico's oil industry workers (PEMEX) and health services for the military (SEDENA) and the National Secretary of the Navy.

In Mexico, there are two supervisory health agencies. The General Council of Health was created by the constitution to be under the direct and exclusive order of the president of the Republic. The SSA is a federal department that is in charge of creating health policy and whose director is the coordinator of the National Health Care System.

The priority programs of the state health sector include the provision of primary-, secondary-, and tertiary-level medical care, maternal child care, mental health care, preventative health care, health education, nutrition, occupational health, drug addiction prevention and treatment, community public health monitoring and control, basic sanitation, environmental health, family planning and social assistance, human resource research and development, and health education material production. These various programs function according to the specific resources available to the particular institutions that carry them out. The specific cases of rehabilitation and mental health programs, which generally benefit only a small population, are found in tertiary care facilities and, as a result, only in large cities.

Although the state claims to offer health care to all Mexican citizens, the budget assigned to the health sector is insufficient to provide medical attention to the entire population. Of the 1989 national budget (247,000 million new pesos), 60 percent was allocated to pay the external debt, leaving 3 percent for education and 1.7 percent for health care.

In Mexico, there are only eight doctors per 10,000 inhabitants, who are primarily located in the larger cities. On average, there exist 1.2 hospital beds for each 1,000 inhabitants, and more than half of these are found in Mexico City and other large urban areas. In 1990, of 86.154 million Mexicans, only 45.835 million had access to health benefits. Private medical resources covered approximately 3.483 million inhabitants, and nearly 30 million people depended on public health services, which primarily consist of vaccination and family planning programs.

In 1991, the National Health Care System provided 13,812 medical facilities, of which 13,040 were dedicated to outpatient care. Of these, 51 percent provided health services to the general population and the remaining only to patients with Social Security benefits. Of the 772 hospital facilities, 28 percent were available to the general population and the remaining services only to patients insured through Social Security. A total of 67,703 documented hospital beds existed, of which 33 percent were available to the general population. The remaining were available only to the population insured through Social Security. The number of physicians and nurses were 97,971 and 141,404, respectively.

In the same year, 151.4 million medical consultations were offered, of which 15 percent were specialist consults and 5 percent family planning visits. The number of hospitalized patients was 3,842,430, with 39 medical consultations for each hospital admittance.

The budget allocation to the various health programs is as follows: Curative medical care receives 81.1 percent of the budget, followed by health care administration and social assistance with 8.4 percent of the budget, preventative medicine with 5.4 percent, and human resource training with 2.8 percent. The areas of research, environmental health, and health education combined receive less than 1 percent of the budget.

The distribution of resources in relation to the population's health care needs is unequally balanced as well. The medical institutions that are part of the Social Security network receive 73.2 percent of the total budget, although they cover only 53 percent of the population. The public hospitals, which cover the general population, receive 26.8 percent of the budget and serve 14.6 percent of the population. (Some sources claim that public health institutions cover 47 percent of the population. Although 47 percent of the population does remain without other health coverage, the actual number of individuals served by the public institutions is closer to 26.8 percent. The remaining segment of the population remains without any access to health care.) Medical services offered to this group are limited. In rural areas, for example, primarily immunization and family planning programs are offered. Peasants rarely have access to secondary medical care. An analysis of the resources allocated to the general population, 47 percent of the Mexican population, shows that only 33 percent of documented hospital beds and 28 percent of hospitals are available to this group.

Since the 1980s, lack of resources available to health institutions has forced the health sector to employ less expensive forms of health care delivery. As a result, the quality of secondary- and tertiary-level hospital care has deteriorated notably. The population has expressed increasing dissatisfaction with the health care services offered by the Social Security institutions. As a result, the state is reexamining its role in the provision of health care services, and privatization has begun to take place.

Private Medicine

Private medicine does not even cover 0.5 percent of the population. Its scope is curative rather than preventative. It is organized through private individual practices or professional group practices. The majority are found in urban areas or other areas with populations of greater than 5,000 inhabitants. Private medical providers also work as subcontractors for Social Security institutions. This practice is primarily found in areas of 100,000 or more inhabitants in which the Social Security institutions only provide basic medical services (internal medicine, pediatrics, surgery, and obstetrics and gynecology).

In the last five years, the presence of private medical insurance has grown. Most of the time they set many restrictions and only cover the major expenses of hospitalizations and surgery. The government has been gradually introducing private insurance into the system by offering it at no cost to particular professional groups (primarily to those who work in academics) who, in the long run, could become private paying clients. At present, these groups have become the privileged few who receive both private insurance and Social Security benefits.

Nongovernmental Organizations

Nongovernmental organizations (NGOs) are groups formed by individuals of diverse ideological, political, and religious orientations who seek a common goal and work within a limited geographic area. The work of these organizations has been favorable to the health status of the Mexican population. They have endorsed and implemented many health care projects sponsored by international agencies. However, the increasing delegation of the responsibility for providing medical care to nongovernment agencies rather than the state has shifted the responsibility for providing medical care from the state to the individual.

Since the 1980s in Mexico, there has been a growing proliferation of nongovernment organizations. There exist a great diversity of those that work in the health area, ranging from those who only provide medical attention to those who advocate popular organization in order to improve the health status of the community. The inability of the government health agencies to provide universal health coverage to the population has allowed NGOs to participate increasingly in the design and application of community health programs.

One of the most visible organizations of this kind is Promotion of Health and Social Service in Popular Education (PRODUSSEP), a health NGO that networks with other health NGOs throughout the country. It is a civil association of physicians, paramedics, nurses, and others involved in organizations dedicated to the health field. Their objectives are to maintain stocks of medicines, medical supplies, and accessible education material for grassroots health organizations throughout the country. They also promote the continuous development of these groups through health education programs and the sharing of knowledge and experience. The association operates basically in four areas of the country, the

Federal District, Oaxaca, Veracruz, and the Southwest, with 28 programs and 40 affiliations. The affiliated groups participate in the organization and elaboration of projects. The board of directors is responsible for the coordination of activities.

The Feminist NGOs

Health issues were among the fundamental concerns of the pioneering feminist groups in Mexico. One of the first and most important of these groups was Communication, Exchange and Development in Latin America (CIDHAL). Other groups, such as the Chopo Women and Network for Maternal and Child Health (REGSAMUNI), have organized exclusively around maternity and sexuality concerns. The consolidation of the feminist NGO movement was facilitated by initial common goals shared by all the groups. One of these goals was that women should be seen as subjects, not objects, of medical practice and government population policies.

The Mexican feminist movement has launched serious criticism of present-day gynecology practice, particularly the loss of control women suffer upon entering health institutions. They have proposed a range of alternatives to the current system. In addition, they question women's health care policy decisions that have been made without women's participation in the definition of such policies. They have proposed alternative strategies in order that women's health programs be by and for women.

The feminist movement and women's groups that work in the health area have pioneered the work related to voluntary maternity and reproductive rights. Their demands include the legalization of abortion, adequate health services for those who choose to terminate a pregnancy, greater access to reproductive health education for women, and access to contraception. They also work toward lowering the mortality rates caused by induced abortions and toward the improvement of the quality of health services for women.

In fighting high maternal morbidity and mortality rates, they have demanded culturally appropriate, short-term, well-defined strategies that will produce concrete advancements in this area. At the present time, there are approximately 30 women NGOs that are committed to this work.

Feminist analysis of family planning policies has also denounced the way in which programs in this area are implemented. In particular, they criticize forced sterilization and enrollment in family planning programs through incentives. Demands for better-quality care and the right to a free and informed choice for women are the result of the analysis of the plans and programs of health care institutions. It was found that these programs are often implemented at all costs in order to fulfill established goals and, as a consequence, to violate women's rights if necessary.

THE INFRASTRUCTURE OF TRAINING AND RESEARCH IN PUBLIC HEALTH

Public health practice in Mexico was linked at the beginning of this century to the campaigns to eradicate yellow fever and smallpox and to control pinta, malaria, and poliomyelitis. The Public Health Institute of Mexico, founded in the 1920s as a public health school under the Health Ministry, was responsible for training management and administrative personnel for the state health sector. Before the school was converted to an institute at the end of the 1980s, it had occasionally been involved in research activities. However, it wasn't able to consolidate specific lines of work nor teams for conducting permanent research. After its conversion to an institute, it began to conduct systematic research.

Beginning in the 1970s, postgraduate programs in public health and medical sociology began to be founded by universities. These were the first of such programs created independently of the Health Ministry. Among the most visible of these is the Master's Degree Program in Social Medicine offered at the Autonomous Metropolitan University, Xochimilco Branch, which focuses on the sociological analysis of the country's health problems. This was the first center whose main objective was to train researchers in the area of public health. Subsequently, new programs were developed, such as the Master's in Public Health at the Autonomous Metropolitan University, Iztapalapa Branch, the Autonomous University of Mexico (UNAM), and the University of Guadalajara. There is also a doctorate program in public health at the Public Health Institute.

MAJOR CHALLENGES FOR THE HEALTH SERVICES

In order to improve the current public health situation, several changes must be made. It is necessary to modernize and increase the efficiency of Mexico's health institutions. A sensible allocation of the small health care budget must be in accordance with the real needs of the various regions. To achieve this goal, modifications in the legal statutes that govern the different institutions must take place. A restructuring of the federal health sector's institutions to ensure that they operate under an efficient coordinating committee will help avoid excessive spending and duplicity of functions.

Decentralization of health services should also take place. Not only should this occur at the state level, but decentralization should be extended to the counties as well. These are political-geographic areas with their own administrative agencies. Such decentralization will encourage rational, efficient spending. However, this option should be analyzed carefully and should be carried out only after an evaluation of those services that have been decentralized in 14 states of the country.

Adequate health planning based on a national system of epidemiological surveillance and subsystems of local and regional epidemiological monitoring is also necessary. Appropriate training must be provided to all qualified health personnel, including traditional health practitioners. Health workers and the general population must be sensitized to the importance of reporting and registering the incidence of illness and death.

It is imperative that research teams be created in the socioepidemiological and health care systems planning area. This will aid in the development of human resources in the health care field who will contribute to the solution to the current health problems. Health care systems planning based on adequate assessment and evaluation of health care issues will also assist in finding solutions to the priority problems of the country's diverse regions and social groups. It must take into consideration the work of NGOs and traditional and popular health practitioners.

Marginalized groups, in particular, demand specific planning strategies. Three of the most important issues relevant to them are nutrition, housing, and basic community services. Historically, they have suffered malnutrition, absence of sewage and other sanitation systems, and inadequate housing. Their health status cannot be improved without addressing these basic needs.

All levels of medical care should be accessible to the entire population, including the marginalized poor. Primary care should be developed at the community level, secondary care should be provided at the regional level, and access to tertiary care should be guaranteed to all when necessary.

It is crucial that medical care meets the actual needs of the groups that it serves in a culturally appropriate manner. This is partially accomplished through health education, which incorporates Western medical understanding with culturally specific traditional and home medical practices. Allopathic medicine is then responsible for solving those problems that cannot be taken care of at this more basic level. Individuals must be referred by their traditional health practitioner or community health worker to the appropriate care facilities in a timely manner.

In addition to health issues associated with extreme poverty, Mexico also faces the health problems inherent in developed countries. The aging of the population presents a new challenge to the health sector, who will require additional resources in order to cover the needs of the elderly. By the end of the century, there will be almost 10 million people over the age of 60, the majority of whom do not receive federal medical or social benefits. Women, in particular, are at risk. Even those who worked throughout their lives find themselves without the resources to live with dignity. The average monthly retirement pension is around U.S.$80. New health policies must incorporate the needs of the elderly into their current programs that currently only emphasize infectious disease and maternal and child health.

Health and the environment must also be considered more seriously in the health policies of the new federal administration. The rural population suffers from a lack of potable water and adequate sanitation facilities. On the other hand, large cities suffer from insufficient water treatment facilities. In some states, there exist almost no water supply systems. These are challenges that demand immediate attention.

Air pollution in large cities, particularly Mexico City, is an increasingly disturbing problem with no short-term solution in sight. The most common pollutants in Mexico City are sulfur dioxide, hydrocarbons, ozone, carbon monoxide, nitrous dioxide, and lead. Industry is not equipped with filters or elimination mechanisms for gas, liquid, or solid contaminants. In spite of antipollution laws, sanctions imposed against polluting industries have been inadequate to control this problem. The gas emissions from cars and buses and, in particular, trucks and public transportation vehicles are also an enormous problem. Several efforts have been made to control emission levels of vehicles through programs such as One Day Without a Car, in which each automobile is prohibited from circulating one day per week, and periodic revision of pollutant emissions. However, pollution levels continue to be dangerously high.

CONCLUSION

The neoliberal policies adopted by the Mexican government in the 1980s have led to a decrease in the federal health care budget. Between 1982 and 1988, the percentage of the gross national product spent on health and social assistance services decreased 2.5 and 1.3 percent, respectively. As a consequence, the government subsidies for the principal Social Security institutions (ISSSTE and IMSS), as well as for those who primarily serve the marginalized poor (SSA, IMSS-SOLIDARIDAD, DIF), have decreased. It is also expected that the recent currency devaluation will cause further cuts in all public services, including health services.

The political economy that diminished the resources available to the health sector has consequently led to a deterioration in the quality of health care services, reflected in a major lack of documentation of morbidity and mortality (the deaths of many Mexicans do not even appear in official statistics); a decrease in the basic resources available for outpatient and inpatient facilities; deficiencies in prevention and health promotion programs for the general population and high-risk target groups; and the resurgence in Mexico of previously controlled or eradicated diseases such as cholera, dengue, malaria, and tuberculosis.

In the current political climate, it is unlikely that short-term improvements will be made in the health conditions of the nation's poor. As an example of the difficult situation, in the indigenous communities of the Chiapas highlands during the 1988–1992 period, the leading cause of death among men between 15 and 55 years of age was gastroenteritis; 70 percent of those who died in 1991 never received any medical attention before their death. These conditions also exist in other areas of the country. They have prompted health officials and the federal government to nominally set goals to improve the standard of living of this segment of the population in hopes of controlling such deteriorating health conditions.

Attention to Mexico's most marginalized groups can no longer be postponed, now that the risk exists of other uprisings similar to that which occurred in Chiapas in January 1994. This is a particularly precarious situation in light of the recent devaluation of almost 100 percent and the resulting political adjustments. It is expected that the unemployment rate will rise—and with it the need for medical care available to the entire population. With these political-economic conditions, it is unlikely that there will be a short-term solution either to the political instability or to the health situation of Mexico.

REFERENCES

Banco Nacional de México (BANAMEX). (1989). *México social 1988–1989, indicadores seleccionados, estudios sociales.* Mexico: Banco Nacional de México.

Blanco Gil, José & López Arellano, Oliva. (1988). De la transición epidemiológica a la epidemiología de la crisis. In: *Política sanitaria mexicana en los ochenta.* Fin de Siglo Editors, S.A de C.V. Mexico: Centro de Estudios en Salud y Política Sanitaria A.C.

De la Fuente, Juan Ramón & Donato Alarcón (Eds.). (1990). *La investigación en salud: Balance y transición.* Mexico: Biblioteca de la Salud, Fondo de Cultura Económica.

Freyermuth, Gracíela & Godfrey, Nancy. (1993). *Refugiados guatemaltecos en México. La vida en un continuo estado de emergencia.* Mexico: Centro de Investigaciones y Estudios Superiores en Antropología Social and Instituto Chiapaneco de Cultura.

IMSS-COPLAMAR. (1983). *Necesidades esenciales en México: Salud.* No. 4, de Siglo XXI. Mexico.

Instituto Nacional de Estadística de Geografía e Informática. (1992). *Anuario estadístico de los Estados Unidos Mexicanos.* Mexico.

Instituto Nacional de Geografía y Estadística. (1989). *Información estadística sector salud y seguridad Social.* Notebook no. 6. Aguascalientes, Mexico.

López Arellano, Oliva & Blanco Gil, José. (1993). *La modernización neoliberal en salud. México en los ochenta.* Xochimilco, Mexico: UAM.

Ravelo Blancas, Patricia. (1990). La salud de la mujer desde la perspectiva antropológica: Una revisión preliminar. In: *Salud Problema.* Vol. 20, Unidad Xochimilco, Mexico: Universidad Autónoma Metropolitana.

Secretaría de Salud. (1991). *México: Información prioritaria en salud.* Mexico: Consejo Asesor en Epidemiología.

Secretaría de Salud. (1992). *La salud de los pueblos indígenas de México.* Mexico: Instituto Nacional Indigenista.

Secretaría de Salud. (1993a). *Estadísticas vitales 1992.* Mexico: Instituto Nacional de Geografía y Estadística.

Secretaría de Salud. (1993b). *Mortalidad 1992.* Mexico.

Soberón, Guillermo, Kumate, Jesús & Laguna, José. (1988). La Salud en México: Testimonios 1988. In: *Problemas y programas de salud.* Vol. 2. Mexico: Fondo de Cultura Económica.

World Bank. (1990). *World Development Report 1990.* New York: Oxford University Press.

PHILIPPINES

Teodora V. Tiglao and Jane C. Baltazar

INTRODUCTION

Public health in the Philippines had its early inception in the late nineteenth century under the Spanish occupation. It flourished during the American occupation, regressed during World War II, picked up the threads after Philippine Independence in 1946, and continued to blossom during the last half of the twentieth century.

Sociodemographic Profile of the Country

The Philippines is an archipelago south of China with a total land area of 300,000 hectares in its 7,100 islands. It was the first republic in Asia (1898) and the first to be granted independence after World War II (1946). It is strategically located and serves as a bridge between the East and the West. The Philippines is mainly an agribusiness and aquacultural country, but it is currently on the brink of being industrialized, which it hopes to achieve by the year 2000.

The population was estimated at 67,898,000 in 1994. The estimated population growth rate showed only a modest decline to 2.4 percent in 1993 from a high of more than 3.0 percent for the period 1960–1970. The fast-growing population exerts a great toll on the economy and on health services. It is envisioned that there will be an annual growth rate of 2.0 percent by the year 2020. The population is concentrated in urban areas. The National Capital Region, or Metro Manila, has a population of 7,948,392, or 13 percent of the total population. While the average population density for the nation was 195.7 per square kilometer, the population density in the National Capital Region was 11,888.3 in 1988.

Figure 1
Estimated Population by Age and Sex, Philippines, 1990

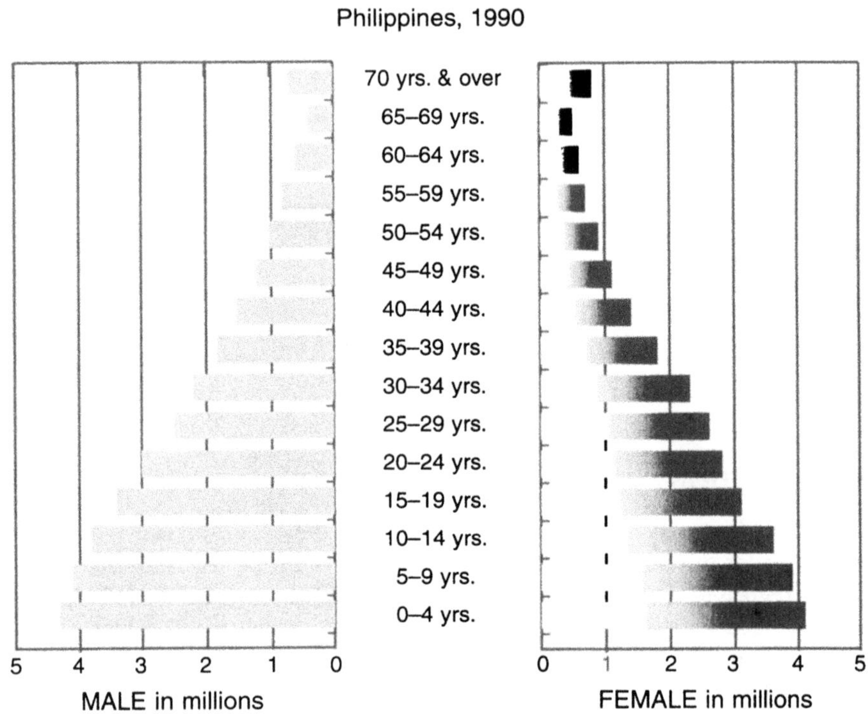

Source: Department of Health Publication 1994.

The age structure of the population has a pyramid shape. In 1990, the age group 0–4 comprised the bulk of the population (13.7 percent). The dependency ratio in 1990 was 73.9 percent, compared with 83.3 percent in 1980, implying a reduction in economic burden borne by the working group. There was a slight excess of males over females (50.3 percent versus 49.7 percent) (Figure 1).

The growth in population is mainly due to natural increase or the excess of births over deaths. In 1990, there were 1.6 million live births or 26.3 for every 1,000 population. The death rate, on the other hand, was 5.1 per 1,000.

One factor affecting population size is emigration and immigration. The National Capital Region has the highest migration rate (0.57 per 100 population in 1988). International migration, while increasing, is an insignificant demographic factor compared with internal migration.

The literacy rate in 1990 was 93.5 percent, highest in the National Capital Region (99.1). Elementary education is free and compulsory. In 1988, the total enrollment was 9.2 million for the elementary school level; 3.4 million for the secondary level; and 1.1 million for tertiary education.

MAJOR HEALTH PROBLEMS FACING THE COUNTRY

The Filipino nation is healthier today than in the 1960s. Life expectancy at birth has risen from 57 years in 1960 to 65 years in 1990. The crude birthrate declined from 32.5 in 1940 to 26.3 in 1990; crude death rate, from 16.6 to 5.1; infant mortality rate, from 135.8 to 57 per 1,000; maternal death rate, from 6.3 to 0.8; and neonatal death rate, from 34.7 to 11.7.

Philippine mortality rates from communicable diseases have progressively declined aggregately at 74 percent over the past 40 years. There has been a change in disease patterns with a decrease in communicable diseases to an increasing incidence of chronic degenerative and lifestyle-based diseases such as cardiovascular diseases, malignant neoplasms, diabetes, acquired immunodeficiency syndrome (AIDS), and multiforms of addiction. In addition, there are emerging diseases caused by increasing urbanization and industrialization such as occupational diseases caused by pollution, traumas, and accidents.

The ten leading causes of mortality per 100,000 population in 1990 were (1) diseases of the heart, (2) pneumonia, (3) diseases of the vascular system, (4) TB (tuberculosis) all forms, (5) malignant neoplasm, (6) diarrheal diseases, (7) septicemia, (8) nephritis, (9) accidents, and (10) measles. Compared with causes of mortality in 1961, diseases of the heart has superseded pneumonia as the number-one cause of death; diseases of the vascular system ranks third, replacing gastroenteritis; malignant neoplasms now ranks fifth, and accidents, ninth (Figure 2).

The leading causes of morbidity in 1990 were (1) bronchitis, (2) diarrheal diseases, (3) influenza, (4) pneumonias, (5) TB, all forms, (6) accidents, (7) diseases of the heart, (8) malaria, (9) measles, and (10) malignant neoplasms (Figure 3).

Infant mortality has declined to 57.0 percent. Among the ten leading causes of infant death, pneumonias still ranked number one, with fetus and newborn respiratory condition as the second cause. Tetanus has disappeared, and bronchitis has moved down from fourth to tenth place. Maternal mortality has declined to 0.8 per 1,000 with hemorrhage as the leading cause, followed by hypertension, other complications, and abortion.

Malnutrition has been a persistent problem, especially among Filipino children, particularly females. Chronic dietary energy deficiency is alarming among schoolchildren (only 65 percent of needed dietary requirements) and pregnant and lactating women (65 percent to 69 percent). Micronutrient deficiencies in iron, iodine, and vitamins have remained high throughout the years. While efforts are being made to promote breast-feeding, it has declined. There are gender and geographic disparities in nutritional status, with females and children suffering from the worst malnutrition level.

Figure 2
Mortality: Ten Leading Causes, Five-Year Average (1985–1989) and 1990

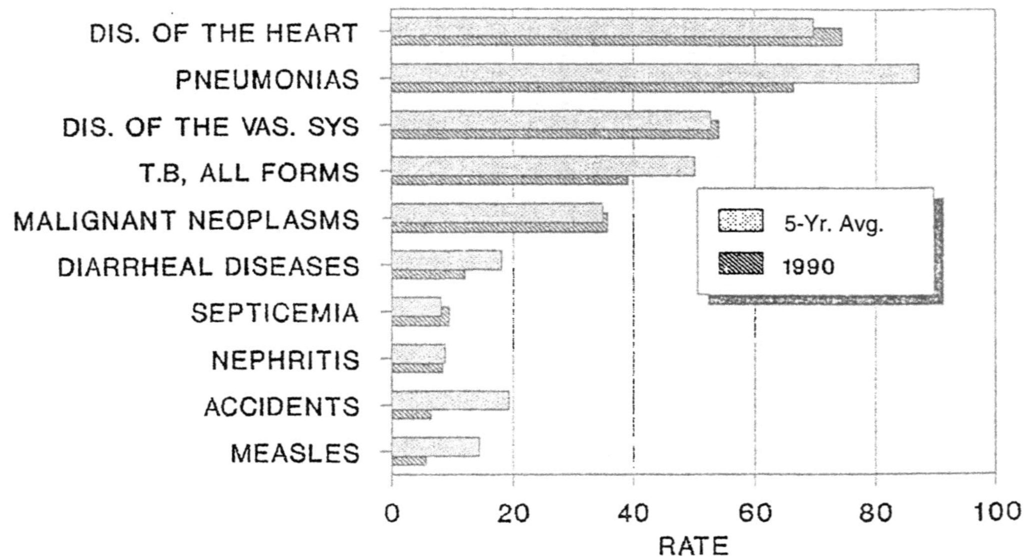

Notes: Rate per 100,000 population; nephritis includes nephrotic syndrome and nephrosis.

Source: Philippine Health Statistics 1990.

Figure 3
Morbidity: Ten Leading Causes, Five-Year Average (1985–1989) and 1990

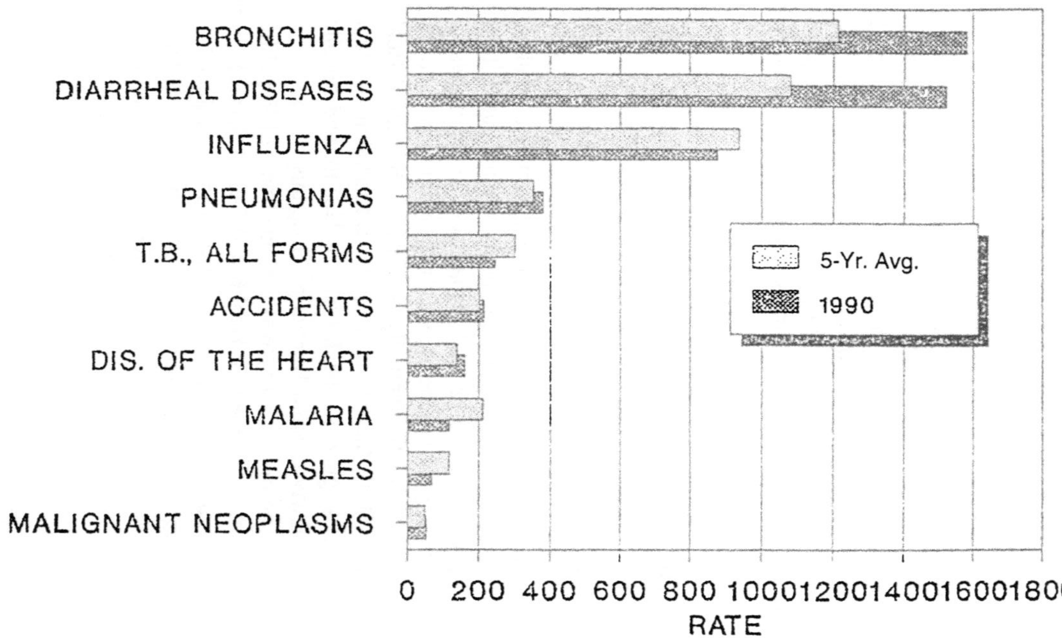

Note: Rate per 100,000 population.

Source: Philippine Health Statistics 1990.

Environmental sanitation and threats from environmental degradation still pose problems in the health of the public. Basic environmental sanitation remains inadequate, especially among the rural and urban poor population. Less than 70 percent of households have access to safe water, and only 73 percent have sanitary toilets. Waterborne diseases and intestinal parasitism, direct results of poor environmental sanitation, are still prevalent.

Destruction of watersheds due to pollution from industrial and domestic wastes has posed threats to safe water sources. Outbreaks of red tide are occurring with alarming frequency in Manila Bay and Eastern Visayas. Massive deforestation due to illegal logging has resulted in soil erosion and siltation and the destruction of crop land and coastal areas. This, in turn, has resulted in food insecurity and migration to urban areas, causing the rise of slums, urban blight and congestion, and crime. Urban dwellers become exposed to risk factors such as air, water, and soil pollution and stress, which aggravate respiratory and gastrointestinal diseases and may cause cardiovascular diseases, malignancies, and accidents.

PROVISION, UTILIZATION, AND IMPACT OF HEALTH SERVICES

Organization of Health Services

While the protection of the health of the people is a multisectoral undertaking, the Department of Health (DOH) is the legally constituted authority responsible for the health of the people. The present Department of Health was established in 1947 soon after Philippine Independence. Its beginning may be traced to the Insular Board of Health, which eventually became the Bureau of Health, during the American regime. With the creation of the Department of Health, public health activities were assigned to the Bureau of Health, and hospital services were assigned to the newly created Bureau of Hospitals.

A significant milestone in its history was the enactment of Republic Act 1082 in 1954 entitled An Act Strengthening Health and Dental Services in the Rural Areas. Rural Health Units (RHUs) were established in more than 1,400 municipalities, each RHU manned by a municipal health officer, an M.D.; one public health nurse; one midwife; and one sanitary inspector. The implementing arm of the project was the Bureau of Health. Prior to the enactment of this act, the concept was piloted in 81 Rural Health Units to test its feasibility.

Following the results and recommendations of a WHO (World Health Organization)/Philippine team survey in 1963 and operations research in 1971–1973, the Rural Health Care Delivery System was restructured. Additional supervisory and treatment responsibilities were given to nurses, and it delegated treatment functions for common ailments to midwives. More midwives were provided to RHUs. The recommendations of said research became the centerpiece of the first national health plan (1974–1977). Twelve Regional Health Offices (RHOs) were established all over the country; district hospitals with a catchment area of three to four municipalities were created; a network of satellite *barangay* (smallest political unit) health stations were constructed, and 250 new RHUs were added. Corollary to this was an expanded and intensive training program for health personnel.

The 1970s saw five significant developments: the proclamation of the Martial Law; the implementation of the first national health plan; the introduction of management by objectives; primary health care; and Medicare. Among the first measures of the Martial Law was the creation of planning units in all departments of the executive branch of the government, of which the Department of Health was among the first.

The restructuring of the rural health care delivery set the stage for primary health care (PHC). Training of *barangay* (village) health workers was initiated in the late 1970s. The thrust was toward more emphasis in the periphery. Management by objectives became part of the managerial process of the department to increase relevance and efficiency of health activities. The year 1981 marked the formal implementation of PHC.

Over 39,000 *barangay* PHC committees were organized and over 350,000 *barangay* health workers trained. Additional *barangay* health stations were constructed and equipped, with the community participating actively. Information, education, and communication (IEC) materials were developed and distributed, herbal processing plants and personnel established, and *barangay* pharmacists encouraged. Finally, to further strengthen the PHC strategy, the Integrated Provincial Health Office (IPHO) scheme was introduced in 1983. Thenceforth, the provincial health officer was tasked with both public health and hospital services for the province.

Nongovernmental Organizations (NGOs)

Establishing linkages/networking with different sectors is one of the essential elements of the PHC. WHO spurred the movement by promoting exchange of information and experiences through country visits, a series of national meetings in its member states, finally culminating in the Declaration of Alma Ata in September 1978.

In the Philippines, Community-Based Health Programs (CBHPs) started in 1973. Three Catholic sisters and a physician nun of the Rural Missionaries decided to set up an alternative health program. The sisters envisioned a program that would train laypeople to meet the health needs for the community and utilize local and indigenous resources for preventive and curative health care instead of the Western-oriented system. Starting with three pilot areas, the movement spread nationwide. As of 1988, it covered 432 villages, 79 towns, and 15 dioceses. Many other groups, sectarian and nonsectarian, have adopted the CBHP approach and utilized it to improve health care delivery in the most neglected communities.

Hospitals

By the time the Americans occupied the Philippines, there were already hospitals established by the Spaniards. These were developed and expanded by the

Americans as new hospitals were organized. The private sector followed suit, particularly those established by Catholic and Protestant missions.

The phenomenal growth of hospitals occurred in 1923 when Act 3114 was passed, setting aside a generous appropriation to aid provinces in the construction, equipment, operation, and maintenance of hospitals. Act 3168 provided that the provinces should contribute not less than 30 to 40 percent of the total cost, the amount depending on the class of the provinces. All provinces were able to establish their own hospitals by the 1960s.

To make hospital services more accessible, Medicare set up small hospitals in the 1980s, 93 in all. In 1987, all these hospitals were absorbed by the Department of Health. By 1992, there were 639 government hospitals with 53,023 beds and 1,103 hospitals with 36,799 beds.

As previously mentioned, for better integration of hospitals and public health services, the provincial health office and the chief of hospitals formed the IPHO. Immediately under this office were the district hospitals (DHs), which were charged with providing hospital services and monitoring the Rural Health Units under their catchment areas (three to four municipalities in one health district).

Quite recently, a new concept has been introduced that transforms hospitals from ''centers of illness'' to ''centers of wellness.'' Emphasis will be on family-oriented programs to address such problems as smoking, cancer, cardiovascular diseases, drug addiction, alcoholism, and a number of communicable diseases such as TB, malaria, and dengue.

Other Public Health Developments

After the Philippine Revolution of 1986, which ended martial law under the dictatorship, the new Constitution of 1987 contained more specific provisions on health, making available comprehensive health care, and emphasized private sector and NGO participation. It retained and maintained the IPHO and DH scheme and supported research. One significant project was the Federal Republic of Germany Agency for Technical Cooperation (FRG-GTZ) collaboration on the health and management information system. Another important development was the passage of the Generic Act of 1988, which mandated generic labeling of pharmaceuticals, generic prescription of doctors, and generic dispensing. It envisioned local generic drug production leading to self-sufficiency.

In 1990, the Magna Carta for Public Health Workers was approved, granting salary increases and fringe benefits to health personnel. This was followed closely by the approval of the Local Government Code (LGC) in 1990. Under the LGC, health care delivery was devolutionized. Prior to the devolution, the Central Health Office had staff functions providing policies and guidelines to the field through the RHOs. Similarly, the RHO had staff functions with technical service and training sections. The RHO monitored health programs. Line functions started at the IPHO, which monitored and supervised the Rural Health Units through the District Health Office. The Rural Health Units were accountable to the Provincial Health Office (PHO) through the District Health Office. Under the Rural Health Units were *barangay* health stations manned by a rural health midwife and assisted by volunteer health workers (BHWs). The midwife screened cases, attended to those she was able to treat, and referred serious cases to the nurse and the doctor at the main health center. Cases that cannot be handled at the RHU were referred to the district hospital or provincial hospital and in some cases to tertiary hospitals. The RHU performed promotive and preventive functions such as immunization, environmental health, prenatal services, deliveries, TB screening, and health education.

After devolution, the Rural Health Units were placed under the mayors of each municipality, while the provincial and district hospitals were placed under the provincial governors. The 13 Regional Health Offices, 45 Medical Centers, and tertiary hospitals were retained under the National Office. So were special programs such as control of malaria, schistosomiasis, tuberculosis, sexually transmitted disease (STD), and leprosy, which were reverted to vertical from horizontal programs.

In 1993, nearly all health personnel, 596 hospitals, and 12,580 centers and *barangay* health stations were devolved to local government units. Under the new scheme, the official link among the health services network became loose, and the DOH was cut off from the peripheral level. The PHOs and district health offices are now administratively under the provincial governor. Similarly, the RHUs are under the mayors. The National Office and the Regional Health Offices can only exercise technical assistance and support when requested; so, too, with vertical programs. The challenge facing the health system is how to maintain the original network and sustain the previous working relationships under the new scheme. Considering that governors and mayors may change after every three-year election, PHO and RHU personnel may be changed, depending on the mood of the elected officials, and program continuity may suffer.

HEALTH CARE FINANCING

The Philippines spent 1.84 percent of gross national product on health care goods and services in 1991. The bulk of this spending (85 percent) was on personal health care, 10 percent on public health programs, and 5 percent on administration. Private individuals financed about half (48 percent) of total personal health care from out of pocket, while Medicare financed some 8 percent. The national government spent some 8 billion pesos (34 percent) for its health program, of which 26 percent went to personal health.

The same estimates also indicate that the DOH financed about 30 percent of the total 23.5 million pesos of health care expenditures. Twenty-three percent went to personal health care, 6.5 percent to public health programs, and 1.2

Figure 4
1995 Presidential Budget

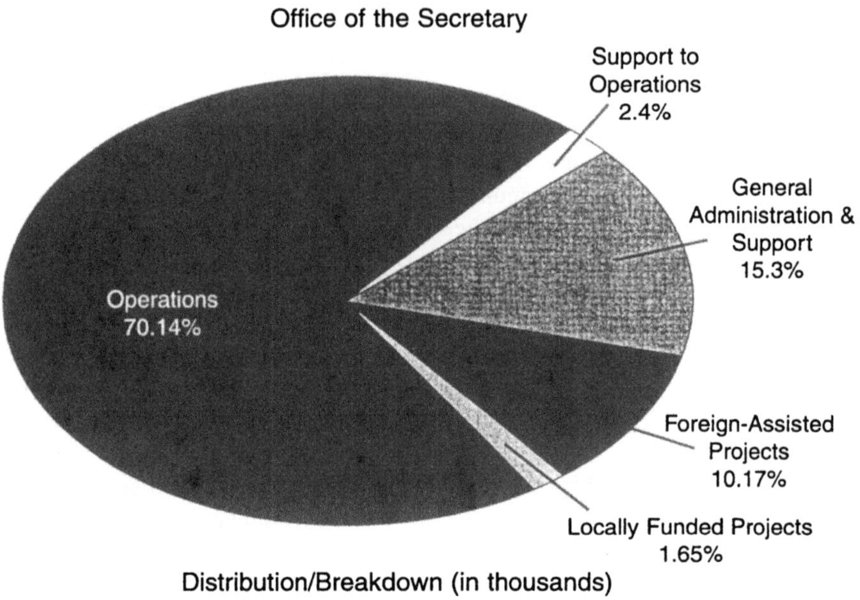

Source: Department of Health Publication 1995a.

percent on health administration. Hence, the national government spent 26 percent for personal health care services and 6.5 percent for public health programs.

The year 1991 was the last year before health functions of the national government were devolved to local governments. With the devolution, it is expected that local government spending for personal health care will increase and be an added strain on its budget unless another financing mechanism is established, such as budgetary support from the DOH.

For 1995 the DOH budgetary outlay was 8 billion pesos and is geared toward redirecting its role and strengthening its program activities to attain its vision of Health for All in the Year 2000. The bulk of the 1995 DOH budget (70.14 percent) went to operations; 15.3 percent to general administration and support; 10.17 percent to foreign-assisted projects; 2.4 percent to support to operations; and 1.65 percent to locally funded projects (Figure 4).

HEALTH INSURANCE

Health insurance in the Philippines is of relatively recent vintage, having commenced only in the 1970s. There are two compulsory health insurance schemes: The Philippine Medical Care Plan (Medicare) and the Employees

Compensation Commission (ECC). The two pay benefits directly to the service provider rather than to the insured.

Medicare has two components—Program I and Program II. Program I, implemented in 1972, covers the regularly employed and their dependents. One third of the members are government employees, and all are covered by the Government Insurance System (GSIS), while the remaining two thirds, privately employed, are under the Social Security System (SSS). Later, retirees and self-employed were added.

As estimated in 1991, Medicare covered 38 percent of the population, but it accounted only for less than 8 percent of the estimated total health expenditure for the year. Premium contribution to Medicare is shared equally by the employee and employer. Basically, benefits are inpatient in nature. Outpatient care benefits are confined to minor surgery, chemotherapy, hemodialysis, and radiotherapy.

Program II, designed to cover non-SSS self-employed and unemployed, has not been implemented except on a pilot basis. Recently, the Senate approved on second reading Senate Bill 1738, the National Health Insurance Act of 1994. The bill, which seeks to provide universal health coverage to all Filipinos at affordable cost, was signed by the president in February 1995. Under this new insurance plan, indigents will receive medical benefits on par with GSIS and SSS members. Monthly contributions of indigents will be shouldered by the national and local governments. The program will take effect within a 15-year phase-in period. Funding will come from national government sources and the DOH. A national Health Insurance Corporation, complemented by Local Health Insurance Offices at the provincial level, will be established to manage the program.

The Employees Compensation Commission, the other compulsory insurance, covers employees under 60 years of age. Its coverage is about 21 percent of the population and grants benefits for conditions that are work related such as disability or death, medical and related services for injury or sickness, and rehabilitation service in case of permanent disability.

Apart from Medicare and ECC, the Labor Code of the Philippines specifies a minimum set of medical, dental, first-aid treatment, and occupational safety obligations to employers. A full-time physician, nurse, and dentist at the company clinic are required, depending on the number of employees.

Voluntary health insurance is estimated to cover 5 percent of the population. In 1988, 102 private companies were involved in health and accident insurance.

Health maintenance organizations have recently begun to appear. Enrollment is less than 1 percent of the population. Its members are mostly those with ability to pay.

THE INFRASTRUCTURE OF TRAINING AND RESEARCH IN PUBLIC HEALTH

Training

The Health Human Resource Development Service of the Department of Health is tasked with formulating plans, policies, programs, standards, and techniques for the effective and efficient manpower development and training of health personnel; designs, implements, monitors, and evaluates training programs; and provides consultative and advisory services to implementing units at different administrative levels.

The other training arm of the DOH is the College of Public Health where health personnel obtain their graduate degrees either as Master of Public Health, Master of Science in Public Health, Master of Occupational Health, or Doctor of Public Health. The college also offers short courses if and when commissioned by the Department of Health, WHO, and other international agencies to conduct some short training courses in the different public health fields.

Research in Public Health

The Research Institute for Tropical Medicine (RITM), the Essential National Health Research, the Philippine Council for Health Research and Development (PCHRD), the National Research Council of the Philippines (NRCP), and the College of Public Health, University of the Philippines (CPH-UP) are the principal research institutions contributing to research in public health.

The RITM, a research facility under the DOH, was inaugurated April 1981. Its primary function is the efficient and economical implementation and performance of research programs on the diagnosis and treatment of tropical and infectious diseases.

The PCHRD is under the Department of Science and Technology (DOST). The council was formally created on March 17, 1982, through Executive Order No. 784, which made it the focal point for health research in the country. The PCHRD's mandate is to lead, direct, and coordinate science and technology activities in health and nutrition. It sets the goals of health research in the country; establishes the implementing mechanism; develops/strengthens research capabilities of institutions through manpower development programs or improvement of equipment and laboratories; monitors and evaluates research; and promotes research utilization.

The NRCP is another research institution under DOST, but unlike PCHRD, which focuses on health research alone, it provides funding for basic research in all the science fields of which health is only one.

The Essential National Health Research of the DOH is of recent vintage. It was established to formulate the health research policy of the DOH; develop, implement, monitor, and evaluate health research programs; set standards/guidelines in health research implementation; and promote intra- and intercoordination in health research.

The College of Public Health also engages in health research. One of the expected functions of the faculty is research; hence, faculty members from the different disciplines have research output. Further, the college also promotes research capability among its students, particularly among the Master of Science and doctoral students.

MAJOR CHALLENGES FOR THE HEALTH SERVICES

1. *Health for all.* How to attain the goal of putting health in the hands of the people by the year 2000 and making health a way of life within the context of the devolved health service delivery system is one challenge. Local autonomy is philosophically and theoretically sound as a step toward putting health in the hands of the people. However, there are many loopholes in its implementation that were not foreseen. One is the continuity of health services. The health care delivery system is now dependent on the management skills, priorities, commitment, and professionalism of the mayors and governors who are changed every election year. Another is the economic capability of the municipality. The economically disadvantaged cannot cope with the demands of health care service delivery. District/provincial hospitals have suffered from lack of supplies, drugs, and the like. Discrepancies in salaries and benefits of health personnel, poor monitoring and supervision, and severing of formal relationships among health personnel at the different hierarchal levels have resulted in inequitable distribution of health services. How to resolve these issues is a real challenge.

2. *Changing disease patterns.* The increasing incidence of lifestyle-based disease such as AIDS, multiforms of addiction, and diabetes; increasing incidence of chronic degenerative diseases, especially cancer, cardiovascular, and endocrine-related diseases; and emerging diseases caused by industrialization and urbanization in addition to persistent communicable diseases will plague the country in the years to come.

3. *The maintenance of health status to meet global standards.* This means reduction in infant, child, and maternal mortality rate, the control of communicable disease, and prevention of noncommunicable disease.

4. *The implementation of the recently approved National Health Insurance Scheme.* This needs to be studied carefully and the management problems well analyzed at the different administrative levels. A National Health Insurance Corporation will be established to govern and manage the program. It will be complemented on local provincial levels by the Local Health Insurance Offices, which will take charge of locally administering and identifying the indigent deserving of government assistance. It is the local level that needs strict monitoring. It is envisioned that the program will take effect within a 15-year phase-in period, which will allow for pilot testing the program to uncover its weak spots.

5. *Making hospitals centers of wellness.* Hospitals should maintain conducive environments, and they must have competent and compassionate caregivers and community-oriented service delivery that is accessible, affordable, culturally sensitive, and responsive. What needs to be done is for local government units to be able to support a healthy hospital. DOH must formulate rules, guidelines, policies, and standards on the maintenance of hospital facilities and equipment and human resource development to upgrade the capabilities of hospital staff and disseminate information through mass media.

6. *How to maintain healthy workplaces.* With growing industrialization and urbanization and with the goal of making the Philippines a newly industrialized country by the year 2000, promotion and protection of worker health and well-being become important issues. This means the need for commitment by concerned sectors/entities to conduct a sustained, coordinated, effective information dissemination and health education campaign on occupational health and safety (OHS) throughout the country; creating greater awareness and responsiveness of all sectors, especially labor and management, on OHS standards and policies; strengthening and operationalizing linkages and cooperation among and between concerned agencies, government and private; and participating actively in any multisectoral OHS undertaking.

7. *Meeting the health needs of the urban poor.* Slums have mushroomed in cities, with corresponding rise in crime rate, drug and substance abuse, poverty and unemployment, prostitution, and sexual harassment. Due to high population density, slums suffer from inadequate health services, uncontrolled communicable and chronic degenerative diseases, inadequate supply of potable water, improper excreta disposal, poor drainage, increased density of rodents and other vectors, and unmanageable traffic. Meeting these problems requires the concerted effort of government, nongovernment, and community/citizen efforts.

8. *Population management.* The Philippines still needs to have faster deceleration of population growth. The family planning program is in place, but there are still many opponents to the program, especially the Church and other pro-life groups. The challenge is for the DOH to be able to reconcile with the Church and agree on an acceptable family planning policy to both. A more aggressive family planning program needs to be in place.

9. *Women's health.* Emphasis on women's health has just been newly conceived. The scope of women's health is wider than that of maternal health, as it not only encompasses the fertile period but includes the risks that women are exposed to from "womb to tomb." This demands a holistic look at women's health within the context of physical, mental, emotional, psychological, and socioeconomic factors. Particular emphasis is placed on disadvantaged women (raped, prostitutes, battered women, victims of incest, overseas contract workers, refugees, and the urban poor). Seen in this light, women's health becomes a very intricate and complex problem and needs a multidisciplinary approach. This means close coordination among different sectors, government and nongovernment. It involves formulation/strengthening of policies for the protection of women. Women need to be educated about their rights and how to be empowered so that they can maintain their self-esteem and fight for what is due them.

10. *Child survival programs.* These need to be sustained and expanded. These include an expanded immunization program, control of acute respiratory infection, control of diarrheal disease, breast-feeding, and improved weaning practices. The continuous supply of vaccines must be maintained, and the coverage of hepatitis B immunization needs to be expanded. The knowledge and skills of health workers in this area need to be enhanced.

If health is viewed as part of a greater scheme of things, then the bigger challenge is that the achievement of its goal—health as a way of life and health in the hands of the people—must go hand in hand with the development of a healthy and sustainable environment and socioeconomic development.

REFERENCES

Alonso, Ruperto. (1994). Medicare Program II, pilot project experience: Issues and concerns. *Technical Brief, Health Finance Development Project*, no. 2 (October).

Cuevas, Bernadette. (1994). DOH 1995 budget goes to Senate. *PISO News, Health Finance and Development Project* (DOH), no. 6 (November).

Department of Health. (1993a). *DOH in '93.* Annual Report. Manila: DOH.

Department of Health. (1993b). *Positioning for Performance Towards Health in the Hands of the People.* Strategy Paper for Philippines 2000. Rev. ed. July 1993. Manila: DOH.

Department of Health, Public Information and Health Education Service. (1994). *Think Health, Health Link.* Manila: DOH.

Department of Health, Research Institute for Tropical Medicine. (1990). *Annual Report.* Manila: DOH.

Department of Health Publication. (1994). *Philippine Health, Today and Tomorrow* (Highlights from the Twenty-five Year Strategic Plan for Health). Manila: DOH.

Department of Health Publication. (1995a). *Primer on Healthy Cities, Think Health, Health Link, 1995-1996.* Manila: DOH.

Department of Health Publication. (1995b). *Primer on Healthy Hospitals, Think Health, Health Link, 1995–1996.* Manila: DOH.

Department of Science and Technology. (1993). *Philippine Council for Health Research and Development.* PCHRD 1993. Annual Report.

Mercado, Remigio D. (1994). *The Philippines Health Care Delivery System* (A Historical Review). Paper commissioned by the Department of Health. Manila.

National Health Statistics Office, Manila. (1988). *Statistical Handbook of the Philippines, 1988 & 1990.* Republic of the Philippines: NHSO.

PCHRD. (1994). *Health Research and Development in the Philippines.* Manila: PCHRD.

Philippine Health Statistics. (1990). *Health Intelligence Service.* Manila: Department of Health.

Quimbo, Victoria. (1994). NHA estimates 1991 total health spending in the Philippines. *PISO News, Health Finance and Development Project* (DOH), no. 6 (November).

Stover, Charles C. (1994). Global budgeting. *Technical Brief, Health Finance Development Project*, no. 3 (November).

Tiglao, Teodora V. & Cruz, W. L. (1975). *Seven Decades of Public Health in the Philippines (1898–1972).* Tokyo, Japan: SEAMIC.

Zaide, Gregorio F. & Zaide, Sonia M. (1995). *History of Asian Nations.* 3rd ed. Metro Manila, Philippines: National Bookstore, Inc.

POLAND

Witold Zatoński and Monika Przetakiewicz-Koziej

INTRODUCTION

Poland lies in the center of Europe, bordering on Russia, Lithuania, Belarus, and the Ukraine in the east, on Germany in the west, and Slovakia and the Czech Republic in the south. The northern border is the Baltic Sea shore. The country occupies an area of about 312,000 square kilometers and has a population of over 38 million people (mid-1990s). The temperate climate of Poland is characterized by considerable variations between the seasons, with cold snowy winters (average temperature in January is −1°C) and hot dry summers (average temperature in July +15.8°C).

The written history of the state of Poland dates back to the second half of the tenth century. From that time, Poland increased its position to become a European power in the fifteenth century. In the Renaissance period, the country witnessed political changes that undermined its status in Europe. After that era, Poland was invaded by its neighbors several times and lost its independence as a result of "the third partition" in 1795. It became an independent state again in 1918 after more than 120 years of foreign domination. During World War II the country was occupied and ravaged following invasions by Nazi Germany and the USSR. The war took a death toll of about 6 million Polish people, half of whom were of Jewish descent. After the war, Poland was ruled by a totalitarian regime affiliated with the Soviets until the national movement of "Solidarity" took over in 1989.

There are now about 18.75 million men and 19.76 million women in Poland, corresponding to a sex ratio of 100 men per approximately 105.4 women. Young people below 25 years of age represent 39 percent of the total population (14.9 million), while people aged 65 and more account for 10.6 percent (4.1 million).

About half of the population (50.4 percent—19.5 million) are people aged 25 to 65. The Polish population is aging. Since World War II the percentage of Poles aged 65 or more has risen from 5.6 percent in 1950 to 10.6 percent in 1993.

Administratively, Poland consists of 49 *voivodships*, or provinces, with populations ranging from a half to a few million people. *Voivodships* are further divided into *gminas*, or communes (basic administrative units), with populations from approximately a few to 12,000 people. There are 2,300 *gminas* in Poland.

The level of education of the Polish population is best illustrated by percentages of students in the various age groups: 87 percent of teenagers in the 15–18 age group attended secondary schools in 1993, while at the same time the percentage of university students in the 19–24 age group was 18 percent.

Present-day Poland is a country whose economy is undergoing the transition from a state-controlled system to a free market. There had been no unemployment in Poland before 1989, and in 1993 the unemployment rate in Poland exceeded 16 percent. Poland is abundant in coal, copper, and sulfur and has developed textile, steel, and shipbuilding industries. Agriculture is also an important sector of the economy, potatoes, rye, wheat, and sugar beet being the main crops.

HEALTH STATUS OF THE POLISH POPULATION

The last 100 years have witnessed tremendous changes in the health condition of the human population. Great Britain is an example of a country with traditionally good health statistics. In 1880, 50 percent of the British people had reached the age of 40, and today only 3 percent die before reaching that age. The proportion of people who survive until the age of 70 has increased from 25 to 70 percent during the last 100 years (Peto et al. 1992). Similar changes have taken place in Poland during a period that can be analyzed. It is worth noting that the risk of dying faced by men and women in Poland in 1931 was very similar in both sexes: for age 40 and under, respectively, 57 and 56 percent; and under 70 years, 84 and 81 percent. In 1991 there was high premature mortality in men, compared with women (the probability of death for men under 70 was 59 percent, for women, 33 percent).

Life Expectancy

During the early 1930s, life expectancy was over 10 years lower in both sexes in Poland than in Germany. After the war, life span increase in both sexes of the Polish population was much faster than in Germany. The life expectancies (of both sexes) in both countries were similar in the 1960s. However, the life expectancy at the age of 0 stopped increasing after the mid-1960s in Polish men and since the mid-1970s in women as well. At the same time, the life expectancy at the age of 45+ dramatically declined in men (from 28.2 years in 1965 to 25.6 in 1991), while it remained unchanged in women.

Infant Mortality

Infant mortality in Poland before World War II was 130 to 140 deaths per 1,000 live births. The mortality rates declined very significantly after the war; the decline has also been observed in the 1980s and 1990s. However, the infant mortality rate in Poland (in 1991 being 15/1,000) continues to be higher than in other western European countries.

Proportional Mortality of Adults

The probability of dying is calculated for the specific age categories. The mortality rate among children aged 1 to 14 years is constantly declining (Figure 1). In the younger-adult age category, 15–39 years, the percentage of deaths in this category in relation to the total number of deaths in both sexes had significantly declined until the 1980s. It has remained unchanged over the last decade. In the older-adult age category, 40–59 years, the percentage of deaths was declining after the war. This trend stopped in the 1970s, and the direction of the trend changed dramatically in men. The percentage of deaths in men of this age category increased from 18.5 percent in 1971 to 23.6 percent in 1991. In women, a temporary increase observed during the latter half of the 1970s was followed by a downward trend (12.4 percent in 1981; 10.5 percent in 1991).

Age-Adjusted Total Mortality Rates, Ages 35 to 64

After World War II, between 1950 and 1965, the mortality rates in the category 35–64 years declined in both sexes by over 30 percent, from 1,720 to 880 in men, and by nearly 40 percent from 780 to 490 in women (Figure 2). This trend was reversed in men in the mid-1960s. In women, the mortality rates stabilized five years later (1970—476; 1991—481). The mortality rate in men has been increasing dramatically. In the early 1990s it reached the level of 1,320, which is higher than the postwar figure recorded in 1950. Following the political changes and the introduction of the free-market economy during the last three years for which death statistics are available, the mortality rates have grown especially high, namely, from 1,185 in 1988 to 1,320 in 1991, which is over 10 percent greater.

Infectious Diseases

The mortality caused by infectious diseases has been on the decline throughout the entire postwar era. This is also the case during the 1980s and 1990s. Infectious diseases are responsible for about 0.6 percent of all deaths. Tuber-

Figure 1
The Probability of Death at a Given Age, Poland, 1960–1992

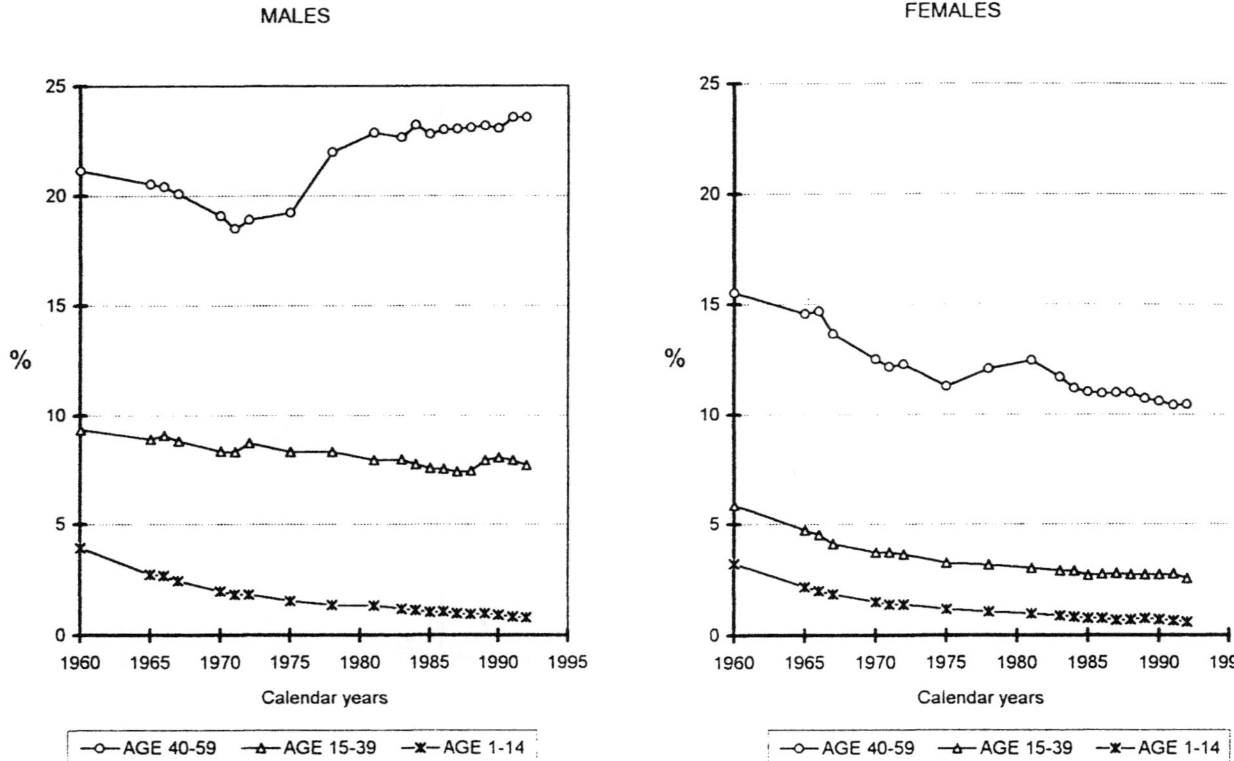

Source: Zatoński 1994.

Figure 2
Age-Adjusted Overall Mortality Rates, Ages 35 to 64, Poland, 1950–1990

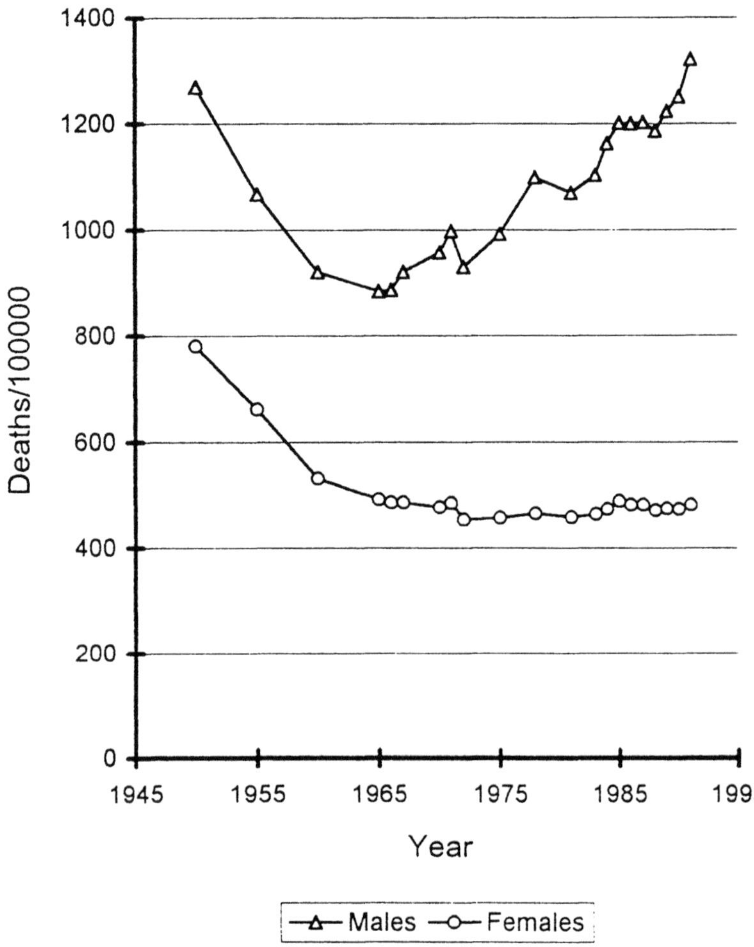

Source: Zatoński 1994.

culosis caused 0.3 percent of deaths among adult men (15–59 years) in 1993. The figures are even lower in adult women (Feachem et al. 1992). Other infectious diseases, for example, meningitis and hepatitis, are these days responsible for a very small fraction of all adult deaths. Deaths from acquired immunodeficiency syndrome (AIDS) continue to be rare in Poland. In 1992, 11 AIDS-related deaths were recorded (8 deaths in 1991) (Magdzik and Czarkowski 1994). Similarly, the mortality of women related to child delivery has been steadily declining and did not present a significant public health problem in the 1980s and 1990s. Infectious diseases among children have also been reduced, owing to effective immunization, among other measures. Also in the 1980s and 1990s Poland continued to be a country with one of the highest immunization completeness rates in the world, a rate corresponding with the result achieved by western European countries (Feachem et al. 1992).

Cardiovascular Diseases

The incidence of mortality from cardiovascular diseases has been declining in all the developed Western countries for about 30 years now. During the same period, the Polish population has experienced a dramatic increase in cardiovascular disorders, especially among men. The risk of cardiovascular death in Polish men aged 15–59 is over twice as high as in West Germany and Sweden (Feachem et al. 1992). Male mortality in the 35–64 age group shows an unusual increase from about 290 in 1971 to about 530 deaths per 100,000 in 1991 (Figure 3). Although the increase in the mortality rate of women is much smaller, the probability of premature death was also higher in relation to the developed countries in 1990 (Feachem et al. 1992).

Cancer

In the early 1960s, cancer mortality in Poland was relatively low in Polish men and women as compared to other European countries (Zatoński and Becker 1988). However, a very dramatic increase in the incidence and mortality from these diseases are observed among men. During the early 1990s, Poland, the Czech Republic, and Hungary belonged to the countries of the highest cancer mortality rates in the age category 35 to 64 in Europe. The increase in the mortality of men results, first of all, from the growing mortality caused by cancer of the lung. This is one of the highest rates in the world. The cancer mortality rates among women over the recent three decades have remained at an unchanged level in Poland. In most European countries, these rates show slightly declining trends. As in men, the mortality rates for lung cancer are significantly increasing in women (similarly as in most European countries). The lung cancer mortality increase has accelerated in Poland during the last 15 years (Zatoński et al. 1993).

Sudden Death Caused by External Factors

This is the third group of death causes responsible for the fact that the mortality of adult Polish men has increased to an unusually high level and continues to go up. The risk of dying from external causes is two times higher than in western Europe (Feachem et al. 1992). The mortality rates in men of the age category 35 to 64 over the 1970s and the 1980s were very high and ranged

Figure 3
Age-Adjusted Mortality Rates from Cardiovascular Diseases, Ages 35 to 64, Poland, 1971–1991

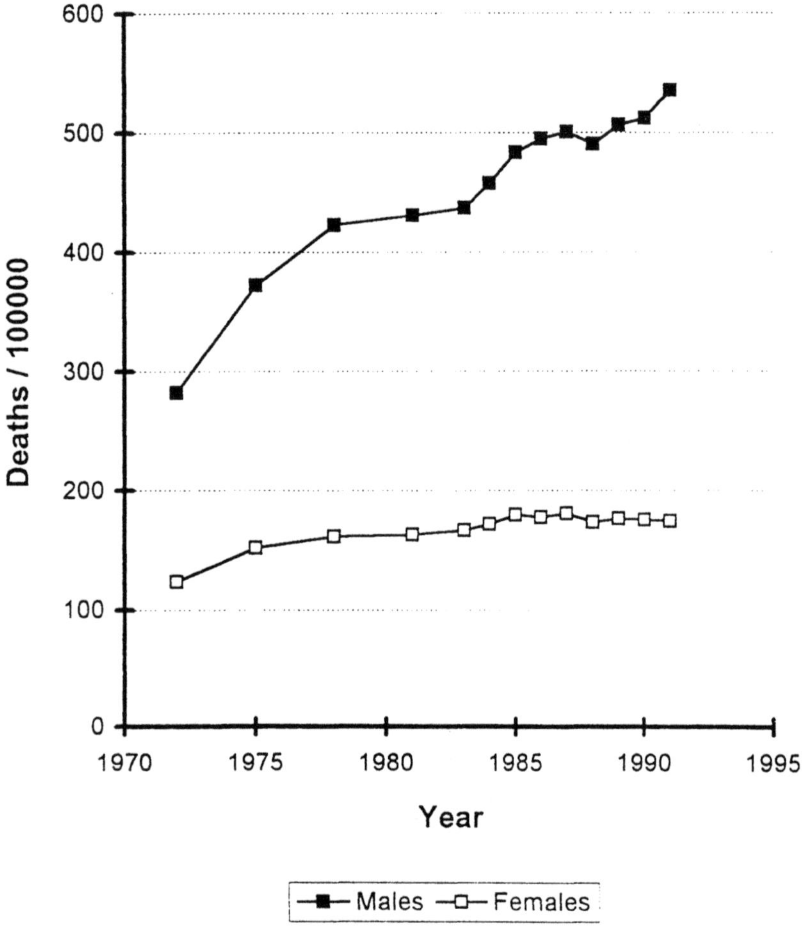

Source: Feachem et al. 1992.

between 130 and 160 deaths per 100,000 yearly (Figure 4). After 1988 (145 deaths), an unusual increase of mortality rates has been observed, reaching 190 deaths per 100,000 in 1991. The number of sudden deaths from external causes continues to be much lower among women, and it is comparable with the picture of other European countries. No increase in this rate has been observed during recent decades as well as recent years.

Figure 4
Age-Adjusted Mortality Rates from Sudden Deaths from External Causes, Ages 35 to 64, Poland, 1971–1991

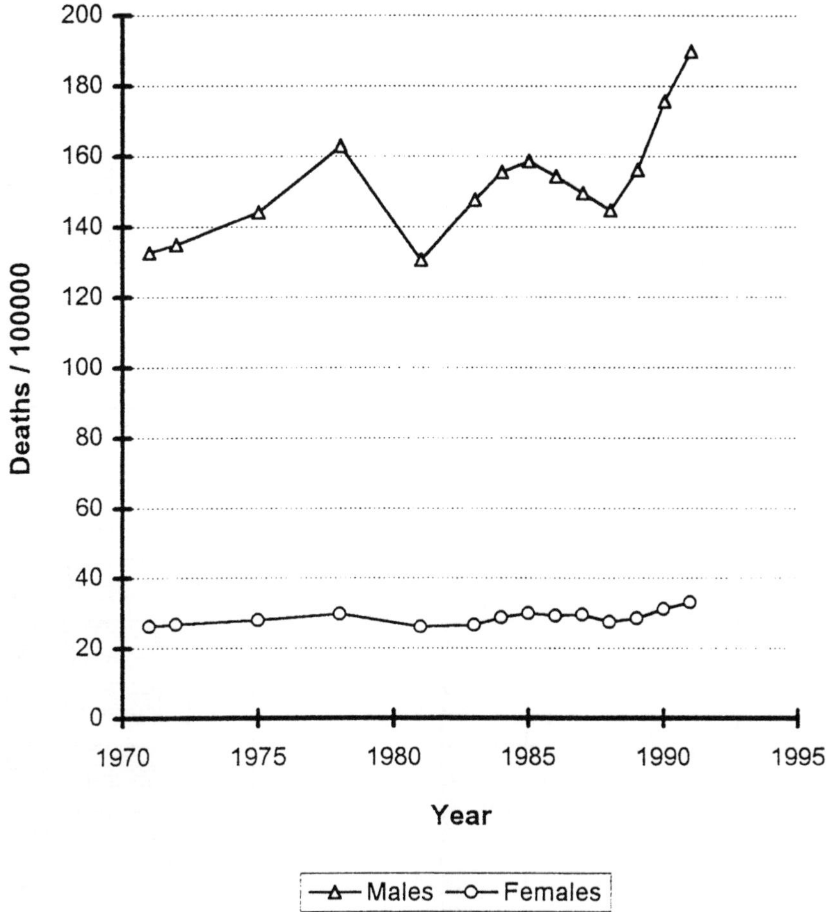

Source: Feachem et al. 1992.

Proportional Mortality in Poland in 1990 in Comparison with Other World Regions

The probability of death in Polish men, when compared with the risk in other world regions, is different for different age categories (Murray and Lopez 1994) (Figure 5). In the age 0–14 category, the probability of death is comparable to

Figure 5
Probability of Dying at a Given Age, by Region and Sex, 1990

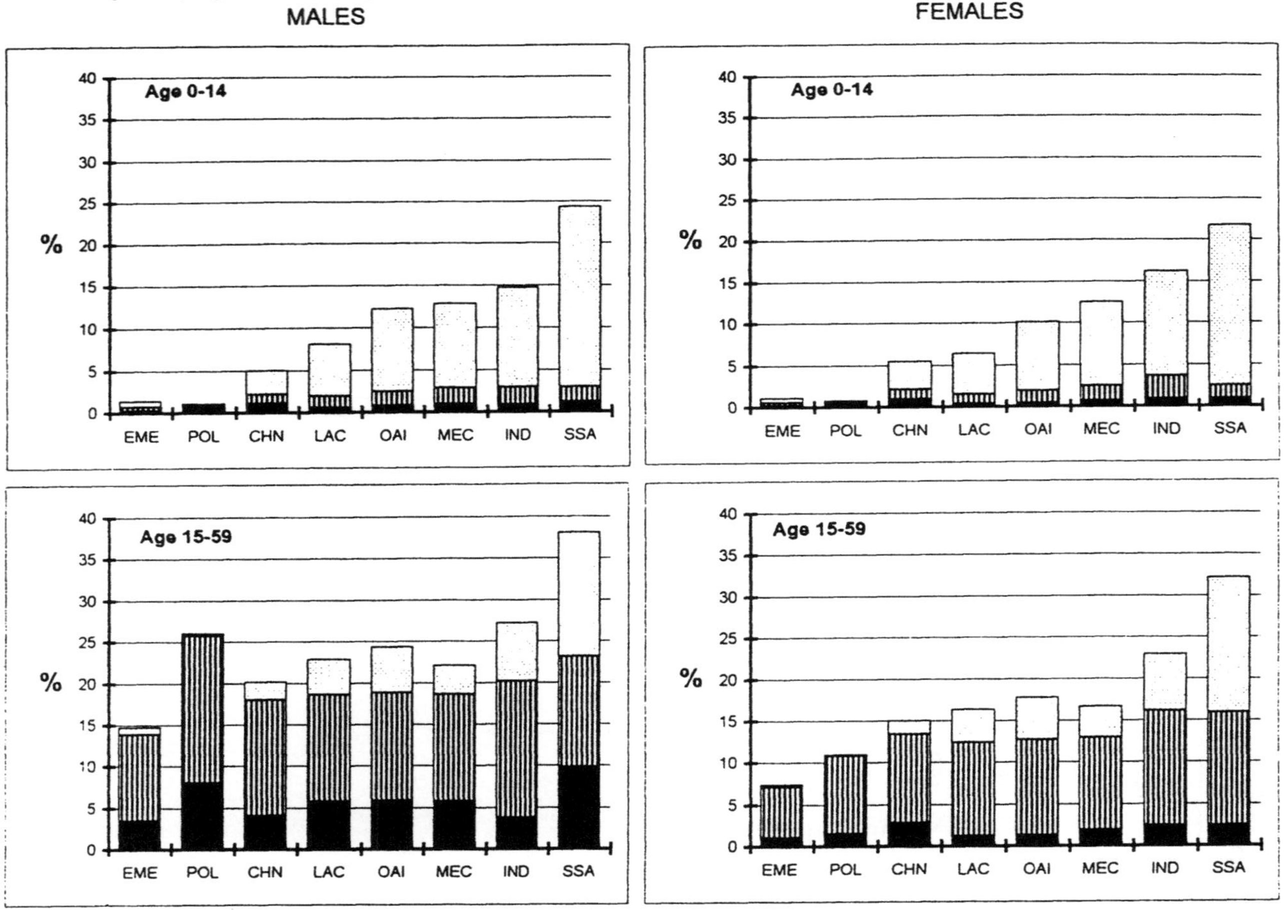

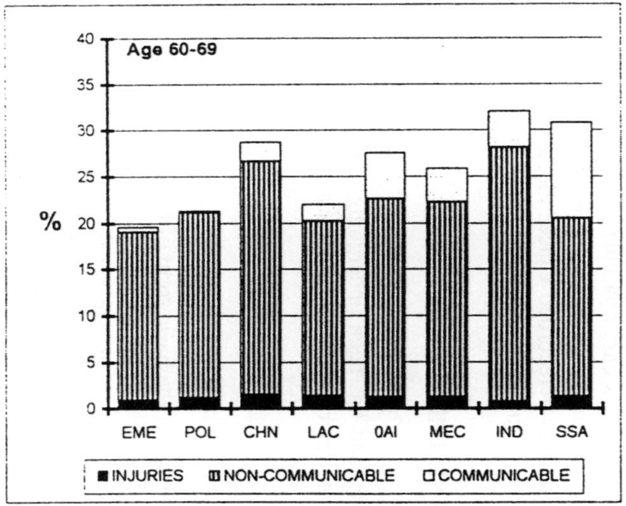

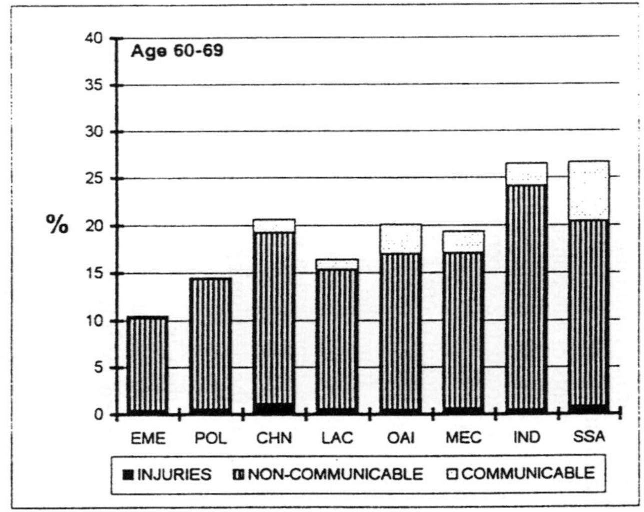

EME - Established Market Economies
CHN - China
LAC - Latin America and the Caribean

OAI - Other Asia and Islands
MEC - Middle Eastern Crescent
IND - India
SSA - Sub-Saharan Africa

Source: Murray and Lopez 1994.

that in the developed world countries. But the chance of a 15-year-old Polish boy (like the chance of boys from most former communist countries) to survive until the age of 60 is lower than in China, most Latin American countries, and India, and higher only than for the inhabitants of sub-Saharan Africa. According to World Bank estimates, in the mid-1980s, over one fourth of all deaths in Polish men occurred in the 15–59 age group (12.6 percent in Sweden, 15.2 percent in West Germany) (Feachem et al. 1992). The main causes of deaths among Polish men of the 15–59 age category are cardiovascular disorders (nearly 30 percent of deaths), cancer (about 20 percent), and sudden deaths from external causes (over 25 percent). Apart from the high mortality related to chronic diseases, another important factor is the high proportion of sudden deaths, of which deaths in road accidents represent a considerable part. The proportion of deaths among Polish men aged 60 to 70 is a little higher than in the developed countries and lower than in the developing world. The probability of death among women is comparable in all the age categories to that in the developed world and significantly lower than in all the developing countries. The main causes of deaths in the population of adult women are cardiovascular disorders and cancer. The mortality caused by infectious diseases is very low (like in men) and comparable with the Swedish or West German rates (Feachem et al. 1992). Also, the frequency of sudden death caused by external factors in women is low and comparable to the developed countries. The growing premature mortality due to cancers (as well as cardiovascular diseases) is a public health challenge in central European countries. The male population of this part of the world has reached the highest ever recorded cancer mortality rate (particularly lung cancer mortality) before the age of 65.

PROVISION, UTILIZATION, AND IMPACT OF HEALTH SERVICES

Since 1989, health service in Poland has been undergoing constant changes. Many of the aspects of the situation described in this chapter are likely to change within the next few years.

Organization of Health Service

For many decades and also after 1989, the basic form of health care in Poland has been national health service organized, controlled, and financed by the state. There is also the traditional private sector. It has become much more active since 1989. Its importance for health care is still insignificant, which is mostly due to a lack of a health insurance institution, both public and private. The role of the private sector is mostly providing consultation. Nearly all the costs of private health care services are covered directly by the patient.

National health care in Poland is organized on a multilevel basis. At the basic level, health care is regionalized and operates within the framework of four main specialties: internal medicine, pediatrics, gynecology-obstetrics, and surgery, as well as dentistry. The basic establishment is a Health Care Unit (HCU). One of its substructures is the Basic Health Care System with district health centers in towns, village and *gmina* health centers in rural areas, and a regional hospital. A village health center employs only a general practitioner, while a *gmina* (about 2,300 in Poland) center also has a gynecological unit and employs pediatricians and surgeons. Another structure within the HCU is the Specialized Health Care System, which also functions on the basis of the four main specialties through a network of specialized outpatient facilities and hospitals. Basic-level health care also includes emergency aid, usually an ambulance service, or the admission room and emergency ward at the hospital. The *voivodship* level (49 *voivodships* in Poland) comprises a multidepartmental *voivodship* general hospital with specialized clinics and departments, *voivodship* specialized hospitals (e.g., providing psychiatric care or rehabilitation services), and specialized HCUs with clinics and hospitals (oncology, psychiatry, mother and child care). Apart from providing treatment, organizing prevention activities, professional training, and consultations, they are also concerned with monitoring prevention and treatment programs being implemented by the HCUs. The next level of health care organizations are regions encompassing a few *voivodships*. Poland is divided into 11 regions, each with a Medical Academy. Medical Academies provide specialized high-level diagnostic services for the home and neighboring *voivodships*. The academies have their own hospitals with outpatient clinics. Apart from the primary tasks (treatment, diagnosis, and consultation), they also carry out research, teach students, and offer specialist monitoring. The national level is represented by specialized institutions that offer research and services and deal with specific health issues, receiving patients from all over the country. These include National Research Institutes run by the Ministry of Health concerned with tuberculosis, oncology, cardiology, occupational medicine, mother and child care, and others. Apart from diagnosis, treatment, consultation, and professional training, they are also obliged to carry out scientific research in order to develop system solutions for a given public health issue. A separate part of the structure of health care in Poland is the sanitation-epidemiology (S&E) service with its rigid hierarchy. It is concerned with threats to public health. S&E workers constantly monitor the working and living conditions of the population. A regional S&E inspector, the head of a regional S&E station, controls the area managed by one HCU. A higher level in the hierarchy is the *voivodship* S&E inspector who executes his duties through a *voivodship* S&E station. The superior position is occupied by the chief sanitation inspector of the country, who is also a vice minister of health.

In 1994, there were 118 persons per hospital bed and 464 persons per one physician in Poland.

Public and Private Health Insurance

Until the present times, the mid-1990s, there has been no health insurance system, either private or public, set up in Poland. The constitutional law giving the whole population free access to medical service financed by the state is still in force. Owing to political reasons, it is difficult to introduce a new system of financing into the health sector. The population is not inclined to lose its free access to medical services. Political parties procrastinate making a decision and bringing in a new system of financing for the health sector. This situation lies in the way of making the system of financing health care more rational. The entire national health service, including a vast majority of the medical services offered, is financed by the state. However, nearly all drug sales have been managed by private companies since 1990. The costs of medication are covered by the state only partly and in the case of certain diseases. It is estimated that now in the mid-1990s about 40 percent of the costs are covered directly by patients. At the same time, taxpayers have to cover the costs of medical services that are becoming more and more expensive. Moreover, a portion of the national health service staff are probably additionally "financed" by their patients. Many patients seek medical consultation in private facilities and pay for it themselves.

Health Care Financing

The national health care system is financed from the state budget. The means are allocated according to the rules of subject financing (i.e., among health institutions rather than tasks). At the *voivodship* level, basic-level establishments (HCUs) and *voivodship*-level institutions (*voivodship* hospitals and specialized HCUs) are financed from local budgets. The central budget of the Ministry of Health and Social Welfare provides funds for institutions subject directly to the Minister of Health, that is, the medical schools, Central Medical Library, the Center for Organization and Economics of Health Care, and others. National Research Institutes of the Ministry of Health have their clinical tasks covered by the state budget, while their scientific tasks are financed by grants from the Committee for Scientific Research. In the future, health service will be financed partly by the state, partly by local governments, and partly by the health insurance fund to be set up. The reform being prepared enumerates two aspects of financial relations between basic and specialized health care. Financial means will directly "follow" the patient and be transferred from the basic-level institution to an outpatient (ambulatory) special care unit or hospital. The transfer of means is determined by the services administered to the patient. Indirect transfer of means will be carried out by the institutions in charge of public finances who will allocate the means among the various levels of health care and the tasks they fulfill and will also monitor their expenditure.

Relation Between Ambulatory and Hospital Health Care

The relations between ambulatory and stationary health care are bidirectional. A general practitioner (GP) or a specialist at the basic level sends the patient to a hospital where patients who cannot be cured on an ambulatory basis receive further treatment. Patients may be admitted to the regional hospital, to a special hospital, to a hospital run by the Ministry of Health, or to the polyclinic of the relevant Medical Academy. Sometimes the patient is sent to a hospital to have a diagnostic test as requested by his physician in an ambulatory health care institution who is not able to perform the test owing to technical difficulties. Ambulatory health service also provides continuation of treatment and/or care for formerly hospitalized persons. The patient's information card contains recommendations for further treatment and rehabilitation aimed at the restoration of mental and physical capacities in people who have overcome the disease process. The distortion of relations between basic and hospital health care are illustrated not only by the distribution of expenditure (20 versus 80 percent) but also by proportions of employees. Only 14 percent of physicians out of the total number of 80,000 professionals work in basic health care institutions. The institutions are also poorly equipped. The staff has a low professional prestige and is poorly paid. A reform of these relations has been theoretically planned since 1989.

Preventive Health Care

In the postwar period, preventive health care has been substantially developed. Particular progress has been noted in infectious disease prevention and control, mother and child care, and occupational medicine. The efficacy of the prevention system in postwar Poland is illustrated by the success in bringing infectious diseases under control, constant reductions in infant mortality (also after 1989), and constant reductions in child and teenage mortality (also after 1989). The system of infectious disease prevention and control and mother and child care was not abandoned after 1989. It still works well. Unfortunately, owing to financial difficulties, the degree of penetration of schools by medical professionals has been reduced after 1989. The most significant changes after 1989 are seen in occupational medicine. With the transfer of ownership into private hands, a large proportion of workplace-based health care establishments have been closed down.

Prevention in the patient-physician relation is generally initiated in basic health care institutions. The duties of basic health care include preventive vaccinations, yearly screening chest X rays, early detection of abnormalities, and active care for infants starting from the sixth week of life as well as the more theoretical tasks of health education and popularization of a healthy lifestyle. Research shows that physicians do not attach importance to educating their patients about the prevention of diseases that are the major causes of deaths. The theoretical knowledge of the methods of cardiovascular disease prevention is not fully utilized by medical professionals in their everyday work. Screening blood pressure measurements, giving advice about healthy eating, encouraging patients to exercise, expressing a negative attitude toward tobacco smoking (about 10 percent of physicians smoke when giving advice), and informing patients about the importance of chest X rays should be the main forms of preventive actions undertaken by physicians in basic health care institutions.

Rehabilitation Service

The rehabilitation process is implemented in two planes: medical rehabilitation and social rehabilitation. It takes place at hospitals, sanitoria, and outpatient institutions. According to a 1994 report by the Social Aspects of Disability Research Group of the Polish Academy of Sciences, there are more than 4.5 million disabled people in Poland. The number rose from 1989 to 1993 by more than 800,000 due to the aging of the society, lowering of health service standard, successful groundless disability claims, and the introduction of an insurance system for farmers. The lack of infrastructure for the disabled and the fact that they are not fully accepted by society, which leads to more difficult access to education (about 60 percent of the disabled complete primary education only, compared to about 3 percent completing university studies), indicates a low level of prosociety education in Poland.

There are a large number of social organizations in Poland that help the disabled, including the Polish Red Cross, the Polish Committee for Social Help, and others. The task of occupational rehabilitation is carried out by the State Insurance Institution, which runs occupational rehabilitation centers; offers training and creates workplaces for the disabled; and produces prostheses, orthopedic devices, and rehabilitation equipment. The number of persons treated at rehabilitation departments in 1993 was 55,000. The number of hospital beds at these departments was 5,700. The rehabilitation departments employed 460 physicians. There were 32 rehabilitation sanitoria and 28 drug addict treatment centers.

Public Health Services

After the war an extensive and quite effective system of S&E services, based on the Soviet model, was introduced in Poland. Its main task was infectious disease prevention and control. In the early 1990s, there are about 500 S&E stations in Poland employing about 22,000 people. The State Sanitation Inspection (SSI) is the basic institution set up to control hygiene in the environment, at work, at schools, and at other educational institutions as well as recreation centers. Its tasks include the protection of human health from noxious factors and prevention of infectious diseases. The SSI performs preventive sanitation control by evaluating projects from the viewpoint of health and hygiene and supervising the implementation of hygiene and health regulations. It also performs ongoing monitoring by controlling the implementation of the principals of hygiene—in the environment, homes, companies, and other institutions, the production process, transport, food merchandising, and storage.

The SSI also carries out epidemiological analyses and evaluations, controls preventive vaccinations, and organizes sanitary protection of the country borders. These tasks are still adequately fulfillled. Some time ago, S&E services took on health education tasks, giving advice and information concerning the prevention and elimination of the noxious influence of physical, biological, and chemical factors and phenomena on human health and popularizing the principles of hygiene, healthy eating, and methods of disease prevention.

In view of the growing excess mortality of middle-aged Polish men, a National Health Program (NHP) was developed, based on World Health Organization (WHO) standards. The program was approved by the first Polish government appointed after independence was regained. The NHP is the first and only document concerned with health promotion and protection on a national scale. The basic premise is that each citizen is also responsible for his/her health, and the state is obliged to create conditions conducive to maintaining and strengthening health. NHP's strategic aim is to stop the increase in, and subsequently reduce the prevalence of, noxious factors and the most important diseases from the viewpoint of their health and social outcome. The health aims of the NHP include reversing the increase in cardiovascular mortality; reversing the increase in cancer mortality, particularly lung cancer; lowering the incidence of traumas and cases of intoxication and reducing postaccident mortality; lowering the incidence of mental disorders and improving the quality of mental health; reducing the prevalence of preventable infectious diseases and also of other diseases related to noxious factors in working and living environments; reducing the incidence of premature births and low birth weight as well as reducing infant mortality; reducing the incidence of disability and making life less burdensome for the disabled; and lowering the intensity of caries in children and teenagers. Unfortunately, due to a lack of funds, the program is being implemented only partially.

Self-Help Organizations

There are 875 charity organizations (including merely 38 supported by the government) in Poland concerned with prevention, rehabilitation, social help, and self-help. They concentrate on specific social groups (disabled children and adults, human immunodeficiency virus (HIV) carriers, drug users, the terminally ill) and differ in the scope of action (the whole Poland, one *voivodship*, a town or a district, quite often one hospital). Their main aims include helping the families of the sick and handicapped, also acting as their representatives; disease-specific training and counseling (e.g., Polish Alzheimer's Disease Foundation); financing research, collecting disease-specific scientific information; financing hospital care, medication, equipment for diagnosis and rehabilitation; maintaining rehabilitation facilities and other institutions; setting up hospices, oncological pharmacies; and organizing home help for the terminally ill.

Set up in 1919, the Polish Red Cross is the most numerous charity with its 2 million members. Their duties include helping the sick at home; running social help institutions; providing financial help and food for the poor; helping refugees and foreigners; spreading health messages; and organizing first-aid courses. The Monar (400 members) runs 18 rehabilitation-adaptation centers for drug users and patients with other addictions as well as for HIV carriers, an ambulance service, and a detoxification facility. ''Amazonki'' Mastectomy Patients Club (200 members) provides psychological support to women prior to and after breast cancer therapy.

Accessibility and Equality of Service

Poland is a country with a high ratio of medical professionals and health care institutions to the number of citizens. Theoretically, there is full access to and equality in health care. Unfortunately, the unclear system of health care financing, badly organized and not suitable to the new economic reality after 1989, is a major obstacle. On the other hand, medical statistics show that despite the limitations, and difficulties, the level of health service is similar to the one theoretically possible for the current level of economic development in Poland.

THE INFRASTRUCTURE OF TRAINING AND RESEARCH IN PUBLIC HEALTH

Graduate Training

Secondary schools include medical schools whose graduates may attend post-secondary colleges or Medical Academies. There are 12 Medical Academies in Poland including 1 run by the army. The academies have the following departments: General Medicine, Dentistry (not in Bydgoszcz), Pharmacy, and Nurse Training (Katowice, Krakow, Lublin, Poznan, Wroclaw). Students of General Medicine have classes at polyclinics and institutes (clinical and theoretical training) as well as in laboratories. The university curriculum includes internships during holidays, also abroad. The curriculum is prepared by the academies (boards of departments). A specified number of hours for obligatory training are mandatory for every academy; for example, students at a General Medicine Department have 5,500 hours of classes including 4,050 hours of obligatory training, 700 hours of practical training, and the rest (750 hours) to be decided upon by the academy authorities. Medical Academies are subject to the Ministry of Education, while the medical activities are supervised by the Ministry of Health and Social Welfare. Nearly 33,000 students attended Medical Academies in the academic year 1993–1994 (the figure for 1990–1991 was 38,000 students). There were nearly 6,400 graduates in 1993, compared to over 5,000 in 1990. The greatest numbers of students (about 4,600) and graduates (about 1,000) were noted for the Silesian Medical Academy; the lowest, in Bydgoszcz (1,000 students and 160 graduates). As for teachers, there were 9,011 in 1993, including 1,190 professors.

Postgraduate Training

The following forms of further education are available for graduates of Medical Academies in Poland: postgraduate internships (supervised by Medical Chambers) and grade I and II specialization and superspecialization training (internships and certificate training courses); postgraduate training courses at the Center for Postgraduate Medical Training; and medical libraries.

Two Public Health Schools have been set up in Poland since 1989, but their scope and potential are still difficult to evaluate.

Scientific Research

Academy polyclinics provide medical care, offer classes for students, and carry out research. There are also other (nonclinical) scientific establishments at Medical Academies. Research tasks in the biomedical sciences are also carried out by scientific research institutes run by the Ministry of Health and specialized scientific institutions of the Polish Academy of Sciences. The Committee for Scientific Research also has a medical science section. Money for research comes also from foreign grants. The number of medical research institutions has increased from 23 (1990) to 26 (1993), but the number of employees has fallen—more than 4,100 (1990), more than 3,600 (1993). More than 650 people received scientific degrees in medical sciences in 1993, compared with about 850 in 1990. The number of postgraduate and Ph.D. students at the Academies has risen from 212 (1990) to 506 (1993). The attendance at the Center for Postgraduate Medical Training was about 15,000 in 1990 and more than 20,000 in 1993.

MAJOR CHALLENGES FOR THE HEALTH SERVICES

In Poland and other new central European democracies that were controlled by the Soviet Union from the end of World War II till 1990, health is one of the major civilizational challenges in their return to Europe. A demographic catastrophe has been taking place in this part of Europe. Despite the doctrine-related free medical service that was available to the society for 40 years, central and eastern European countries have witnessed a rise in the premature mortality of middle-aged men (35–59) that has not been recorded in any other part of the world (Murray and Lopez 1994). The chances of a 15-year-old boy living in a central or eastern European country surviving until the age of 60 are twice as low in comparison with western Europe and North America and worse than in a majority of developing countries including China, Latin America, or even India. Only the male population of sub-Saharan Africa has a higher premature death rate at the middle age (Murray and Lopez, 1994). The increasing trend in premature mortality in men from central European countries (Czechoslovakia, Hungary, Poland) started around 1960 to 1965. It had been preceded by a remarkable success in combating infectious diseases and a dramatic fall in infant mortality in this part of the world in the years from 1945 to 1960 (Zatoński 1994). The epidemic of chronic diseases (myocardial infarct, lung cancer) that has been spreading since the mid-1960s was mostly due to lack of access to and understanding of the achievements of the medical sciences, political control of the development of epidemiology, concealment of statistical data, unavailability of modern technology (computers), and lack of communication (mass media) between the scientific community and politicians and the public. As a result, contemporary methods of epidemiological analysis, including the application of modern computer-aided methods of disease monitoring—the key to understanding the situation and preparing modern remedy programs—could not be developed in this part of the world until the early 1990s.

The development of modern public health policy (not only curative medicine) in this part of the world is all the more important as it is unlikely that economic growth itself can effect improvement of the health status in these countries. More and more data show that above a certain level, the gross national product (GNP) is weakly related to the health status. The postcommunist countries may serve as a good example, as the lowest premature mortality in adult men is observed in Albania—the least economically developed country in the region (a World Bank estimate sets the risk of dying between the ages of 15 and 59 years in Albania at 14.2 percent; in former Czechoslovakia, 22.8 percent; Poland, 25.0 percent; and Hungary, 27.7 percent) (Feachem et al. 1992).

Poland and other eastern European countries are examples of the results of the lack of a modern public health policy. The results can be seen in chronic man-made diseases in the middle-age population, especially male. Since the end of the war, the Polish state has pursued a protective policy toward alcohol and tobacco. Tobacco consumption has kept Poland among the "world leaders" for the last 20 years. In 1974 the percentage of men who had never smoked was 18 percent. Cigarettes contained on average 25 to 30 milligrams of tar and 2.0 to 2.5 milligrams of nicotine. Most cigarettes sold did not have filters (Zatoński and Przewozniak 1992). Hence, at the beginning of the 1990s, more than 40 percent of deaths in men aged 35 to 69 are attributable to tobacco smoking (Peto et al. 1992). Similarly, alcohol consumption has been increasing steadily in the postwar period (Sieroslawski 1992). Apart from alcohol's role in the etiology of some chronic diseases, it is probably responsible for a considerable part of sudden deaths caused by external factors. The Polish diet is characterized by high caloric content, high animal fat content, and low levels of seasonal consumption of fresh fruit and vegetables. Apart from lifestyle-related factors, other factors such as occupational exposure at work (obsolete, unsafe technologies and working conditions) and environmental pollution potentially contribute to the increase in mortality in the adult population. The attributed risk linked to environmental pollution seems to be generally overestimated. Environmental pollution does not appear to be an important risk factor in cardiovascular diseases or to be responsible for sudden deaths caused by external factors. According to epidemiological research, environmental pollution is likely to exert a small impact on cancer mortality in Poland (similarly to other central European countries) (Zatoñski et al. 1995). Epidemiological observations in Poland show that only a small fraction of cancers is attributable to pollution. The attributed lung cancer mortality risk of air pollution is estimated to be 5 to 9 percent (Jêdrychowski et al. 1990).

Analysis of the development of public health problems in eastern Europe is also important for the development of ideas for public health. It is commonly known that health is influenced by three main external elements: lifestyle, broadly defined working and living environment, and health care organization. Although this thesis has been universally accepted in theory, the emphasis in efforts to improve health is placed on the development of curative medicine and on treating illnesses that already manifest. The fact that health service alone is able to secure good health for the nation to a limited extent only is best illustrated by analysis of mortality trends in Poland and other eastern European countries (Zatoñski 1994). In the period when the number of medical professionals, beds in hospitals, the accessibility of curative medicine, and new treatment techniques were constantly growing (1960–1980), these countries experienced growing mortality in middle-aged men on a scale unprecedented in the history of man in times of peace. The increase in mortality is mainly due to an epidemic of chronic diseases. With a lack of a comprehensive public health policy, the dramatic yearly increases in chronic disease incidence in middle age have made it impossible to guarantee good health care for the entire population. The number of new cases has been growing more rapidly than health service capacity, resulting in health service professionals and their patients becoming more and more frustrated. It is connected with the need for more and more financial means and a lower standard of service due to the increased number of patients. Treatment techniques are designed to repair bad health and have little to do with risk factors—the causes of diseases, especially chronic ones, that are substantially man-made. The causes of premature mortality, resulting from tobacco smoking, alcohol consumption, eating too much food rich in animal fats and only limited amounts of fresh fruit and vegetables, obesity, little physical activity, and possibly some psychological and social factors, cannot be conquered by treatment techniques offered by curative medicine.

Like the developed European countries, Poland needs a multifactorial health program to overcome its health crisis. This program, just like the one implemented in Finland in the early 1960s, should combine diverse elements of the government public health policy, antipromotion policy on tobacco and alcohol, nutrition policy based on scientific findings, better safety on roads, health education, the development of sports, and the well-oriented activities of curative medicine.

REFERENCES

Feachem, R., Kjellstrom, T., Murray, C., Over, M. & Phillips, M. (Eds.). (1992). *The Health of Adults in the Developing World.* Oxford University Press: World Bank.

Jêdrychowski, W., Becher, H., Wahrendorf, J. & Basa-Cierpalek, Z. (1990). A case-control study of lung cancer with special reference to the effect of air pollution in Poland. *Journal of Epidemiology and Community Health,* 15, 213–224.

Kupsc, W. & Jasiñski, B. (1991). *Sytuacja epidemiologiczna w zakresie chorób ukladu krazenia w Polsce I–IV* (Cardiovascular diseases in Poland—an epidemiological approach). Instytut Kardiologii.

Magdzik, W. & Czarkowski, M. (1994). Choroby zakazne w Polsce w 1992 roku (Infectious diseases in Poland in 1992). *Przeglad Epidemiologiczny,* 47, 1–2, 45–48.

Murray, C. & Lopez A. (1994). Global and regional cause-of-death patterns in 1990. *Bulletin of the World Health Organization* (Geneva), 72(3), 447–480.

Peto, R., Lopez, A., Boreham, J., Thun, M. & Heath, C., Jr. (1992). Mortality from tobacco in developed countries: indirect estimates from national vital statistics. *Lancet,* 339, 1268–1278.

Sieroslawski, J. (1992). *Spozycie alkoholu i polityka wobec alkoholu w ocenie spolecznej. Raport z badañ ankietowych* (Public opinion view on alcohol consumption and alcohol policy. A public opinion poll report). Warsaw: Instytut Psychiatrii i Neurologii (Psychiatry and Neurology Institute).

Zatoñski, W. (1994). *Stan zdrowia Polaków* (The health of Polish population). Medycyna po Dyplomie (Postgraduate Medicine, Polish version). Vol. 3. Warsaw: Ariel.

Zatoñski, W. & Becker, N. (in collaboration with Gottesman, K., Mykowiecka, A. & Tyczynski, J.). (1988). *Atlas of Cancer Mortality in Poland, 1975–1979.* New York, Springer-Verlag.

Zatoñski, W. & Przewozniak, K. (Eds.). (1992). *Zdrowotne nastêpstwa palenia tytoniu w Polsce* (Health consequences of tobacco smoking in Poland). Warsaw: Ariel.

Zatoñski, W., Pukkala, E., Didkowska, J., Tyczynski, J. & Gustavsson, N. (1993). *Atlas of Cancer Mortality in Poland, 1986-1990.* Warsaw: Interspar.

Zatoñski, W., Smans, M., Tyczynski, J. & Boyle, P. (Eds.). (1995). *Atlas of Cancer Mortality in Central Europe.* Lyon: IARC Scientific Publications no. 134.

RUSSIA

Valery E. Tchernjavsky

MAJOR HEALTH PROBLEMS FACING THE COUNTRY

The Russian Federation is one of the largest countries in the world. It stretches from the Baltic Sea in the west to the Pacific Ocean in the east. It occupies a total area of 17,075,400 square kilometers. The country covers several climatic regions, from polar in the north, through subarctic and humid continental to subtropical in the south. The Russian Federation has a population of 148,325,600 and consists of Russia and 17 autonomous republics (Bashkir, Buryat, Chechnja, Ingushetija, Chuvash, Dagestan, Kabardino-Balkar, Kalmyk, Karelia, Komi, Mari-El, Mordovia, North Osetia, Tatarstan, Tuva, Udmurt, and Yakut).

The health status of the people of the Russian Federation has been declining in past years. Since 1985 the number of births in Russia has dropped by 33.2 percent. The 1992 fertility rate was 10.7 per 1,000 population, 35.5 percent less than in 1985. The population of the Russian Federation has decreased by 1.5 percent since 1991. Life expectancy at birth dropped from 69.2 years in 1990 to 67.5 years in 1992, while life expectancy for urban males decreased by 2.8 percent. In Russia the maximum level of life expectancy in 1986 was 66.6 years for males (Figure 1) and in 1988 was 76.6 years for females (Figure 2). This indicator in Russia, in the sixties, was appreciably below those in Western countries, but for the first time in the last decade, this parameter has not reached 60 years for males. On the other hand, it is impossible not to notice an increasing gap between male and female life expectancy. In 1993, it has reached almost 13 years.

Prior to 1985, maternal mortality was calculated per 10,000 childbirths with at least 28 weeks of pregnancy, so that later data are not comparable. Since

1985 the maternal death rate has dropped by 5.9 percent. The 1992 infant mortality rate was 18 per 1,000 live births—3.4 percent up from 1990.

Since 1980 the official neonatal mortality rate has risen by 25 percent in Russia as a whole and by 88.5 percent in its rural areas. Early neonatal mortality rates have increased by 32.4 percent and more than twice, respectively. This phenomenon may be due to inaccurate reporting of neonatal deaths in the 1980s. Since 1971 the general death rate of the Russian population has gone up by 41.7 percent, and the age-adjusted rate (European standard), by 10.5 percent. The higher age-adjusted rate is due to an increased rural death rate in the 55–64 age group. Since 1985 in the 15–24 age group, the death rate for urban adolescents and young adults has grown by 34.8 percent, with a 51.9 percent increase in the death rate for urban young females.

Between 1990 and 1992 the death rate for children (aged 1 to 14 years) went up by 3.2 percent; for adolescents and young adults (15 to 24 years), by 17.5 percent, and for adults (25 to 64 years), by 14.6 percent. The highest increase in the death rate (23.6 percent) was registered among 15- to 24-year-old men in the cities as compared to a 4 percent decrease in the death rate for 1- to 14-year-old women in the villages.

Since 1981, there has been a 12.6 percent increase in the age-adjusted death rate for most causes; the highest increase (31.5 percent) has been registered in deaths from malignant neoplasms (Table 1). Table 1 shows all age-adjusted death rates for selected causes of death.

Since 1990 the homicide rate has soared by 60.3 percent, and deaths due to traffic accidents, by 31.4 percent. Plummeting standards of living, soaring rates of unemployment, and other social problems ranging from rising divorce rates to worsening alcoholism are all contributing to a disturbing new trend in Russia: rising rates of suicide. If 1992 saw a shocking number of suicides with over 46,000 reported instances, then 1993 was even worse with 53,000 taking their own lives. The 1993 figure translates into 38.0 per 100,000 (in 1992 it was 26.5). For comparison, the figure for England in 1993 was 9.0 per 100,000. Suicide levels were greater in regions of Russia with more acute drops in standards of living and higher rates of unemployment, divorce, and alcoholism. The northern regions of Russia, the Urals, and eastern Siberia witnessed up to 50.0 suicides per 100,000.

Since 1985 the morbidity rate for salmonellosis, pediculosis, scabies, Russian spring-summer encephalitis, and diphtheria has increased by 150 to 250 percent. The decreased official rate for viral hepatitis is attributable to inadequate statistical reporting of morbidity, particularly in the case of types C and D. Since 1990 there has been an increase in follow-up cases of syphilis, gonorrhea, psychic disorders, and narcotic and other drug abuse registered with health and preventive care institutions and a decrease in the number of follow-up tuberculosis (TB) patients. In connection with the introduction of new legislation on psychiatry providing for strictly voluntary resort to specialized medical aid and a transition to anonymous statistical registration of so-called borderline cases,

Figure 1
Life Expectancy at Birth for Men in Russia and Some European Countries, 1958–1993

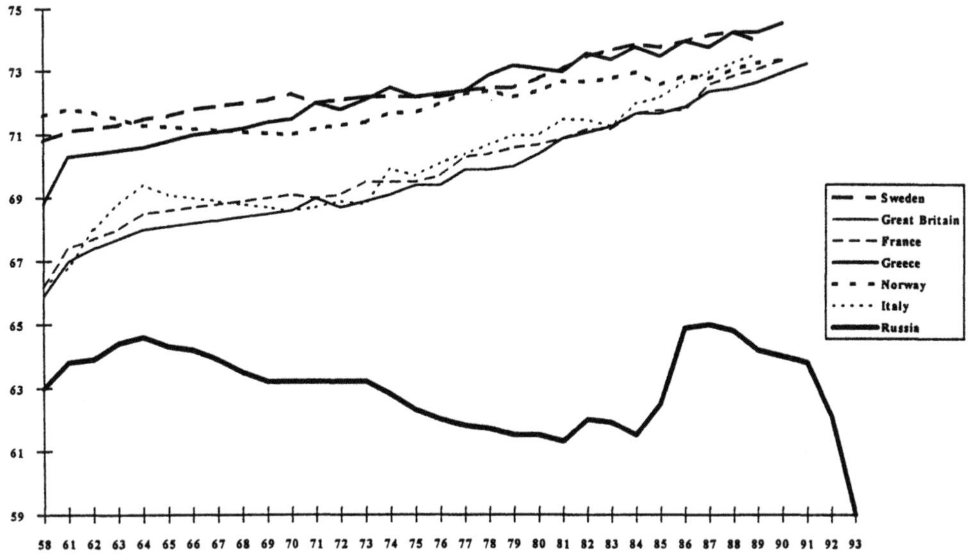

Source: National Center for Health Statistics 1995; Tchernjavsky 1994.

Figure 2
Life Expectancy at Birth for Women in Russia and Some European Countries, 1958–1993

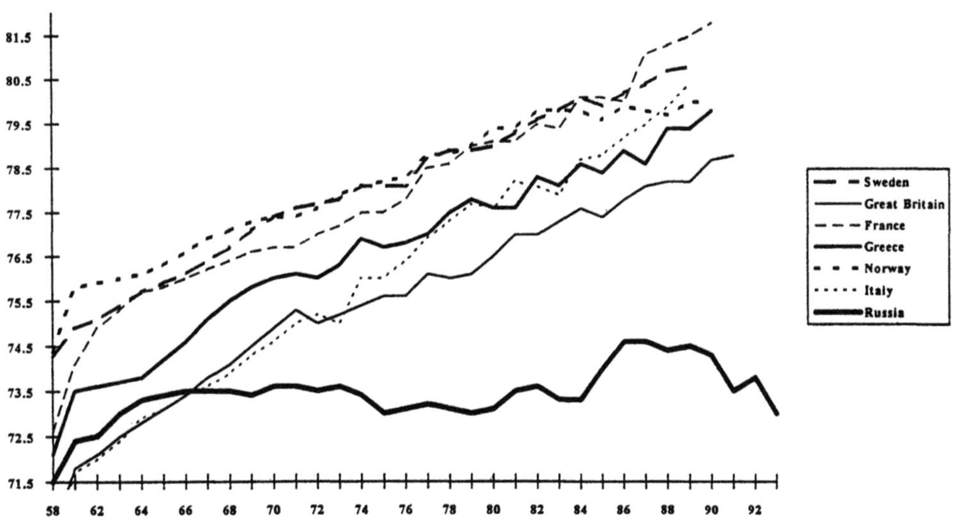

Source: National Center for Health Statistics 1995; Tchernjavsky 1994.

Table 1
Age-Adjusted Death Rates for Selected Causes of Death, by Sex: Russian Federation, Selected Years 1981–1993

Sex and cause of death[1]	*1981*	*1991*	*1993*
	Deaths per 100,000 population		
All causes			
Total	1,233.9	1,198.1	1,474.5
Male	1,821.0	1,699.0	2,128.0
Female	903.9	889.6	1,041.0
Diseases of the heart (390–398, 401–429)			
Total	389.4	332.5	401.9
Male	540.3	467.4	576.2
Female	315.8	256.1	296.4
Cerebrovascular diseases (430–438)			
Total	245.9	242.2	277.6
Male	297.9	282.3	328.7
Female	222.8	221.0	248.5
Malignant neoplasms (140–208)			
Total	151.6	197.6	207.8
Male	264.3	309.5	322.4
Female	96.5	136.9	143.2
Malignant neoplasms of the respiratory system (160–165)			
Total	39.3	50.4	51.5
Male	95.8	116.9	117.6
Female	10.1	11.5	11.6
Malignant neoplasms of the breast (174)			
Female	14.2	19.8	21.4
Pneumonia and influenza (480–483, 485–487)			
Total	13.4	7.2	15.4

Male	21.6	11.8	27.1
Female	8.3	4.2	6.8
Chronic obstructive pulmonary diseases (490–496)			
Total	28.5	33.0	39.5
Male	49.4	64.7	78.6
Female	20.0	18.9	20.8
Chronic liver diseases and cirrhosis (571.0–571.3, 571.5, 571.6)			
Total	12.4	14.0	18.6
Male	20.3	19.6	25.8
Female	7.8	10.7	13.9
Motor vehicle accidents (E810–E825)			
Total	---	25.8	25.0
Male	---	42.6	40.7
Female	---	10.8	11.0
Suicide (E950–E959)			
Total	---	26.9	38.0
Male	---	47.6	68.9
Female	---	10.1	12.1
Homicide and legal intervention (E960–E978)			
Total	---	15.1	29.7
Male	---	24.1	47.5
Female	---	6.7	13.2
Other external causes (E800–E807, E826–E949, E980–E999)			
Total	---	74.8	133.0
Male	---	126.6	221.7
Female	---	29.5	52.8

[1]Cause of death codes are from the *International Classification of Diseases, Ninth Revision.*

Note: Age adjusted using as standard population the European standard 100,000 population prepared by the World Health Organization.

Source: National Center for Health Statistics 1995.

the number of follow-up cases of alcoholism and alcoholic psychoses has tended to decrease on a short-term basis. Since 1990 the morbidity rate for female syphilis has soared by 160 percent and for male gonorrhea, by 40 percent. The rate of human immunodeficiency virus (HIV) infection and morbidity has declined due to the fact that there have been no more cases of large-scale HIV infection in health centers in the last few years.

PROVISION, UTILIZATION, AND IMPACT OF HEALTH SERVICES

Health Care Delivery System

There are three main levels of health care delivery system in Russia:

- Primary care is presented in rural areas by feldsher-midwife stations with nursing personnel, rural doctors' ambulatories, and district and central district hospitals (polyclinics departments). For urban areas, polyclinics are the main health institutions of primary health care.
- Secondary care is presented by different kinds of hospitals: central *rayon* (district) hospitals and *oblast* (provincial) hospitals. In addition to the above, there are also specialized hospitals affiliated with large industrial enterprises and the particular ministries, providing services for respective employees and their families.
- Tertiary care is the most complex care and is offered at large and highly specialized hospitals associated with research institutions in the respective fields. Since 1990 the number of physicians per 10,000 population has declined by 4.7 percent and that of nursing personnel, by 7.5 percent, with a marked drop in the number of feldshers (a type of nursing personnel in Russia) (by 19.4 percent) and midwives (19.7 percent) (Table 2).

Since 1990 the number of hospital beds per 10,000 population has declined by 4.8 percent primarily due to a reduction in the number of specialized beds: by 38.8 percent for drug patients, 20 percent for infants, 7.9 percent for orthopedic patients, 6.4 percent for patients with infectious diseases, and 6.1 percent for TB patients. This group has declined by 13.8 percent since 1990, when it accounted for 16.2 percent of the total number of hospital beds. Since 1990 the number of residents per physician has grown by 7 percent, and per hospital bed, by 5.2 percent. Since 1985 the number of visits to physicians per resident has declined by 18.9 percent, and the number of persons given emergency medical aid in outpatient departments or at home, by 11.2 percent. Since 1985 the rate of inpatients (per 100 residents) has decreased by 17.6 percent. As a result, inpatient bed occupancy has declined by 9.9 percent, particularly in infectious disease hospitals for adults and children (by 19.1 percent and 13.8, percent respectively), maternity homes (18.5 percent), and psychiatric and psychoneurological hospitals (13.2 percent). The length of stay in hospitals has decreased

Table 2
Number of Providers per 10,000 Population, by Specialty

Provider type	*1985*	*1990*	*1991*	*1992*	*1993*
			Personnel per 10,000 population		
All physicians[1]	45.1	46.9	44.3	44.7	45
Family practice and internal medicine	10.8	11.5	11.1	11.3	11.4
Pediatrics[2]	22.9	24.5	23.3	23.5	22
Obstetrics and gynecology[3]	4.8	5.2	4.9	5	4.7
Surgery	4.7	5.6	5.2	5.3	5.4
Ophthalmology	0.9	1	1	1	0.9
Otolaryngology	0.8	0.8	0.8	0.8	0.8
Orthopedic surgery	---	---	---	---	---
Neurology	1.1	1.2	1.2	1.2	1.2
Psychiatry and narcology	1.2	1.5	1.3	1.4	1.3
Dentists	4.6	5.1	4.9	4.8	5.2
Nursing personnel, total	120.6	122.6	114.1	113.6	111.7
Physician assistants (feldshers)	26.5	27.9	23.8	22.5	20.3
Midwives	23.5	20.3	16.6	16.3	16.8
Nurses[4]	60.5	67.1	62.6	63.4	63.5
Laboratory assistants (feldshers-laborants)	4.7	5.7	5.9	4.9	6
X-ray technicians	1.5	1.9	1.7	1.7	1.5

[1]Includes dentists and both active and nonactive physicians who are not retired, residents and interns, sanitary-epidemiological doctors, dentists, and physiotherapists.

[2]Per 10,000 children.

[3]Per 10,000 females.

[4]"Nurses" refers to all types of nurses.

Source: National Center for Health Statistics 1995.

for World War II veterans and military servicemen (by an average of 21.7 percent) and for other patients in adult and children's infectious disease hospitals (12 to 13 percent), children's TB hospitals (11.7 percent), and regional, territorial, and republican adult hospitals (10.9 percent). The rate of patients who have had medical operations (per 1,000 population) has dropped by 19 percent.

So far in Russia, out-hospital care is provided by so-called polyclinics (outpatient clinics) that serve 60,000 to 80,000 people. They are staffed by district therapists or pediatricians and different specialists. They have relevant diagnostic and supporting services and equipment. Almost 86 percent of all patients receive complete examinations and treatment in the polyclinics. The creation of such primary care centers has been aimed at two goals: to make the primary care *acceptable* and *specialized.* But therein lies the contradiction: If care is widely acceptable, it cannot be specialized; on the other hand, specialized care cannot exist in the framework of primary health care.

To address this contradiction, it was necessary to redefine the stages of primary health care, and we came to the idea of the general practitioner (GP)/family doctor. It's interesting to note that before the Revolution of 1917 in Russia, there was a system of primary health—so-called *zemskaj medicina*—where the "*zemcki* doctor" actually was a GP. Unfortunately, later on this system was destroyed, and it is only now being restored in our time.

Role of Primary Health Care Personnel in Disease Prevention

The Public Health Institute in Moscow in collaboration with other research and training health institutions was designed as a special program of transition to the new system of primary health care adopted by the Ministry of Health and Medical Industry of Russia that is now in the process of implementation. This program contains the following parts:

1. Education and training—undergraduate and postgraduate training of GPs (necessary volume of knowledge, vocational program, requalification of district therapists and pediatricians, etc.). For regulation of doctors' and nurses' activities in the framework of general practice in 1992, Special Order 237 was prepared and approved by the Ministry of Health and Medical Industry of Russia and outlined educational programs for GPs, their rights, duties, responsibilities, and so on. According to this order, regional health bodies were beginning GP preparation in two ways: (1) undergraduate specialization for two to three years in basic medical education and (2) postgraduate training at the Medical Academies, institutes, and faculties of postgraduate training, large hospitals, and polyclinics. Highly qualified specialists with a lot of experience may train in personal programs. Questions of license distribution are under consideration.
2. Legislative support for GPs. Taking into consideration the particular role of the GP in primary health care, two special articles were entered into the Law on Health Care in Russia: One concerned primary health care; and the other, the general practitioner/family doctor.

3. Connection of GPs with the other specialists (for definition of medical technology standards).
4. GPs' quality assessment. The Donabedian approach is used here: structure standard (resource)—technology standard (process)—outcome standard.
5. Information system for GPs (information about patients, diagnostic services, specialists, pharmaceuticals, etc., and return information from medical doctors for statistical needs). A computing medical advice system should be designed on the basis of the experience of highly qualified experts in various spheres of science and practice.
6. Organization of nursing personnel work.
7. Organization of interaction with social services and community. In the frame of primary medical-social care, we consider as key directions the following:
   - Prevention of chronic noncommunicable diseases and formation of healthy lifestyles at the individual, family, and community levels.
   - Dynamic control of quality for preventive work.
   - Design and implementation of a complex of diagnostic-treatment and rehabilitation measures for patients with detected health disorders.

According to the proverb "Prevention is better than cure," our concept of preventive improvement suggests not only the future development of health services but also the GP's orientation toward personal preventive measures at the level of the family and encouraging healthy lifestyle. At present the rendering of primary medical-social care is provided by general practitioners/family doctors with special vocational training, practical nurses, and social workers. General practitioners/family doctors are responsible for providing medical services to all age groups, family planning (genetic family diseases, psychological, psychiatric, juridical, and other issues at the level of family), health education, and so on. Their psychological help may be demanded for solving individual problems of loneliness or family relationships in different periods of marriage. Legal aspects of their work consist of helping to set up pensions and benefits; protecting the rights of disabled people, pregnant women, and mothers with many children; and rendering opinions in cases of guardianship, care, and adoption. Among the duties of general practitioners/family doctors are certain preventive and sanitary-hygienic measures: doctor's and nurse's home visits; definition and struggle with personal health hazards (nutritional imbalance, alcohol abuse, smoking, physical inactivity, etc.), implantation of healthy lifestyle; detection and follow-up of families with risk factors; extending personal hygiene; dealing with problems of individual and community sanitation and hygiene.

The results of our investigations showed that preventive work consumed more than half of all GPs' time; yet even more prophylactic measures have been demanded during home visits. To alleviate this demand, nursing personnel should be more involved in preventive work with the local population.

General practitioners/family doctors have to define level and type of necessary medical-social help, register social risk factors in the family, provide help within their competence, attract resources from other health care services and local municipalities, and integrate all of this to promote family health. GPs have to pay more attention to juveniles, pregnant women, mothers with many children, elderly and aging people, persons at risk (industrial, social-hygenic, social-psychological), and drug and toxic abusers. Taking into account the magnitude of the GP's duties, it is very important to have reliable assistants and the co-operation of all member of the primary health care team: qualified general nurses, social workers, psychologists, and others.

Community Participation in the Organization of Health Care

It is widely known that one of the normal functions of primary health care is to draw individuals, families, groups, and local authorities into the planning and organization of primary medicosocial care. According to the conception of primary health care development adopted in Russia, it is necessary to radically change the direction of activity of the health institutions to provide not only preventive and curative (rehabilitation) care but also medicosocial and psychological care.

Reorganization of primary health care in Russia includes the creation of general practitioners who must solve a wide range of patient problems: medicosocial, psychotherapeutical, psychological, juridical, and so on. In this way, the complex problem of integrating the medical and social service of the patient may be solved. GPs, in their activity, closely collaborate with municipalities, social services, public education bodies, enterprises and offices where patients work, offices of trade, and living (home-aid) services. With GP recommendations, employers provide appropriate labor conditions for pregnant women, for persons with different chronic diseases, and for employees after traumas. There are prophylactic centers—so-called sanatorium-prophylactoriums of different types (gastroenterologic, cardiac, neurologic, etc.)—attached to industrial enterprises. In these prophylactic centers, patients receive treatment without being absent from work. Special groups of patients are formed by GPs to help lonely, aging people, disabled persons, chronic patients, mothers with many children, and so on.

In addition, these patients have access to trade offices (for food delivery), canteens (for delivery of semiready products, free-charge meals), and drugstores (for purchase and delivery of pharmaceuticals). Recently, different religious organizations have contributed to the organization of medicosocial help. They train home and hospital nurses and fund construction of hospitals and houses for the disabled and elderly. These services are rendered free of charge. At the same time, there are official service boards in many Russian cities that provide social and home help. The social service system also offers a wide spectrum of free services. Since 1987, Russia has set up regional centers for the social care of pensioners (medicosocial offices), intended for both full-time and temporary care (including payment) of the elderly and aging in hospitals, as well as at-home care. Regional social bodies are responsible and fund regional centers, but it is the general practitioners who refer patients to them.

The health care offices control quality assessment and the sanitary-epidemical situation at the regional centers. There are special committees for social help, charity, and philanthropy in the Russian Parliament and on the regional level. In recent years, a considerable volume of medical and social help was provided by the different charity funds, for example, the whole net of organizations and offices under the auspices of the Fund of Charity and Health. Funds of this kind are found in almost all Russian regions and of course in Moscow and St. Petersburg. In addition, there is an international fund that includes the funds of all the countries of the former USSR. Fund activities are very variable. Among them are providing constant and urgent social help; building houses for disabled and elderly people; constructing disabled vehicles plants, orphanages, and boardinghouses; providing special programs such as those for oncological patients and the program "Anti-AIDS"; helping families with a disabled child; distributing foreign humanitarian aid; and supporting everyday philanthropic cultural help (concerts, performances). The funds are subsidized through the assignment of large-enterprise profits and different voluntary donations. They have close contact with religious institutions in Russian and certainly with regional health care bodies and offices.

THE INFRASTRUCTURE OF TRAINING AND RESEARCH IN PUBLIC HEALTH

In spite of many circumstances, the years 1992–1994 saw increasing research in different areas of public health and increasing support for the policy and practice of health care reforms in the Russian Federation. Many institutions, centers, and departments operate in the area of public health research in Russia: the Public Health Institute "MedSocEconomInform"; Semachko Research Institute on Social Medicine; and more than 80 chairs and Departments of Social Medicine and Health at medical universities, medical academies, and medical institutes.

MedSocEconomInform, as the National Coordinational Center of Social Hygiene, Health Care Organization and Health Informatics in Russia, was set up in 1991 for research and management of Russian public health research databases. This database consists of 61 topics of research on public health, such as health policy and strategy (health legislation, national and regional health care reform, primary health care, hospital care); health economics (health insurance schemes); quality assurance; investigation and monitoring of health status of different groups of the population; mortality and morbidity; and social-hygiene problems of the population (alcohol and drug abuse, smoking, stresses, conditions of work). One important problem of fundamental and applied research is achieving international cooperation in this field because the area of public health and health protection is so vast. In light of cuts in government subsidies and the downturn in the number of commissions received from the Ministry of Health, the approach in 1992–1994 was more strongly market oriented.

The additional efforts put into establishing new relations, and aimed at private sector interest in research, produced satisfactory results. Our informational computer system organizes public health research, providing an overview of the country's overall scientific progress, as it tracks data on scientific teams, their provision of resources, and activities in all the various fields of public health.

The database promotes, on one hand, the development of science and, on the other, better implementation of scientific results. This system, based on Russian environmental data, has six components: (1) to input the basic, raw scientific data; (2) to include data on the criteria of quality with proper explanations, indexes, gradations, and so on; (3) to propose models and algorithms that include standards of quality on scientific research; (4) to formulate and explain appropriate recommendations (approve, finish off, decline) based on generalized indexes; (5) to choose and to monitor every unit of information from the whole database; and (6) to analyze and generalize expert input.

This system is used within national programs and for monitoring the realization of separate tasks and projects. MedSocEconomInform carries out research with these mentioned goals in mind. Classification of regions in Russia was performed on the basis of mortality rates (including those due to noncommunicable diseases) and life span. To analyze the health status of the population, the following parameters were calculated: average age of death due to basic causes (cardiovascular, oncological, respiratory, digestive and infectious diseases, accidents, poisonings, injuries) as well as "nonsurvived" person-years of expected life span related to early death from these diseases. The "Medical & Demographical Situation Description in Russia" was prepared considering the above classification. Investigation was performed to assess mathematical and statistical models of environmental factors' impact on birthrate mortality and morbidity rates, and the like, based on specific computer algorithms of quantitative evaluation of endogenic and exogenic components of these processes.

On the basis of losses in the working-age potential of the Russian population due to early death (using a new approach combining a cohort concept of population and methods of potential demography), the top priority directions were established in the development and introduction of health care programs on different levels of management, including priorities in the formation of programs aimed at reduction of basic noncommunicable diseases. Calculation of parameters was performed on the basis of a set of application programs. "Demometrics" were used for calculation of parameters characterizing the survival of the population under study as well as prognostic assessment of the age and sex ratios of the population. "Demometric/tables" is a calculation of table parameters of mortality. This program allows one to calculate more than "values" from mortality rate tables by causes of death (mainly, noncommunicable diseases) and parameters of surviving. They include average expected life span in various age groups, probability to "survive" to a certain age in cases of mortality rate change due to certain causes of death, and others aimed at investigation of the mortality rate effect on the demographic situation.

The Russian Health Care Reform Program is based on the evaluation of priority population health problems, social-economic conditions and their trends, the experience of Russia and other countries in the development of a health care system, World Health Organization (WHO) recommendations, objectification of the initial data regarding health and the health care system, the conclusions of experts, and interview of the population. It should be noted that in 1991–1992 almost 60 percent of those interviewed were not satisfied with medical care, and in 1993, this share increased due to the high cost of drugs and medical service. In addition, a nonadequate level of quality of medical care was taken into account. The priority directions of the developing health care system were identified in the program. They are based on the evaluation of losses in society due to early death, for which the health care system is responsible. Then the different types of medical care responsible for the losses were identified; stage and adequacy of their development were estimated; main defects in their functioning were identified; and measures for overcoming them were established.

On the whole, five basic priorities were established—to improve primary health care (general practice/family doctor), reanimation and intensive care, quality of health care, quality of personnel, and drug supply. On the strategic level, a transformation from "treatment" to "preventive" is recommended; and at the strategy level, emphasis should be removed from hospital and general health care to primary and general health care, from quantity to quality.

This is the general conception of health care reform in Russia. At present we are endeavoring to reform the health care system in Russia on the basis of health insurance. This conception of reform also includes incorporating the general practitioner into the primary health care concept. The problem is to design a juridical base, organizational principles, and a system of incentives to remunerate GPs. Now we are nearly through with the work on the system of targeting GPs to the medical problems of patients and forming risk groups based on detection of risk factors.

With regard to the medical information situation in Russia, it now reflects statistics representative of the entire country. It was approved by a special order of the Ministry of Health Care concerning the development of health care information in Russia. This order is the next step in carrying out a federal information program on health care (1990). During the last three years, on the federal level, information systems have been created on state medical statistics, resource evaluation of medical institutions, medical staff registration, analysis of patient complaints, planning and management of scientific research, registry of patients suffering from disasters such as Chernobyl, and so on.

In the polyclinics, there are computer systems, urgent aid stations, and specialized service offices (psychiatry, traumatology, oncology, etc.). The creation of systems on medicodemographic monitoring, urgent aid in extraordinary situations, health insurance regulations, and others is under way.

There is a whole network of information computing centers all over Russia; computing centers number about 100 on the regional level. The Public Health Research Institute, on the federal level, is among them. One national program of import is Health Care Information in Russia During 1993–1995 Years. This program can be divided into federal and regional levels, based on the financing of the projects. On the federal level, one can mark the following main projects:

- A computer monitoring system on the population's health.
- A united information computer system on urgent medical care in extraordinary situations.
- A united information computer system for collection, analysis, and transmission of medical statistics based on the telecommunications network.
- Expert computer systems for quality assurance and specialized health care services.
- A computer database on drugs and medical equipment.

These projects are financed by the state budget through the Ministry of Health and Medical Industry, and the State Committee on Information. In addition, there are a lot of programs that need to be designed at the regional level with financing from local resources. For example:

- An information system for health management at the regional level. A regional-level monitoring system of medicodemographic processes.
- Information systems for polyclinics (outpatient clinics), hospitals, urgent care, health insurance, different specialized workstations.
- Expert support systems (diagnostic, prognostic, preferred treatment, etc.).

MedSocEconomInform takes part in some of these projects, in particular concerning the design of:

- A system on health care quality and effectiveness and managers' workstations for experts from the Ministry of Health and Medical Industry itself.
- A system of planning, organization, analysis, and supervision of scientific research in the institutes working under the responsibility of the Ministry of Health and Medical Industry.
- An information system for the evaluation and prognosis of the health of the population in accordance with social factors, the environment, and so on.
- An information system–database for improving medical aid (cure-preventive measures) on the different directions of health care on the federal level; the research carried out by us will help to formulate a conception of public health for the Russian Federation during the transition and later.

MAJOR CHALLENGES FOR THE HEALTH SERVICES

The socioeconomic reform in Russia associated with the fall of the Soviet Union in 1991 targeted decentralization, democratic decision making, private ownership, and market economy approaches. In health care, there is a turn to general practice as a key element of reform. For the time being, there are some priorities for health care in Russia that are extremely important for running reform.

Health Economics and Health Service Management

This involves the effective distribution and delivery of existing resources within the existing budget and without any additional support. There is no doubt that the management malaise prevalent in the former Soviet society is equally apparent in the medical field and making grossly inefficient use of scarce resources.

Maternal and Child Health

This includes contraception by means other than abortion, the spacing of pregnancies and postnatal infection, immunization of infants, and infant and child nutrition and development. Gaping deficiencies in all these areas are currently disastrous for the next generation and represent a fearful legacy for the future. Maternal mortality in Russia remains on a high level (four to five times more than in developed countries), and there is no downward tendency. The reasons for maternal mortality in Russia are unique and absurd, as there are no other countries where so many women have died from out-hospital abortions, gestational toxicosis, and hemorrhage. According to experts' conclusions, maternal mortality could be prevented in 60 percent of all cases.

It is well known that abortions have a negative effect on women's health and outcome of future pregnancies and childbirths. In 1990, there were 3.9 million abortions; in 1991, there were 3.6 million abortions—twice more than the number of childbirths in the same time period. There are 100.3 abortions per 1,000 fertile women, one of the highest rates in the world (in the Netherlands, for instance, 5.0; Canada, 10.2; Finland, 12.8). Concurrently, abortions in 40 percent evoke different complications that influence women and child health. One of the main reasons for the high level of abortions is that women are not being provided with modern means of contraception. Contraceptives in Russia are used by only 18 percent of women, in comparison with 50 to 60 percent in the developed countries.

Russia occupies one of the top spots in the world involving women in public production (90 percent). But 3 million women are working in industry under unfavorable labor conditions; almost 250,000 women are working in manufactures under particularly hard or unhealthy conditions (more than 50 percent are textile, chemical, or oil-chemical enterprises). A considerable number of women work at night (39 percent).

In the last ten years, newborn morbidity has increased twice; and in 1991, the share of newborn children with physical and psychic disorders (every fifth) also increased. Investigations show that up to 60 percent of children of early age have manifestations of rachitis, hypotrophy, and diathesis, and more than 10 percent have anemia.

In 1991 and 1992 we observed in Russia an increase in infant mortality, which reached a level of 18 per 1,000 newborn children on a backdrop of a sharp decrease in the birthrate. According to certain investigations, this figure is low and the actual figure is not less than 22 per 1,000 live births. Currently, 35 percent of newborns in Russia are healthy (the rest, unhealthy), and by the year 2000, this share will decrease to 13 to 15 percent. Among schoolchildren, 60 percent have at least one chronic disease.

Infection Control

Every year in Russia, more than 40 million cases of communicable diseases are registered including 25,000 lethal outcomes. First, there are the so-called usual mass infections. In 1991, more than 800,000 cases of acute intestinal infections were registered—about 110,000 cases of salmonellosis (in the United States, with more population, about 50,000 a year) and 284,000 cases of virus hepatitis (United States, 50,000 to 60,000 a year). In the last ten years, the virus hepatitis B morbidity rate has doubled and increased to 15 percent, after blood transfusion. So far, only sporadic cases of extremely dangerous infections such as cholera have been seen (1965, 1971, 1990).

Tuberculosis, once announced as a disappearing illness, has reappeared once again, with a morbidity rate of 30 per 100,000 people. It spreads particularly among far north native people, residents of mountain and taiga areas, and risk groups such as the homeless, prisoners, and alcohol and drug abusers. Among them, tuberculosis morbidity is 20 times higher than in other groups. Since 1989, we have observed a tuberculosis increase in children. However, these data cannot be considered as full and exhaustive. In addition, the number of cases of diphtheria with lethal outcome has increased in both children and adults.

Increasing numbers of refugees and the concomitant unsanitary living conditions produce an increasing incidence of itch and louse infestation. The absence of simple conditions to promote hygiene threatens outbreaks of typhus.

Infection adds unnecessary costs to medical care and deprives people needlessly of their health. It is alarmingly prevalent in abortions; after childbirth, other operations, and burns; and among the community at home through lack of hygiene, poor diet, and deficient immunization programs. Public, medical, and nursing education in infection control techniques and behaviors is a relatively cheap and highly effective and topical requirement.

Medical, Nursing, and Public Health Education

There is a vast discrepancy between health sciences and practice. Medical education is directed toward diseases but not toward prevention and holistic approaches. There is a need for training and development of qualified staff for the health care system in Russia and particularly for general practitioners and nurses.

The Care of the Elderly

According to our data, the necessity for medical service for the aging population was 50 percent greater than for people in middle age, and the hospital need for people over 60 years was three times greater than for the population as a whole. About 4 percent of all observed elderly needed special help. Additional social aid was demanded for 17 percent of patients 80 years and more, due to sickness of both husband and wife (32.1 percent), absence of family members (46.4 percent), and loneliness (24.5 percent). The main figure serving the elderly population is the GP. Those in the 60–64 age group were visiting the GP in 43.5 percent of all their visits; those of 80 years and older, 63.4 percent. The care of the elderly is a universal problem confronting governments and populations everywhere, not only in Russia. It is a growing concern that will not go away and requires attention. But this attention is even less likely to be forthcoming in light of the stretched circumstances confronting Russia.

NOTE

This chapter would not have been possible without the long-term and permanent support of my colleagues from MedSocEconomInform: Prof. Yuri M. Komarov, Mr. Sergy M. Ermakov, Dr. Yuri A. Korotkov, and Prof. V. Kudrina. Special thanks for editing go to Mrs. D. Olivier.

REFERENCES

Banoob, S. N. (1993). Public health around the nation and world—Russian health care reform. *FJPH* (5) (Summer–fall), 22–24.

Ermakov, S. P. (1986). Demographic models of processes of reproduction of a health of the population. In: *Methods of Research.* Moscow: Aidea. 133–150.

Ermakov, S. P. & Kiselev, A. A. (1992). Economic aspects of health: world health. *Statistics Quarterly*, 46, 50–60.

Feachem, R. (1994). Health decline in eastern Europe. *Nature*, 367, 311–314.

Komarov, Y. M. (1994). Lessons for others. *International Journal of Quality Health Care*, 6 (1), 27–53.

National Center for Health Statistics. (1995). Vital and health statistics: Russian Federation and United States. Hyattsville: U.S. Department of Health and Human Services.

Russian Federation. (1991). *Nursing and Midwifery Profile*. Copenhagen: WHO/EURO.
Tchernjavsky, V. E. (1991). *Health Manpower Development in Central and Eastern European Countries*. Report on WHO Consultation. Copenhagen: WHO/EURO.
Tchernjavsky, V. E. (1994). Russia and USA: Two ways to strengthening health of nations. *Medicinskaja Gazeta*, 60, 4.
Tchernjavsky, V. E.& Liashenko, T. S. (1994). *Research on Public Health in Russia in Transition*. FICOSSER, Third General Conference, Helsinki. 171–172.
Weselowsky, T. (1994). Suicide rate rises. *The Moscow Tribune*, 4.

SOUTH AFRICA

Carel B. Ijsselmuiden

South Africa became a democratic country on April 27, 1994. This momentous date, in the words of the new minister of health, "marks the end of the first phase of our struggle for democracy. The central struggle now is to fight poverty. South Africa exhibits the worst of social outcomes: destitution for the majority amid plenty for the minority" (Zuma 1994).

This short description of South Africa lies at the core of this chapter. The current health situation is sharply polarized, as is the provision of health services. To compound this, the quality of data available to examine the health status of South Africa's population and to document improvements therein are poor. The recent democratic transformation heralds major changes in the manner in which society is organized, including the ways in which resources for the promotion, maintenance, and restoration of health will be distributed.

This chapter should be seen in this context of rapid transition. The first major changes will occur in the provision of basic services, water and sanitation, housing and education, and, hopefully, employment. Similar rapid changes will take place in the provision of health services, with an emphasis on accessible primary health care and a deemphasis on tertiary care, and in the financing of the health care system to ensure free basic services for high-risk groups and affordable basic services for all. With time, these adjustments should result in changes in health status, away from a situation in which the major causes of mortality and morbidity are related to socioeconomic deprivation toward one where morbidity and mortality patterns will show smaller differentials between groups and will show evidence of a shift toward chronic diseases and diseases of lifestyle. A revision of this chapter in a few years' time is thus likely to produce an entirely different picture of health and health services.

GEOGRAPHY AND DEMOGRAPHY

South Africa is situated at the southern tip of the African continent. Its weather varies from subtropical in the north and east to Mediterranean in the south. Although the country is well endowed with natural resources such as minerals, coal, and gold, one essential resource is in short supply, namely, fresh water. Rainfall in the northern, central, and western areas occurs only during summer and is often sporadic. The country is prone to serious droughts in all but the coastal areas. It has been estimated that South Africa's fresh water supply is sufficient to sustain a maximum of 80 million people. As the current population is estimated at about 42 million people, and the population growth at about 2.5 percent per year, fresh water may become a critical commodity by 2020. The current population density is relatively low at 33 persons per square kilometer. There are vast areas, however, of uninhabitable land.

From colonial to apartheid rule, the population was classified into four "race" groups. Most health and other government data are presented using this classification so that it is not possible to describe the South African reality without reference to this legislative and ideological categorization. The relative proportions of these groups in the population are Indians, 2.6 percent; Blacks, 76.1 percent; Coloreds ("mixed race"), 8.5 percent; and Whites, 12.8 percent.

The population is relatively young. Children under the age of 5 years account for 14 percent, and the group aged below 15 years for 40 percent of the population. Those aged 65 years and above constitute only 3.7 percent of the population. The population pyramid drawn for the White population closely resembles those of industrialized nations, while for Blacks it more closely resembles those for developing nations. The population structures for Indians and Coloreds are intermediate to these. Literacy in the Black population is 60 percent for men and 45 percent for women, but improves with decreasing age. Literacy in the other groups approaches 100 percent.

An average of 58 percent of South Africa's population is urbanized. Nearly 95 percent of Whites and Indians, 80 percent of Coloreds, and 50 percent of Blacks are urbanized. The rural-urban migration is high, and it is expected that 80 percent of South Africans will live in an urban environment by the year 2000, mostly in informal settlements or "squatter camps" around established towns and cities.

South Africa is truly a multicultural society. In addition to the language and cultural subgroups within the Indian and Colored communities, there are among the Black population nine main ethnic groups, while the White population is composed of members of at least eight cultural and language groups. Recently, immigration from African countries north of South Africa, from countries around the Pacific, and from eastern European countries has added to this cultural diversity. There are now 11 official languages and a multitude of religious institutions, among which the Christian faith is the largest.

South Africa's economy is built on agriculture, mining, many types of manufacturing, construction, and service industries, as well as a large public service. The large primary and secondary industries are comparable in quality and sophistication to similar industries worldwide but do not provide sufficient employment for the rapidly growing population. Total unemployment is estimated at 40 percent of the economically active population. The economic growth over the past decade has been below the rate of population increase, and unemployment may therefore worsen. The annual per capita income is estimated at $2,500, an average that masks extreme economic disparities. Because of its relative wealth in terms of the African continent, there is an enormous influx of legal and illegal immigrants into the country, mostly for economic reasons. Presently, it is speculated that there are 2 to 10 million illegal immigrants in South Africa.

MAJOR HEALTH PROBLEMS FACING THE COUNTRY

Table 1 provides information on mortality and life expectancy in 1988 (Van Rensburg, Fourie, and Pretorius 1992). Given the low quality of the population register and of the system of notifications of deaths and births, these figures are likely to be inaccurate, especially in relation to the rural Black population. Nevertheless, when grouped, they provide a reasonable picture of proportional mortality in the various groups and, consequently, an indication of relative priorities for intervention.

Infectious Diseases

Infectious diseases are still the most common cause of mortality in young children. Infantile gastroenteritis, acute respiratory infections, and measles are the most prominent of these. In very young children, neonatal syphilis is the cause of failure to thrive and of early death in approximately 1,000 children annually, while human immunodeficiency virus (HIV) infection is rapidly surpassing this number. Other infectious diseases that are common include hepatitis A (up to 80 percent of rural children in populations surveyed were infected by age three), hepatitis B (up to 10 percent of the adult Black population are carriers), typhoid fever (especially in rural areas where nearly 800 cases and 13 deaths were notified in 1994), malaria (in the northern and northeastern parts of the country where 5,100 cases and 6 deaths were notified in 1994), and meningococcal infections. Reductions in childhood vaccine–preventable conditions, except measles, have been achieved and sustained. There was 1 notification of diphtheria and 9 cases of neonatal tetanus in 1994. There were no cases of poliomyelitis. Pertussis was not notifiable in 1993, but 45 cases were notified after it became notifiable in 1994.

Tuberculosis. Tuberculosis (TB) was introduced into southern Africa at the beginning of colonization. The mining industry was, however, the major trigger of TB as an endemic disease in South Africa. A peak was reached in the 1960s, after which there has been a gradual and consistent decline to 45,000 notifica-

Table 1
Major Causes of Mortality (per 100,000 population), Infant Mortality, and Life Expectancy at Birth by Population Group and Sex in South Africa, 1988

White			Asian			Coloured			Black		
Total	M	F	Total	M	F	Total	M	F	Total	M	F
Diseases of the Circulatory System			Diseases of the Circulatory System			Diseases of the Circulatory System			Accidents, poisoning, and trauma		
312.1	341.5	283.1	201.2	241.2	161.7	189.0	183.9	194.1	114.8	179.4	44.7
Neoplasia			Accidents, poisoning, and trauma			Accidents, poisoning, and trauma			Symptoms, signs and ill-defined conditions		
150.2	161.9	138.5	72.6	116.1	29.8	136.9	211.7	64.3	114.4	118.8.	109.6
Diseases of the Respiratory System			Endocrine, Nutritional, Metabolic Diseases, and of the Immune System			Neoplasia			Diseases of the Circulatory System		
100.3	105.8	94.9	63.5	56.4	70.4	104.9	127.8	82.8	80.0	76.5	83.8
Accidents, poisoning, and trauma			Diseases of the Respiratory System			Diseases of the Respiratory System			Infectious and Parasitic Diseases		
84.6	125.1	44.7	56.1	74.2	38.3	104.7	128.4	81.8	77.7	88.3	66.2
Signs, Symptoms, and ill-defined conditions			Neoplasia			Perinatal Conditions			Diseases of the Respiratory System		
53.6	46.8	60.3	51.4	52.9	49.9	71.2	79.9	62.7	57.7	67.2	47.3
Life Expectancy at Birth (years)											
	67.7	75.5		64.4	71.6		58.5	66.2		58.9	65.9
Infant Mortality Rate (/1000)											
7.3			12.7			36			54.3		

Note: Note that the first cause of death is a category marked "accidents, poisoning, and trauma," which is largely determined by violence and homicide-related deaths. Violence is also the major cause of under-five mortality in townships such as Soweto. Also noteworthy is that the second major category of deaths in Blacks is a category labeled "symptoms, signs, and ill-defined conditions," which effectively indicates that the access to quality health care for Blacks is so low that many causes of death are undiagnosed or that notifications of such deaths are completed by police departments who do not have the expertise for medical diagnosis.

Source: Adapted from Van Rensburg, Fourie, and Pretorius 1992, 138.

tions in 1987. Since then, partly due to coinfection with the human immunodeficiency virus, TB has rapidly increased to over 80,000 notifications in 1994. Multiple-drug resistance is now a serious challenge to tuberculosis control.

HIV Infection and AIDS. HIV infection and acquired immunodeficiency syndrome (AIDS) were first diagnosed in 1983 in two White males, while the first infection in a Black person was diagnosed only in 1985. The impending epidemic was largely ignored until recently. Currently, the overwhelming number of HIV infections occur in Blacks and are mostly heterosexually transmitted, although vertical transmission from mother to fetus is also a significant route of infection. No comprehensive, nationwide database exists, but it is estimated from surveys of antenatal clinics and other, more targeted studies that about 800,000 persons (2 percent of the population) are HIV positive. However, only 2,143 cases of AIDS were notified during 1994, and the cumulative total of AIDS notifications at the end of 1994 was 5,864. Notification is done anonymously through laboratories, as neither HIV infection nor AIDS is legally notifiable. Current estimates are that up to 1 million children may be orphaned through parental HIV infection by 2010. Other sexually transmitted diseases are very common and often remain untreated.

Chronic Diseases

Protein-energy malnutrition is common in children, more so in the rural Black population. A survey of primary school entrants in 1994 showed that between 4.6 percent (Gauteng) and 20.9 percent (Northern Cape) were underweight for age (national average was 9 percent), while between 7.1 percent (Gauteng) and 19.2 percent had stunted growth (national average was 13.2 percent) (Zuma 1994). Micronutrient status, for example, vitamin A, is, on average, in the low-normal range, while iodine deficiency is rarely diagnosed.

The most common causes of morbidity and mortality in adults include myocardial infarction and other hypertension-related conditions, especially in Whites, Indians, and Coloreds. Hypertension, and related cerebrovascular disease, is becoming increasingly common in the urbanizing Black population. Diabetes mellitus occurs in 13 percent of the Indian population, and familial hyperlipemia requiring medical treatment occurs in 16 percent of Whites of African descent. Cancers are an important cause of mortality. The most prominent forms are breast, lung, cervical, and colon cancer. While esophageal cancer is not a major cause of mortality, there is a high incidence in the southeastern parts of South Africa, with an incidence rate of 50/100,000 (Jaskiwiscz, Marasas, and Van der Walt 1987). Proportional mortality from cancer is 21 percent in Whites, 11 percent in Indians, 15 percent in Coloreds, and 10 percent in Blacks (Sitas and Pacella 1994).

Mental Health

Epidemiologically accurate morbidity and mortality data in mental health are not available. Given the excessive, but largely underresearched, effects of political, domestic, and criminal violence in South Africa, it is widely assumed that the prevalence of mental health problems exceeds that usually found internationally: that is, 15 to 20 percent of the population suffer from disabling mental health conditions, and 1 to 3 percent suffer from a severe disorder. Services are mostly medical only and are biased in favor of institutional rather than community care. The number of psychologists and psychiatrists in the public sector and in rural areas is extremely low. For example, the Northern Cape, the Northern Transvaal, and the North West Provinces each have one public sector psychiatrist for a combined population of 9 million people. Traditional healers tend to play a major role in mental health care, reflecting in part cultural beliefs and in part lack of access to other care. The traditional and modern health sectors remain independent of each other, and though proposals on cooperation have been made, no definite plans for such cooperation are in place. The integration of mental health with primary health care is seen as essential for improved mental health care.

Environmental Hazards

The need for economic growth places environmental considerations as a secondary priority except where industrial or developmental activities impinge on protected nature areas. Major environmental problems are, however, experienced in parts of the country due to industrial air pollution around major centers, acid rain over the northeast of the country, toxic waste disposal around urban centers, the processing of toxic waste from industrialized nations (although this has been formally halted since the new government was elected), and contamination of South Africa's coastal waters. The mining industry has caused major surface deposits of chemically polluted crushed rock in so-called slime-dams, but these deposits and their potential risk to surface and drinking water are relatively well controlled. Extensive crop spraying against pests is practiced, but its health impact has not been well researched. To contain malaria, DDT (dichlorodiphenyltrichloroethane) spraying inside houses in rural areas is employed in large areas in the north and northeast. The few studies that have been done on DDT spraying do not show lasting deleterious health effects. A most serious environmental problem relates to deforestation due to using wood for fuel and protected areas for the erection of informal settlements. Open fires and use of paraffin instead of wood add to child morbidity and mortality in rural areas through burns and through paraffin inhalation–induced chemical pneumonitis.

PROVISION, UTILIZATION, AND IMPACT OF HEALTH SERVICES

The health services are, at present, under intense review, and it is not possible to predict in detail the outcome of debates in this regard. The following section will therefore describe aspects of the current system and indicate the direction of changes that may be anticipated.

Organization of Health Services

The public health services in South Africa are divided into three tiers: national, provincial, and local or district services. The restructuring of separate departments of health for different "races" has resulted in one central Ministry of Health and nine provincial health departments.

South Africa's new ("interim") constitution places the responsibility for health care with the provincial legislatures. The aims of this new public health service are the following:

1. To reorient the services from a curative, tertiary care–focused system to one centered around primary health care.
2. To ensure that all people will have access to "basic" health services.
3. To ensure that special risk groups, children under the age of six years, pregnant mothers, and elderly persons, will have access to free health care.
4. To decentralize health services to the "district" level; it is as yet not clear how "districts" will be constituted in terms of existing local authorities.

The national Ministry of Health is responsible for policy and standards development, monitoring, programs for health problems of national relevance, the development of a national information system, human resource development, and international liaison.

The provincial health departments are charged with the coordination of services within each province, the delivery of regional hospital services, emergency services, and services that are more efficiently provided at provincial level. The provincial services function under a provincial political head to increase accountability to the electorate.

District health departments are envisaged to become the main direct service providers of public primary care services. In larger districts this will probably include the provision of general, nonspecialist hospital services, while in smaller districts curative care may be limited to ambulatory care only. Virtually all promotive and preventive services will be delivered at district level, although provincial and national support may be added. It is intended to have multisectoral committees within each district to ensure optimal interdepartmental and intersectoral cooperation. Out of the more than 600 local authorities in South Africa, only 15 had a full-time medical officer of health, the rest being headed by environmental health officers with the assistance of part-time, private medical practitioners. The capacity for program management and implementation at the local level is therefore low and poses a major challenge to the restructuring of the nation's health services.

There are 24,000 registered medical practitioners, 7,000 of whom are specialists, and both groups show a skew geographical distribution, being based predominantly in urban centers. The density of medical personnel varies from

13 to 15/10,000 population in the Western Cape and Gauteng Provinces to 2/10,000 in the Northern Transvaal, averaging about 1:1,500. However, in various rural areas, this ratio can be as low as 1 doctor per 30,000 population. In 1985, 88 percent of medical practitioners were White; 7.7 percent, Indian; 2.2 percent, Colored; and 1.3 percent, African. Although shifts in intake of medical students have increased the number of Africans in medical education, in 1991 only 300 of the 1,300 graduating medical doctors were "non-White," and only 120 were African. In 1985, only 17 percent of nonspecialists and 6 percent of specialists were women. There are 150,000 registered nurses (1:280), of whom up to 40 percent are no longer practicing. Two thirds of nurses work in the public sector. There are 4,000 dentists (1:10,500), 9,000 pharmacists (1:4,700) and 25,000 other health professionals (Van der Linde 1995a). There are 834 hospitals, providing 2 to 8 beds (average 4.1) per 1,000 population (Rossouw 1994).

Public and Private Health Care Financing

Private, for-profit medical organizations were encouraged to develop by the government from the late 1970s. Until then, with the exception of general practitioners and the mining health sector, there was a virtual national health service covering the entire country. Although access to the national health service was unequal in that Whites and urban residents had far greater access, the system did not place restraints on the care available once a person had entered the system. The growth of the private sector over the last 15 years has created a situation in which 81 percent of the population are dependent on the public sector, while the private sector covers 19 percent of people. Yet the private sector consumes 55 percent of all health care expenditure. This has resulted in a major drain of skilled staff from the public to the private sector due to salary differentials and differentials in the quality of working environments. The private, for-profit health care sector in South Africa consists of three main groupings: general practitioners; organizations providing medical care, insurance, or managed care; and an industrial health care system available mostly in the mining sector. Except parts of the mine medical system, the private sector is concentrated in urban areas. The government is intent on forging cooperation between the public and private sectors rather than nationalizing health care.

The per capita public expenditure on health demonstrates historical inequities with R360 ($100) per capita in the Western Cape region to R147 ($41) in the Northern Transvaal region. Overall, South Africa spends 6.4 percent of its gross domestic product (GDP) on health (McIntyre and Dorrington 1990).

The current public health care system is financed through tax revenues and, to a limited extent, through user fees. Modifications now being discussed include permanent "health levies" and a national insurance scheme that will be sufficient to guarantee an adequate "basic" health care package. It can be anticipated that a private, largely curative sector will remain, especially in urban areas, that a basic package of health care will include most preventive and promotive services and curative medical services of an ambulatory nature, and that for more advanced curative care within the public sector a waiting list or quota system of rationing will be employed.

Academic Centers

South Africa has eight academic complexes graduating about 1,100 medical doctors annually. Some of these universities are world-renowned; others were creations of apartheid, that is, to train Black health workers. Government subsidies to these centers vary greatly, both directly and through research funding administered by statutory research bodies. Given that 75 percent of the public health budget is spent on hospital and academic centers, given the drive toward a primary care–focused health system, and given little expansion capacity of the health budget, it is inevitable that allocations to academic centers will be reduced. Ministry of Health funding for academic centers was reduced by 5 percent for the 1995–1996 financial year, and further cuts are likely. These global reductions were not effected within a framework for academic care and human resource development but rather as part of an overall reduction of government expenditure. It is, therefore, unclear how many of the medical schools will remain, but significant rationalization is likely (Van der Linde 1995).

Preventive Services

Preventive services are currently delivered mainly at the level of local authority health departments, and this will remain a primary function for the new district health authorities. Routine services include well-baby clinics, antenatal clinics, family planning services, sexually transmitted disease services, immunization services, and school health services. Screening for hypertension, diabetes, breast and cervical cancer, and tuberculosis is, with exceptions, not well developed nationally. In the case of tuberculosis, a large nongovernmental organization and the mining industry provide screening services. Because of the fragmented nature of preventive service provision, there is no information on actual expenditure. It is estimated that 5 percent of public health expenditure is spent on preventive care (McIntyre and Dorrington 1990). Given the new priorities in health, this amount is likely to increase, through, for example, free care for children, pregnant women, and the elderly and through the Primary School Nutrition Program, a breakfast program for primary schools in poor areas.

Nongovernmental Organizations (NGOs) in Health

There is a plethora of NGOs active in health. A large number of NGOs were initiated to provide primary care or to advocate change and equity under the previous government. This group is now undergoing major changes and is at risk of dissolving because much of the leadership has joined the new governmental structures; because the prime reason for its existence, namely, opposition to the apartheid government, has disappeared; and because international donors are urged to donate through the government's Reconstruction and Development Program rather than directly to NGOs. The other part of the NGO sector consists mostly of local or regional health and welfare organizations. Since 1994, the NGO sector has been supplemented by the large international health and development organizations that, until recently, were officially not operating in South Africa. As in many other countries, the NGO sector has played a major role in AIDS advocacy and gay rights. It is also active in the fields of tuberculosis, reproductive health, drug and alcohol abuse, and the relief of famine and drought. In addition, church-related primary care clinics provide clinical care and basic health promotion to over a million people countrywide.

Other Services

Rehabilitation services are severely underdeveloped across South Africa. Virtually 80 percent of all physical therapy, for example, is provided within the private health sector, which is urban based and is generally accessible only to those with medical insurance. Salary discrepancies between public and private sectors are mainly responsible for this. Similarly, occupational therapy and speech and hearing therapy have a presence in academia and in the private sector but are not widely available in the public sector. Training and education for blind and deaf persons is effected virtually entirely through the private sector and through nongovernmental, nonprofit, state-aided councils and other organizations.

INFRASTRUCTURE OF TRAINING AND RESEARCH IN PUBLIC HEALTH

Education in Public Health

Training in public health has been limited to doctors, nurses, dentists, and environmental health officers. Each of the eight medical schools has a small department of community health, which, collectively, graduate 5 to 10 specialists a year after a four-year course. Within the pediatrics and obstetrics training at medical schools, there are options to focus on public health in community pediatrics or in obstetrics. Nurses have community health as part of the four-year basic qualification and can subsequently obtain master's or doctoral training in community health. This mode of preparing public health professionals is entirely inadequate. Not only are insufficient numbers of staff trained, but the training is also not available to graduates outside this narrow range of health professions. And, in addition, training is done within professional groups in virtual isolation from other public health professionals and is available either at a very introductory level or as a four-year specialization. The training in public health is likely to undergo major changes with the development of at least two, but possibly three, Schools of Public Health. Both the Transvaal School of Public Health and the Western Cape School of Public Health focus on postgraduate training in public health that is open for all those whose work impacts on public health. The major educational efforts are centered around short courses and around a Master in Public Health degree that allows for a high degree of individualization of coursework through modular and elective approaches to teaching. Both initiatives are multiinstitutional in nature and attempt to integrate the educational, research, and service aspects of public health practice.

Research in Public Health

In addition to the academic centers, there are several national or statutory research and service institutes that strengthen the public health capability of South Africa. *National institutes* refer to units within the Department of Health that deal with specialist areas. There is the National Institute for Virology (NIV), which conducts virological research and training and produces vaccines; and the National Institute for Occupational Health (NIOH), which caters to toxicological, clinical, and epidemiological research and training in the field of occupational health. A private mining industry–funded counterpart is the Medical Bureau for Occupational Diseases (MBOD).

Statutory councils refer to research councils set up under an act of Parliament that are largely funded through an annual government grant and whose board is appointed by government. Relevant to public health are the Medical Research Council (MRC), which currently spends about 50 percent of its budget on "essential national health research"; the Human Sciences Research Council (HSRC), which is focusing on psychological, social, and policy research; and the Council for Scientific and Industrial Research (CSIR), which, in terms of health, focuses mostly on environmental issues, although it is not a major component of this council's activities. The MRC has the smallest allocation of all the research councils, on the order of R44 million ($12 million). Also in health research the tension between the public and private sector is acute: The budget for pharmaceutical industrial research alone is more than twice the annual budget of the Medical Research Council.

Besides a great number of private sector laboratory and pathology services, two other research and service institutions exist: the South African Institute for Medical Research (SAIMR) and the South African Blood Transfusion Service (SABTS). The SAIMR provides routine laboratory and pathology services throughout hospitals in South Africa, conducts microbiological research, and produces some bacterial vaccines. The SAIMR is legally a private, nonprofit company. The SABTS is the largest blood transfusion service in the country, providing blood and blood products of high quality.

An epidemiological service, with responsibilities for surveillance, reporting, and outbreak control, is available at the national Department of Health, but it is inadequately resourced. Expansion of this service in the future is likely.

MAJOR CHALLENGES FACING THE HEALTH SERVICES

Achieving Equity in Health and Health Care

The reduction of the enormous discrepancies between the Black and White, rural and urban, and poor and rich sections of the population is the single biggest challenge facing the South African health care system in the immediate and longer-term future. The drive toward equity will affect all aspects of the health system. On the one hand, there is a shortage of at least 1,400 primary care clinics, and an ambitious clinic-building program was started within six months after the inauguration of the new government. On the other hand, the already understaffed public services have to extend still further to provide services in these new facilities. Quality assurance of primary care is one major area to be developed to ensure that with increased coverage the quality of services will be improved as well.

Basic services such as adequate water supply, sanitation, food, and housing will arguably bring about the largest immediate reductions in South Africa's mortality and morbidity. The government's Reconstruction and Development Program is aimed at providing just these services as a major short-term priority. The challenge to the health services is to effectively cooperate across government departments and across societal sectors to optimize efforts.

The status of academic medicine in South Africa is at risk. In the past, the academic centers brought excellence in medical education when measured by world standards but did little, if anything, to bring health and health care to those in need. The imperative of the new order is to bring health and health care to all and to redefine excellence in terms of relevance to the country's health needs. This shift will put major demands on academic staff but can potentially result in a renewal of medical and public health education (Van der Linde 1995).

Merging private sector activities with the aims of the public health service, including arriving at a financing mechanism that will ensure adequate staff and quality care in the public service, will require great leadership in both sectors. Currently, the doctor:patient ratio in the private sector is 1:685, while that in the public sector is estimated at 1:1,855, illustrating the attractions the private sector offers to medical personnel and indicating the difficulty in reducing this differential.

Managing the Health System

The current curative sector in the public health service consumes at least 75 percent of the public health budget. Yet this sector was built largely on ideology, not on sound health planning. Consequently, there are extensive and expensive duplications, there are major gaps, and there has been a long-standing underdevelopment of management expertise and information management in the health care system. For example, there is virtually no public hospital or clinic that can adequately cost procedures or treatments, that can specify the main causes for admission or death with any certainty, or that knows in much detail the profiles of diseases and deaths in the communities they serve (Rossouw 1994). Similarly, there is no functional health information system other than one for notifiable conditions. Most data are obtained from ad hoc studies, and few comprehensive national data sets are available and being maintained.

The establishment of an effective health information system has been identified as a priority but will face major hurdles before being implemented. Given that there is no tradition of information-based decision making, not only are many skills lacking, but also the training capacity to develop these skills is lacking. Additionally, a tradition of integrating services, research, and academia needs to be developed for the optimal generation and use of information. Finally, the training of large numbers of district, provincial, and national health managers will be required for the establishment of an effective health management infrastructure. Given that the current status of health management training is inadequate, the rapid development of Schools of Public Health and other modes of training is essential.

A particular feature of many sectors, including the health sector, in South African society today is the absence of adequate labor relations mechanisms. In the years running up to the first democratic election in 1994, many groups and individuals considered the wider societal goal of freedom from racial oppression as their first aim, and the more narrow goal of their particular sector or profession as secondary to this. This was, and is, often aggravated by obsolete labor relations approaches. Consequently, strikes in the health sector are common. The achievement of many of the goals of the new government in the health sector will depend on how well politicians are able to put in place credible and effective mechanisms to deal with the problems and grievances of health workers. In view of current and contemporary history, especially in view of the amalgamation of 14 departments of health for different "races" and different "homelands," this will be a major task indeed.

Dealing with Increased Expectations and Demands

In promoting primary health care as the new orientation of South Africa's health system, the government not only wishes to promote equity and health but intends to reduce costs. While in the very short term such a reciprocity may be seen, worldwide evidence points to a direct relationship between increased health care coverage and increased health care costs, at least in part due to increasing demand for care not previously sought and for more advanced care about which there was no awareness in the past. In other words, while coverage with more primary care clinics is clearly a priority now, the quality of the service may become a major source of dissatisfaction with potential political consequences in the near future. Since a similar pattern is likely to occur in all other societal sectors, including particularly education, housing, and employment, the additional health care demands generated by improved coverage may remain unmet. Already health care consumers, even the poor, often prefer to use expensive care in the private sector because of discomfort in the public health care system. Innovations in community care, in contributory health financing, and in quality assurance, health personnel training, greatly improved resource management, and the establishment of a just labor relations mechanism are essential ingredients toward solving these problems, and such interventions need to be initiated now.

Decentralization of Health Services to District Health Authorities

One of the intentions in the public health sector is to decentralize health care to the district level, with the aim of making health services more accountable and responsive to communities, and to promote intersectoral cooperation in health. The obstacles to this are large. First, in all sectors of public life in South Africa, there has been a tradition of centralization that is not easy to change. Second, the new (''interim'') constitution makes no provision for districts as separate entities so that there is no legal imperative to pursue implementation. And third, management capacity at the local authority level is often too low to manage a health care system effectively and efficiently.

As interim measures, subprovincial structures are being constituted that straddle more than one district. This effectively creates a fourth tier of government, at least in the health sector. Similarly, larger local authorities may be divided into more than one district, creating possibly even a fifth tier of government and leading to extremely complicated lines of public authority that may effectively negate the intended increase in community participation. Debates on this matter are clearly not resolved, but, in a nutshell, the challenge to the health system is to superimpose a model of health services delivery that has worked well in developing countries onto an existing infrastructure that is in many places relatively sophisticated and to make it achieve its goal of community responsiveness and control despite the inherent risk of further bureaucracy.

AIDS and Tuberculosis

While many conditions of deprivation can be reduced or eradicated with correct spending in the Reconstruction and Development Program and in targeted health sector programs, two major diseases constitute a major threat to South Africa and its health services. Predictions based on several models have it that within the next 20 years up to 24 percent of South Africa's population may be

HIV positive, that 1 million or more children may be orphaned due to parental AIDS, and that, at current rates of hospitalization and treatment, up to 75 percent of the total health care expenditure will be spent on HIV-related disease. Besides a major upgrading of the nation's response to HIV infection, which has now been initiated, further policy development on community care, on hospitalization and treatment of infected persons, and on the care of orphaned children will have to be made soon to prevent a social disaster.

Tuberculosis has increased significantly since it reached its lowest level in 1987, presumably fanned by the HIV epidemic. In addition, multiple-drug-resistant tuberculosis is increasing to a level of 5 to 10 percent of all infected cases. Although no economic analysis has been done in terms of future health care costs, South Africa's health care program will have to make substantial provision in the short term to achieve some measure of control over tuberculosis. The past approach was to "muddle on," while a new approach, in principal based on World Health Organization guidelines, has yet to be defined.

Violence and Trauma

Criminal and domestic violence, combined with very high traffic mortality and incidents of politically inspired violence, have created a situation in which violence and trauma are the main causes of adult mortality in South Africa at present. In particular areas such as large townships, violence has also become the main cause of child and adolescent mortality. The public health care sector has a major role to play to document its effects on health, its costs to society and to the health care system, and to lobby for and facilitate change. The challenge to intersectoral cooperation is probably nowhere so great as in finding solutions to these problems, and it is in this arena that the ability and motivation to work across departmental, professional, and public-private sector barriers will be tested most severely.

Tobacco and Alcohol Use

As anywhere else in the world, tobacco use is a major cause of premature illness and death and of substantial losses in industry and overexpenditures in the health sector. Smoking is increasing in the Black and decreasing in the White population. The new government has taken firm steps to institute education and counseling efforts, to legislate sales of tobacco and the advertisements for tobacco products, to gradually raise taxes on tobacco products, and to declare smoke-free environments. As yet, these comprehensive steps are too new to have an impact, but given the commitment of the government, it can be expected to produce healthy results in the near and distant future, even in a country with a powerful tobacco lobby. Alcohol abuse is a major source of ill health and excess mortality across the country. The Colored community is probably most affected, which is historically connected to work on wine farms where remuneration was provided in part in the form of wine.

NOTE

I am grateful to Linda Richter, William Pick, Werner Coetzer, and Melvyn Freedman for their critical comments. The responsibility for the contents of this chapter is, however, entirely mine.

REFERENCES

Jaskiwiscz, K., Marasas, W. F. O. & Van der Walt, F. E. (1987). Oesophagus and other main cancer patterns in four districts of Transkei 1981–1984. *South African Medical Journal*, 72, 27–30.

McIntyre, D. E. & Dorrington, R. E. (1990). Trends in the distribution of South African health care expenditure. *South African Medical Journal*, 78, 125–129.

Pick, W. M. (1994). The development of human resources for health in South Africa: Ethical dilemmas post apartheid. In: Aoki, K. (Ed.). (1994). *Ethical Dilemmas in Health and Development*. Tokyo: Japan Scientific Society Press. 93–115.

Priorities in the Departmentt of Health. (1995). *South African Medical Journal*, 85, 14–15.

Rossouw, W. (1994). A review of hospital services in South Africa in four parts: Part 1. *Epidemiological Comments*, 21, 133–148.

Sitas, F. & Pacella, R. (1994). *Incidence and Geographical Distribution of Histologically Diagnosed Cancer in South Africa*. Johannesburg: South African Institute for Medical Research.

Van der Linde, I. (1995a). Head counting of physicians shows decline. *South African Medical Journal*, 85, 18.

Van der Linde, I. (1995b). Medical schools: Smaller and more, no less. *South African Medical Journal*, 85, 17–18.

Van Rensburg, H. C. J., Fourie, A. & Pretorius, E. (1992). *Health Care in South Africa: Structure and Dynamics*. Pretoria: Academia. 252–292.

Zuma, Dr. N. C. Dlamini, Minister of Health. (1994). Budget vote in the national assembly, 20 October 1994.

TANZANIA

Cyril Pervilhac, Martin Alilio, and Peter Kilima

MAJOR HEALTH PROBLEMS FACING THE COUNTRY

Infectious Diseases

Despite the emergence of noninfectious diseases with the ongoing epidemiologic transition, infectious diseases remain the main problem in Tanzania. The present data are limited to routine epidemiological data and hence do not reflect the people's perception of the diseases. About 90 percent of the causes of outpatient attendance in Dar es Salaam are due to infectious diseases (City Medical Office 1993). Communicable diseases clearly dominate (Table 1), as confirmed with more reliable data on morbidity available from the Dar es Salaam Urban Health Project. In Tanzania in general, using the scarce data available, infectious diseases still constitute more than 80 percent of the burden of diseases (Mmuni et al. 1994).

Control programs (Expanded Programme on Immunization, TB [tuberculosis] and Leprosy Control, Diarrhoeal Diseases Control, and AIDS [acquired immunodeficiency syndrome] Control) have been established that focus more on infectious diseases.

Chronic Diseases

The general assumption that in developing countries chronic diseases are not a problem is proving to be a fallacy. Recent studies carried out in rural and urban Tanzania by the Adult Morbidity, Mortality and the Urban Health Project show that noncommunicable diseases like cardiovascular diseases and diabetes are on the increase. In a surveillance area in Dar es Salaam, chronic diseases

Table 1
Top Ten Infectious Diseases in Dar es Salaam, 1993

Infectious Disease		Morbidity	Percentage
1	Malaria	489,413	27.48
2	Upper respiratory tract infections	222,103	12.48
3	Diarrheal diseases	152,891	8.59
4	Skin diseases	112,382	6.31
5	Pneumonia	77,230	4.34
6	Eye diseases	60,874	3.42
7	Intestinal worms	59,235	3.33
8	Gonorrhea	35,266	1.88
9	Ear diseases	27,491	1.54
10	Schistosomiasis	18,887	1.06
11	All other conditions (including noninfectious)	525,053	29.58
12	Total	1,780,825	100.00

Source: City Medical Office 1993.

have been shown to be among the top ten common causes of mortality in adults (Gilson, Kilima, and Tannes 1995). These findings are in line with findings elsewhere (World Bank 1993) where noncommunicable and chronic diseases are among the top ten causes of death.

Mental Health

Drug abuse is on the increase in Tanzania, with exact figures not available. Cannabis, heroin, and mandrax are spilling into the streets of Dar es Salaam from drug trafficking through the Tanzanian ports, as shown by the increase in seizures by police in recent years. Alcohol is a problem both in rural and in urban areas.

There is insufficient information regarding the morbidity of mental health in Tanzania and elsewhere in East Africa. The clinical picture is marked by prominence of acute psychoses, many cases of schizophrenia, prominence of a tendency to transfer blame (projective and persecutory ideas), and a tendency for hysteria or transient psychotic states to arise in the presence of physical and emotional stress (Bitanyi 1992).

Research, intervention, and support in modern institutions for mental health problems are still much needed in Tanzania, and traditional healing still functions as an important referral system used by the rural population.

Effects of Gender and Social Class

Health problems affect both men and women but in different social and physical ways. The extent of gender differences in Tanzania is not well known. Poor health for women, related in some cases to general malnutrition and infection as well as to complications of pregnancy and childbirth, explains the high level of maternal mortality and morbidity. These conditions also occur in the context of poor socioeconomic situations where education, health, and other social services are lacking. Some of these underlying causes have their roots in social-cultural beliefs and practices that adversely affect the status of women in Tanzanian society (Alilio 1993).

As a result of the interaction between different social and ecological factors, there is an apparent health inequality in Tanzania. Differences in the sheer availability of care—and to some extent, the quality of care available—in different localities provide a channel through which social inequality penetrates the health system. A second channel is the structure of the current health care system, which is seen as being based on the values or assumptions and preferences of the middle class. As a result, inadequate attention is paid to the particular problems and needs of those who are less able to express themselves in ''acceptable'' terms and who suffer from a lack of command of resources, time, and money (Macintyre 1986).

Health Situation of Immigrants and Refugees

In addition to the high birthrates, and the decrease in death rates, net migration may play a major role in the rapid population growth of Tanzania (TFNC 1992). However, information on immigrants is scarce.

Tanzania has remained a host to a number of refugees from eastern and southern African countries (UNHCR 1989). In the mid-1960s 36,000 refugees from Rwanda settled in western Tanzania following political and ethnic strife. Then, in the early 1970s another major influx came as a result of events in Burundi, as well as from Uganda, Mozambique, Namibia, South Africa, Angola, and Zimbabwe (TNFC 1992). More recently, approximately another half a million arrived from Rwanda (UNHCR 1994), with the biggest refugee camps in the world located in the Kagera Region.

An increase in the refugee population has a number of effects on the host communities, such as increases in the demand for and price of food and shelter and environmental damage. Health hazards can be numerous and have dramatic consequences: The introduction of endemic diseases such as cholera, AIDS, malaria, or bloody diarrhea change the prevalence and severity pattern of diseases among the host community.

Population Development

Tanzania's population growth rate of 3.4 percent per year is one of the highest in the world. Forecasts estimate that the present population of more than 24 million people will grow to 36 million by the year 2000. Approximately 85 percent of the population live in rural areas and 15 percent in urban areas. Given the high growth rate, Tanzania has a young, broad-based population structure, with more than 47 percent of the total population below 15 years of age (Ngallaba et al. 1993). By the turn of the century, nearly one third of the population is expected to be urban. In some areas, villagization policies adopted by the Tanzanian government in the 1970s have concentrated the rural population in limited geographical areas. Although there is land surplus as a whole, land has thus become a relatively scarce resource (DANIDA 1990).

There are big differences in mortality rates between regions in Tanzania. Similarly, there are some differences between rural and urban areas due to the varied socioeconomic conditions and access to medical facilities between regions.

Nutritional Problems

Malnutrition in Tanzania is reflected by the high rates of morbidity and mortality among children under 5 and women, particularly those who are pregnant (Tanzania Food and Nutrition Centre 1992). With a fertility rate of 6.3 (Ngallaba et al. 1993), Tanzanian women, like average African women, go through many cycles of pregnancy and lactation. Between 20 and 45 years of age, women are bearing children at very short intervals, breast-feeding them, and at the same time continuing to perform energy-consuming workloads. About 5 percent of children under 5 are estimated to be severely malnourished (City Medical Office, Health Annual Report, 1993), and a recent baseline survey done (not yet published) by the Tanzania Food and Nutrition Centre (TFNC) in collaboration with the World Bank will shed new light on the current nutritional status in the country.

The major nutrition problems are protein-energy deficiency (PED); iodine leading to iodine-deficiency disorder (IDD) (Kavishe 1994); vitamin A leading to vitamin A deficiency (VAD) and xerophthalmia; and micronutrient deficiencies of iron leading to iron-deficiency anemia (IDA). Malaria appears to be the single most important factor related to the geographical variability in the prevalence of anemia (Mpanju 1992).

TFNC spearheads most of the efforts to improve the nutritional status in Tanzania and, with other sectors, facilitates the attainment of national nutrition goals toward reduction of malnutrition, prevention of low birth weight, reduction of high maternal mortality, reduction of anemia (all types), and elimination of micronutrient deficiencies.

Environmental Hazards

In the 1990s, the ''environmental lobby'' has been slowly emerging in Tanzania (Mascarenhas 1994). Following the formulation of Environmental Guidelines in 1991, recently published *Strategies for the Promotion of Environmental Health* (Ministry of Health and World Health Organization n.d.) covers the whole spectrum of the hazards in a brief but bleak situational analysis.

In 1971, legislation was passed to supply potable water to people within 400 meters of a source. However, to rehabilitate old water schemes and to provide for the expansion of water supplies to keep up with population growth would require twice what is presently allocated (The Government of the United Republic of Tanzania and United Nations Children's Fund 1990).

Fuelwood and charcoal provide over 90 percent of national fuel consumption. Almost all rural households depend completely on wood for their fuel, and most poor households in urban areas use charcoal for cooking. In most societies in Tanzania, women collect fuel (The Government of the United Republic of Tanzania and United Nations Children's Fund 1990).

In parallel, the average national population density has steadily increased over the past decades with a constant decline in the per capita availability of land; an unevenness of distribution is reflected in 65 percent of the population occupying 36 percent of the land.

PROVISION, UTILIZATION, AND IMPACT OF HEALTH SERVICES

Organization of Health Services in Tanzania

Since the decentralization of government administration in Tanzania in 1972, a fairly complex administrative and structured health care system management has evolved in which district health managers have been found to be frustrated with the organizational structure of the government health system (Gilson, Kilima, and Tanner 1995).

The administrative setup to implement the Primary Health Care (PHC) Strategy (The Government of the United Republic of Tanzania 1992) is divided into 20 administrative regions (from 670,000 to 1,700,000 each), which are further divided into 104 districts. The latter are subdivided into divisions, wards, and villages.

If classified according to funding sources, the health care system in Tanzania comprises two subsystems. The first is the public health care sector, which is financed to a large extent by central government through taxes and other government incomes. Public health care services range from small rural dispensaries to the main referral hospitals in big towns. The other subsystem is that of nongovernmental organizations (NGOs) and the private sector. It includes the provision of care by religious organizations, mainly Christian missions and charity organizations that also charge patients for their services. Apart from charity and religious organizations, a private sector operates for-profit. Drugstores (chemists' shops) are rapidly increasing in number.

The interaction between the subsystems is complex, and the boundary between them is hard to define. The picture becomes even more complicated when looked at from the way patients use these resources (the pattern of health seeking).

"Organizing and managing urban health services" (Harpham and Tanner 1995) is complex, as documented with comparative examples of decentralization in different large cities of the world, including Dar es Salaam. The important role of involving local governments and municipalities in implementing health care in comparison to relying on the traditional high degree of medicalization of urban health projects alone is being recommended (Tanner and Harpham in Harpham and Tanner 1995).

Public and Private Health Insurance and Health Care Financing

There is a monopoly of formal insurance in the country at the moment in the hands of the National Insurance Corporation (NIC), which offers group health insurance to employers. In 1992 nearly 2,000 employees were covered, plus 2,550 dependents (Abel-Smith and Rawal 1992). A form of semiinsurance is offered by the Tanzania Occupational Health Services (TOHS), a nonprofit-making company, for partial health insurance. In July 1991, the Parliament of the United Republic of Tanzania enacted a law on cost sharing. Up to then, public health services were given free, and consequently, public and private health insurances have not yet fully developed. This should encourage the development of private insurances as one of the options for health financing, in addition to earmarked taxes.

Presently, studies by the Ministry of Health (MOH), in the context of Health Sector Reform (the United Republic of Tanzania, Ministry of Health 1994), to identify different options for cost sharing are in progress. The system of cost sharing is based upon fixed fees for services, payable directly to the hospital as a first step. Different approaches are being developed and tested in various regions of the country. The existing sources of funds for health care financing are mixed: central government, donor agencies, and clients. Several exemption mechanisms for indigent people are being tried out, as a study documented that in NGO hospitals and dispensaries in Tanzania 68 percent and 40 percent of patients, respectively, were unable to pay their full fee (Mujinja and Mabala 1992).

Relation Between Ambulatory and Hospital Health Care

Most common medical conditions can be treated in relatively simple facilities—hence, the concept of primary health care (PHC) with the village health workers (VHWs) and the village posts, with the referral primary health facilities or dispensaries (Heggenhougen et al. 1987). The district secondary hospital is often a remote place even four or five kilometers away where no transports are readily available, in addition to being difficult to access due to bad road conditions.

In a qualitative study in a rural district of Tanzania (WHO/TDR 1994), traditional healing services are utilized, along with modern services, as a parallel health system. They are sought when modern services are considered fallible, too expensive, or useless, for provisional care, or the "last chance" in cases of extreme illness where modern services have failed.

Community Health Workers (CHWs) often lack the means to execute their activities. Primary health facilities and dispensaries in rural districts in turn lack equipment and drugs. As informed by villagers during the same qualitative survey (WHO/TDR 1994), ill patients must often walk long distances, back and forth, between health posts, dispensaries, hospitals, and drug shops before beginning their treatment, often bypassing the primary level of care to go directly to the hospital level. The lack of incentives for personnel to perform well is detrimental to the quality of the services. Acceptable standards of health units need to be improved, such as the patient flow, waiting areas, and rooms both for privacy and for more comfortable child delivery (Kilombero District Health Support 1994).

The referral patterns from one level of care to the other are not well known and are presently being studied in some health systems research carried out by the MOH.

Preventive Health Care

The major causes of morbidity and mortality in Tanzania are preventable diseases. This fact gives special importance to preventive services in Tanzania. Preventive health services comprise mainly preventive and health promotional activities, coupled with environmental sanitation.

Preventive health services, important as they are, still receive a comparatively minimal budget within the health sector. This hampers the implementation of most health preventive activities. Health preventive and promotion activities comprise mainly health education, vaccination, and safe lifestyle promotion. Environmental health is mainly centered on environmental sanitation. Most of these activities are undertaken by the preventive health staff who are trained health officers. Preventive services at the national level are headed by the Preventive Directorate of the MOH. At regional and district levels these services are under the general jurisdiction of the Regional and District Medical Officers.

Rehabilitation Services

Rehabilitation services can cover various subjects ranging from rehabilitation following accidents and injuries to nutritional rehabilitation. Due to the magnitude of the problem in Tanzania, the services described here are restricted to the latter only.

The hospital-based nutrition rehabilitation unit (NURU) policy in the 1970s showed clearly that it is the home conditions of the malnourished child that determine the success of rehabilitation measures rather than the functions and facilities of the NURUs. Since 1986, TFNC has promoted the use of a community-based system with the focus on the immediate factors in the child's home environment (TFNC 1993). This approach has been using the support of extension workers, parents, guardians, and community leaders (United Nations Children's Fund [UNICEF]–supported Child Survival Protection and Development Programme). Following this, communities in 1,200 villages in 31 districts have improved their own capacity to assess and analyze problems affecting children and women and have taken action to improve their nutritional status (TFNC 1992). In many places, severe malnutrition is decreasing and has dropped to below 2 percent (The Government of the United Republic of Tanzania and United Nations Children's Fund 1990).

Public Health Services

The government provides most of the health services (60 percent) in the country. Due to the increasing demand on health services and the toughening economic situation, the government, which assumed a major role in service provision, could no longer afford to provide free services. Because of lack of financial resources, most of the health units became run-down and had no drugs, and the staff morale deteriorated as time went by. This situation has led to the government review of its policy and hence the introduction of cost sharing in 1991.

The general strategy is still in line with the PHC strategy. The government is undergoing a social sector reform that includes the health sector (The United Republic of Tanzania, Ministry of Health 1994). In the health sector the aim is to target resources to services that have greater impact on the health of the community. Organizational and service delivery reform areas are being addressed in order to facilitate equity and quality. In achieving this, the government seeks to collaborate with the private sector to foster an appropriate public/private mix and reciprocity between government and private health services.

The organization of the health services delivery system centers around the government's ability to play its role effectively, from being a main provider to a facilitator. The introduction of user charges and the relegalization of private medical practice for-profit as alternative means to health care delivery are examples of the positive changes the MOH is promoting.

Self-Help Organizations

Self-help groups in Tanzania can be grouped into three classes according to the mode of formation. The first includes groups emerging spontaneously with no support or guidance from outside the group members. Most of such groups deal with economic activities (perform all kinds of activities including carpentry, crafts, farming, fishing, and masonry). In most cases, however, they also provide most of the informal social security needed by their members. They are formed because members cannot operate individually due to lack of facilities and capital. The number of these types of self-help groups in the country is very large, but their numbers are not known due to the fact that very few are formally registered or have any formal affiliations with government authorities (Alilio and Tembele 1994).

The second type of self-help groups includes those formed due to outside influences, especially NGOs. Some work directly in health promotion, while others focus on both health-related activities as well as economic activities. They also include religious-based groups dealing with a whole range of activities (weaving, flour milling, and animal keeping).

The third type of self-help groups is those formed through government involvement. They include cooperatives and those organizations that are affiliated with the ruling party, especially youth groups and women's groups. They mainly deal with public health issues like provision of health education and support in the provision of safe water supply systems. They occasionally provide loans (e.g., cooperatives) in cases of life-threatening emergencies.

Accessibility and Equity of Health Services

Following the introduction of the Arusha Declaration in 1967, Tanzania had a public health care strategy in which government took the responsibility of providing health care free up to recently, with the main focus on primary health care. This approach was based on the principal of equity and improved access in which care is provided according to need rather than ability to pay. It involved the construction of dispensaries in the rural areas, training local middle cadre manpower, providing salaries for staff, and financing other recurrent costs, including equipment and pharmaceutics, from public funds. Local resources were to be mobilized to construct local health facilities through community involvement.

This strategy has improved access to health care facilities from a situation where only 20 percent of the country's population had a dispensary within a 10-kilometer catchment area in the 1970s to a situation where, in the 1980s, about 70 percent of the entire Tanzanian population now lived within 10 kilometers of a dispensary.

The question of quality of services and equity is still far from being addressed. An improved use of the Health Management Information System (HMIS, Ministry of Health 1993) may contribute to this effort. Studies on community satisfaction with primary health care (Gilson, Alilio, and Heggenhougen 1994) that have looked into the equity and quality of health services suggest that the quality of care is poor and the marginal groups—for example, the very poor, especially women—have varying access to the available services (The United Republic of Tanzania 1992a).

THE INFRASTRUCTURE OF TRAINING AND RESEARCH IN PUBLIC HEALTH

The thrust of public health training in Tanzania has been invested in midlevel training of paramedical health personnel in nursing schools, health officer schools (sanitary officers), and medical assistant training centers. These categories of personnel have worked on public health at the grassroots, secondary, and primary health care levels. However, they have often had little recognition for their accomplishments and function with limited resources and difficult working conditions. In public health training, the Muhimbili College of Medical Sciences (former Faculty of Medicine) through the Community Medicine Department has been playing a major role in supporting the PHC development of the 1970s and early 1980s with its training outputs.

However, at the present time, the college has approximately 40 medical graduates per annum, a modest output in comparison with some of the neighboring countries that produce over 100 medical doctors per year (Kilama 1992). These graduates are trained mainly to support a clinically based service rather than a public health or research career. The Institute of Public Health has been struggling to maintain the present much-needed diplomas in public health (a three-year Master of Medicine in Community Health and a two-year Master of Science in Tropical Diseases Control). Several push factors encourage the applicants to look beyond Tanzania for training in public health: The local degree does not have the prestige of an international Western degree, nor recognition on the international market; the instructors are struggling with lower salaries and complement those with external consultancies, decreasing their availability to students; the curriculum needs updating; and finally, the facilities (teaching, libraries, etc.) are poor. The pull factors, on the other hand, are difficult to compete with: Northern facilities are attractive, with well-equipped schools offering a Master of Public Health; despite high registration fees, these schools are finding sponsors through international organizations; and finally, they have few incentives, with their own economic and survival dilemma, to strengthen the southern institutions.

Tanzania has pioneered and still does pioneer some very important public health research, from Robert Koch in the nineteenth century to the very recent malaria vaccine trials (Alonso 1994).

The National Institute for Medical Research (NIMR), established in 1979, is one of the leading research institutions among various others (the Tanzania Commission for Science and Technology, the Health Systems Research Unit of the MOH, the Muhimbili Medical Center, and the Faculty of Arts and Social Sciences of the University of Dar es Salaam). The proceedings of the *Essential National Health Research* (NIMR and COSTECH 1992) document the "Past,

Present and Future Medical and Public Health Research'' (Bitanyi 1992) and the ''Constraints to Health Research in Tanzania'' (Kilama 1992) as well.

MAJOR CHALLENGES FOR THE HEALTH SERVICES

The following five major challenges for the Tanzanian health services in the 1990s are heavily linked to political, historical, social, and economic factors.

Political Changes

After intensive domestic discussion, the government came to an agreement with the International Monetary Fund (IMF) and World Bank on a series of adjustment programs. Based on those, a policy framework (PPF) for 1992–1993 to 1994–1995 has addressed, for the first time, policy issues in the social sectors alongside policy issues in the macroeconomy. Over time it is expected that the increase in the share of public sector resources going to education, health, water, and other social sector support services, as a percentage of total expenditure, will rise gradually from 25 percent in 1992–1993 to 40 percent by the mid-1990s and be maintained at around 43 to 45 percent thereafter (The United Republic of Tanzania 1992b; The Government of the United Republic of Tanzania 1993). However, other sources (UNDP and The United Republic of Tanzania 1992) are less optimistic on the subject. Under the Priority Social Action Program (PSAP), it is stated clearly that for the foreseeable future budgetary constraints on the level of the central government will not permit large increases in the allocation of funds to social sectors. Instead, it envisages a combination of budgetary shifts, user charges, community participation, and improved management and accountability in the use of meager resources as realistic and sustainable strategies to revive and improve social services.

Demographic and Health Challenges

Tanzania may just be starting its demographic transition with a decline in mortality and a gradual decline in fertility during the last 20 years; for example, the cumulative fertility of women ages 15 to 34 decreased from 5.7 to 4.6 during this period (Ngallaba et al. 1993).

The epidemiological challenge of Tanzania is in addition to the common infectious diseases, the new pandemic diseases that are related to human immunodeficiency virus (HIV) infection, and the transition to noncommunicable diseases.

The burden of HIV and AIDS is falling more on females than on males because of their responsibilities in caring for sick people. In addition, there is evidence that more women are getting infected with HIV. There is an increase in drug-resistant disease strains of malaria (antimalarial drugs), upper respiratory infections (URIs), and diarrheal diseases (*Shigellosis dysenteriae* type 1 with complete resistance to common antibiotics). In addition, noncommunicable diseases or chronic diseases (cardiovascular diseases, cancer) are increasing from the continuing demographic transition with the aging of the population.

Ecological Challenges

The current poor management of existing natural resources such as land, water, and natural vegetation leaves a lot to be desired. Common water shortages, affecting the electrical supply (hence, the national industrial production as well), excessive pollution of groundwater with both agricultural and industrial chemicals, and poor waste disposal are some examples of common ecological challenges that need to be overcome. The current food shortages are also an important consequence of poor environmental management (poor land use, deforestation).

Organization of Health Services and Health Care Financing

The main challenge in the future of the health services and health care financing will be to implement *Proposals for Health Sector Reform* (The United Republic of Tanzania, MOH 1994). Those forceful recommendations and reforms are based on well-described organizational, managerial, financial, public/private mix, research, nutrition, and population issues. The *National District Health Planning Guidelines* (Kielmann, Mwadime, and Msanga 1993) for the use of the district health management teams are already a step in the direction of decentralization, and their use and applications will need to be encouraged and supported.

Cost-recovery mechanisms and insurance schemes are being presently organized in light of the declining resources in the government. To what extent these will be efficiently managed remains a challenge for the MOH, which is presently working on operational research in various regions of the country.

Accessibility to and equity of health services are also dependent on the population's ability to buy the health services, but growth in income has been lagging behind. In the 1970s, several shocks struck and impoverished Tanzania: severe and protracted droughts, the war against Idi Amin in Uganda in 1978, the breakup of the East African Community, increased prices of oil imports, and declining terms of trade. As a consequence, socioeconomic development suffered a downward spiral between 1979 and 1984, with a real per capita income declining by an average of 2.4 percent annually. Rural and urban households suffered from falling real incomes and shortages of essential commodities, and average income levels have remained very low, at an estimated $110 per capita.

Health Research Challenges

The various research institutions of Tanzania have attempted to determine health research priorities that are more demand driven (Mwaluko 1990). In the early 1990s, a concept of essential national health research (Kilama 1992) emerged to identify intersectoral areas for research collaboration, to improve the local communication and utilization of results, and to establish linkages between Tanzanian researchers, research clients, and policy/decision makers.

However, the government allocation to health research is meager, including low development expenditures, giving evidence that the development of Tanzanian institutions in undertaking research in human health is not a priority. The dependency on foreign donors is growing, and "donor fatigue," combined with the influence that donors may have on the choice of research projects undertaken by national institutions (Kilama 1988), still illustrates the weaknesses in the system.

In conclusion, these global political, historical, social, and economic factors will influence how much Tanzania will be able to meet its major challenges for improving its health services and reaching its goals for the year 2000.

REFERENCES

Abel-Smith, B. & Rawal, P. (1992). *Health Sector Financing Study for the Government of Tanzania*. Second Report: National Health Insurance. July.

Alilio, M. S. (1993). *Gender and Acceptance of Technologies for Tropical Disease Control. Impregnated Bednets for Malaria Control.* International Development Research Center, Technical Report.

Alilio, M. S. & Tembele, R. (1994). *Kilombero District Health Support: Social-Cultural Assessment.* Consultant Report.

Alonso, P. (1994). Randomised trial of SPf66 vaccine against *Plasmodium falciparum* malaria in children in southern Tanzania. *Lancet*, 344, 1175–1181.

Bitanyi, H. F. (1992). Past, present and future medical and public health research. In: *Tanzania ENHR*. Report on the First Workshop, Arusha.

City Medical Office. (1993). Health Annual Report. Dar es Salaam: City Medical Office.

DANIDA. (1990). *Tanzania: Environmental Profile.*

Gilson, L., Alilio, M. & Heggenhougen, K. (1994). Community satisfaction with primary health care services: An evaluation undertaken in the Morogoro region of Tanzania. *Social Science and Medicine*, 39 (no. 6), 767–780.

Gilson, L., Kilima, P. & Tanner, P. (1995). Local government decentralization and the health sector in Tanzania. *Public Administration and Development*, 14, 451–477.

The Government of the United Republic of Tanzania. (1992). *Primary Health Care Strategy* Document). Ministry of Health and DANIDA.

The Government of the United Republic of Tanzania. (1993). *The National Programme of Action (NPA) to Achieve the Goals for Tanzanian Children in the 1990's.* The National Coordinating Committee for Child Survival, Protection and Development (NCC/CSPD).

The Government of the United Republic of Tanzania and United Nations Children's Fund. (1990). *Women and Children in Tanzania: A Situation Analysis* (Report). Dar es Salaam.

Harpham, T. & Tanner, M. (Eds.). (1995). *Urban Health in Developing Countries. Progress and Prospects*. London: Earthscan Publications.

Heggenhougen, K., Vaughan, P., Muhondwa, E. & Rutabanzibwa-Ngaiza, J. (1987).

Community Health Workers: The Tanzanian Experience. Oxford and Nairobi: Oxford University Press.

HMIS, Ministry of Health, United Republic of Tanzania. (1993). *Health Management Information System (HMIS).* Implementation Plan 1992–1996.

Kavishe, F. (1994). Control of iodine deficiency disorders: The Tanzanian experience. *News on Health Care in Developing Countries,* 8, 3.

Kielmann, A. A., Mwadime, R. M. & Msanga, G. P. (1993). *National District Health Planning Guidelines.* Modules 1–3. Prepared for Ministry of Health. Eschborn, Nairobi, and Dar es Salaam.

Kilama, W. L. (1988). *Overcoming Research Barriers: The Response of Tanzania's National Institute for Medical Research.* Proceedings of the 2nd African Dental Research Conference, Morogoro, 28 September–1 October 1987. Division of Dentistry, Muhimbili Medical Center. Dar es Salaam.

Kilama, W. L. (1992). Constraints to Health Research in Tanzania. In: *Tanzania Essential National Health Research.* Report on the First Workshop, Arusha.

Kilombero District Health Support. (1994). *Workshop Proceedings.* Planning Workshop 3, 11–14 October. Ifakara.

Macintyre, S. (1986). The patterning of health by social position in the contemporary Britain. *Social Science and Medicine,* 22 (4), 399–415.

Mascarenhas, O. C. (1994). Environmental Issues and Poverty Alleviation in Tanzania. In: Bagachwa, M. S. D. (Ed.). *Poverty Alleviation in Tanzania: Recent Research Issues.* Dar es Salaam: University Press.

Ministry of Health and World Health Organization. (n.d.). *Strategies for the Promotion of Environmental Health.* Development of Health Programs in Tanzania.

Mmuni, K., Kikuli, R., Matee, W., Mwengee, W., Rugemalira, J., Fox, T. & Burns, M. (1994). The burden of disease: Cost effectiveness and health policy. Paper presented to the Eastern Regional Workshop Series. 17–19 August. Nairobi, Kenya.

Mpanju, W. (1992). *Women in Tanzania.* A paper presented to the Social Science and Medicine Annual Meeting. Nairobi.

Mujinja, W. and Mabala, S. (1992). Experiences and Lessons Learned. In: The World Bank (Ed.). *Better Health in Africa.* Washington, D.C.: The World Bank.

Mwaluko, G. M. P. (1990). *Issues and Problems in Identifying Health Research Priorities in Tanzania.* Proceedings of the TPHA Annual Scientific Conference.

National Institute for Medical Research (NIMR) and Tanzania Commission for Science and Technology (COSTECH). (1992). *Essential National Health Research.* Tanzania ENHR. Report on the First Workshop, 24–26 February. Arusha.

Ngallaba, S., Kapiga, S. H., Ruyobya, I. & Boerma, J. T. (1993). *Tanzania Demographic and Health Survey 1991/1992.* Bureau of Statistics Planning Commission. Dar es Salaam.

Tanzania Food and Nutrition Centre (TFNC). (1993). *TFNC's 20th Anniversary 1973–1993.* Dar es Salaam.

Tanzania Food and Nutrition Centre (TFNC), World Health Organization. (1992). *The Food and Nutrition Situation in Tanzania.* Country Paper for the International Conference on Nutrition, Rome, December 1992.

United Nations Development Programme (UNDP) and the United Republic of Tanzania. (1992). *Status of the Social Dimensions of Adjustment (SDA) Project in Tanzania.* SDA Activity Report for January 1991–June 1992. Prepared for the first joint review meeting on the Tanzania SDA Project, September 1992. Dar es Salaam.

United Nations High Commission for Refugees (UNHCR). (1989). *Refugees and Refugees Assistance in Tanzania.* General Information Paper. P.M.O. Dar es Salaam. (mimeographed)

United Nations High Commission for Refugees (UNHCR). (1994). *Information Bulletin.* Issue no. 14, 25 November 1994. Dar es Salaam.

The United Republic of Tanzania. (1990). *Safe Motherhood Strategy for Tanzania* (Strategy and Plan). Dar es Salaam.

The United Republic of Tanzania. (1992a). *Safe Motherhood Strategy for Tanzania* (Activities and Plan of Action). Prepared by Safe Motherhood Task Force under the Guidance of the Ministry of Health with the Assistance of Family Care International.

The United Republic of Tanzania. (1992b). *Summary of the National Program of Action (NPA) for Children in the 1990s in Tanzania.* Prepared for the International Conference on Assistance to African Children, Dakar, Senegal, 25–27 November 1992. Dar es Salaam.

The United Republic of Tanzania. Ministry of Health (MOH). (1994). *Proposals for Health Sector Reform.* (draft)

WHO/TDR. (1994). *Workshop on Qualitative Research Methods.* Report on the Field Work in Kikwawila Village. (unpublished)

Willet, W. (1990). *Nutritional Epidemiology.* Oxford: Oxford University Press.

World Bank. (1993). *Investing in Health. World Development Report.* Washington, D.C.: World Bank.

THAILAND

Somjit Supannatas

MAJOR HEALTH PROBLEMS FACING THE COUNTRY

Public health development in Thailand has progressed significantly when considering different health and social indicators such as the maternal mortality rate, the crude death rate, the infant mortality rate and morbidity, and child deaths. Deaths related to pregnancy and birth delivery have been reduced significantly. However, some disease patterns are on the rise.

Causes of morbidity and mortality have shifted more toward the noncommunicable diseases—that is, heart disease, hypertension, cancer, and mental health problems. Accidents, suicide, and drug addiction have become more common. The mortality pattern has changed dramatically due to the transition of demographic and economic development.

Infectious Disease

Prevalence of preventable diseases such as pneumonia, diphtheria, tetanus, rabies, leprosy, and sexually transmitted diseases (STDs) appears to be generally on the decline (Table 1). Malaria, which used to be the leading cause of mortality in Thailand in the 1990s, has been reduced significantly. Diarrhea is still a major public health problem with increases each year. Tuberculosis and pneumonia are expected to increase, however, as sequelae of increasing human immunodeficiency virus (HIV) prevalence in the country.

Morbidity caused by infections shows small variations by geographic regions but remains within the disease categories including enteritis and diarrhea, hemorrhagic fever, bacillary dysentery, typhoid fever, and upper respiratory infection (URI).

Table 1
Rate of Infectious Disease

Disease	1987	1988	1989	1990	1991	1992
1. TB	10.2	8.2	7.6	7.0	6.5	6.3
2. Bacterial disease	7.9	6.6	6.7	6.7	7.7	8.0
3. URI	12.6	12.6	13.8	13.0	13.9	14.4
4. Pneumonia	8.5	6.3	7.1	6.8	7.0	7.2
5. Notifiable infections	9.7	10.0	9.4	8.5	8.2	8.6
6. STD	-	0.1	0.0	0.0	0.0	0.0
7. Parasitic infection	-	1.6	2.1	1.8	1.5	1.6

Source: Division of Health Statistics 1992.

Chronic Disease

Heart disease and accident have become major causes of death at present (Table 2). For heart disease, hypertension, drinking and smoking, and stressful lifestyle are considered to be the main risk factors.

Cancer is found to have increased within this decade. Liver cancer and lung cancer are the leading causes of death in males, while cervical cancer and breast cancer are the principal causes of cancer death in women.

Another noncommunicable disease cause of death is accidents. There is evidence that most accidents are related to drug and drinking behavior. Heroin (number four) was the most popular drug being used. In big cities such as Bangkok, Chiangmai, and Hadyai, most cases of drug addiction are found in the slum areas. Opium was found to be common in the north and northeast; marijuana was common in the central and northeast. The pattern of drug use is changing to greater use of amphetamines, minor tranquilizers, and sleeping pills. Among juveniles, volatile inhalants (such as paint thinner, lacquer, and glue) are increasingly popular since they are cheap and can be accessed easily.

A recent survey reported to the policymakers of the Ministry of Public Health found that perception of illness was reported the least (37 percent) by the northern region people and the most (50 percent) by the central region people. The age group that reported the most sickness was the 0–9 years old group, and the least sickness was reported in the 10–25 years old group.

The urban population reported illness less than those who lived in the rural area. Injury was reported by males more than by females. Cause of injuries include slipping (40 percent), cuts (30 percent), motor vehicle accidents (11

Table 2
Rate of Chronic Disease

	1987	1988	1989	1990	1991	1992
1. Pulmonary /Heart	40.3	42.0	47.5	49.8	52.5	53.56
2. CA	31.5	33.5	36.2	39.5	41.2	43.5
3. Heart failure	26.9	23.8	25.7	28.5	28.0	27.9
4. CVA	9.5	9.5	10.4	10.5	11.1	11.8
5. Accident	8.6	10.4	12.4	15.3	18.3	20.1
6. Motor V. traffic Accident	8.3	9.9	12.0	14.9	17.9	19.2

CA = Cardiac arrest.
CVA = Cardiovascular accident.

Source: Division of Health Statistics 1992.

percent), and occupational accidents (10 percent). Rate of smoking was found to be higher in the male population than in the female population. For the male population, those who live in the southern region reported smoking the most. Some 80 percent of smoking behavior starts at 10 to 25 years of age. The rate of smoking in pregnant women was found to be 7 percent.

Approximately 900,000 diabetes mellitus patients were estimated in 1994, representing 2 percent of the whole adult male population and 2.8 percent of the whole adult female population. Most of the patients live in Bangkok. Around 2.1 million people were estimated as having hypertension. This amounts to 5.2 percent of the whole adult male population and 5.7 percent of the whole adult female population. Of this 2.1 million, 60 percent have symptoms that are minor, and 40 percent are moderate and severe cases. Approximately 10 percent of the general population does not know that they have hypertension. Known cases of hypertension were found the most in the central region (11 to 13 percent), followed by Bangkok (6 to 9 percent) and the northern and southern regions least. Urban populations have more cases of hypertension than the rural population. Hypercholesterolemia was found more in females than in males. Almost all of those who have hypercholesterolemia do not know that they have it. Most of the reported cases of hypercholesterolemia were in the southern region, while the northeastern region was reported to have the least (7 to 10 percent).

Mental Health

The population is now facing mental health problems due to the fast pace of Thai society, which has a severe impact on adjusting and adapting to new lifestyles. Thai culture has implicitly held a negative value toward mental health services such as counseling, group therapy, support groups, and self-help groups. Statistics revealed that people in the north have a high percentage of neurosis and of attempting suicide when compared to other regions. Neurosis was reported highest in Bangkok. Men have shown a higher rate than women. People in the north have the highest rate of suicide, and people in Bangkok have the lowest rate. Mental health and drug-addicted treatment services are provided at the regional hospitals and regional mental health centers throughout the country.

Age, Gender, and Social Class Effects

Thailand has reduced the growth rate from 6 births per woman in the mid-1960s to about 2.2 births per woman in late 1980. The aged population increased from 2.5 million in 1980 to 3.4 million in 1990 and will grow to 10 million by the year 2000, a growth increase of about 200 percent since 1990. The population under 15 years has decreased from 36.2 percent in 1975 to 33.3 percent in 1989. The working group population (15 to 59 years old) has increased 2 to 3 percent each year, while the elderly population has increased the most (6.1 percent).

Women are entering the labor force more often than before, and the parental role has changed gradually to rely on both husband and wife rather than on the wife alone. Legally speaking, the family has not allowed women to be equal. According to Book Five of the 1976 Commercial Code, a husband may file for a divorce from his wife if she commits adultery; however, the wife cannot sue her husband on the same grounds. Increasingly, women are choosing not to marry. An intersexual comparison of percent never married from 1970 to 1990 showed significant increases in female celibacy.

Social class partitions exist in Thai society only implicitly. Royal family and government officers used to have a higher class than others. However, this social class distinction has diminished. At present, people can shift their social class through many channels such as changing their education level or generating higher incomes. However, in 1992, Thailand Development Research Institute had given the estimate that a quarter and fifth of the population, respectively, were living below the poverty line of 20,705 bahts per year for a rural family and 31,260 bahts for an urban family. Moreover, about 30 percent of students go on to secondary school after completing their compulsory education. Of this group, 5 to 6 percent enter university. Therefore, it is still unclear how social class changing by these criteria will affect Thai society at large.

Refugee Health Service

Due to political turmoil in Cambodia, Vietnam, and Laos during the year 1975, thousands of refugees took refuge in Thailand, mostly along the border. Those refugees were very sick and malnourished. They brought with them malaria and other infectious diseases. At the beginning, the Thai Red Cross started

Table 3
Population Growth Rate

Per hundred (%)

	1985	1986	1987	1988	1989
Whole Kingdom	2.40	2.27	1.71	2.02	1.69
North	1.07	0.95	0.91	1.38	1.32
North east	2.40	2.72	1.79	1.96	1.67
Central	3.12	2.70	1.92	2.64	1.72
South	2.24	2.59	1.64	2.15	1.97
Bangkok	3.65	1.97	2.57	1.92	2.03

Source: Office of the National Economic and Social Development Board 1992.

health services for those refugees. Gradually, hundreds of thousands of refugees from Indochina arrived in Thailand, and they were housed in several camps and the health situation worsened. To tackle the health situation of the refugees, many nongovernmental organizations (NGOs) and United Nations extended their helping hands for health services care.

Thailand has a policy to act as the transit area before these refugees will be accepted by the third country or before they make the decision to go home. Supports given to these refugees include shelter, food, cloth, and medicine. Public health and medical service have been provided by different organizations. The ICRC (International Committee of the Red Cross) has a 100-bed hospital with good medical equipment and qualified health personnel.

In addition, the Thai Red Cross has also provided outpatient services. Christian Outreach provides maternal and child health service including an immunization program; the IRC (International Rescue Committee) has looked after general environmental sanitation. The FPIA (Family Planning International Assistance) and CBERS (Community Based Emergency Relief Services) have been responsible for the family planning program. Some of these organizations have had to abandon their services recently owing to monetary and other difficulties.

Population Development

Thailand's population stands at an estimated 60 million (1994). The achievement of population policy and the National Family Planning program, which was initiated in 1971, have resulted in the reduction of the population growth rate (e.g., from 2.4 percent in 1985 to 1.69 percent in 1989) (Table 3). The change in sex-age structure population distribution or pyramid, or the proportion of children, has been reduced compared to the increase in adult and old-age population groups. The general fertility rate in the south is the highest (79.6,

Table 4
General Fertility Rate

Per 1,000 population

	1985	1986	1987	1988	1989
Whole Kingdom	79.7	75.1	68.3	60.8	61.5
North	60.0	70.1	60.2	53.9	52.4
North east	85.0	76.8	71.0	61.6	60.4
Central	72.1	67.2	63.8	59.5	61.3
South	107.0	101.6	87.3	78.1	79.6

Source: Office of the National Economic and Social Development Board 1992.

1989); it is higher than the national general fertility rate (61.5). The north has the lowest (52.4) (Table 4).

The percentage of population growth rate by region shows that Bangkok has the highest growth rate (2.03, 1989), which is higher than the national growth rate (1.69, 1989) (Table 3). The birthrate is four times that of the death rate in 1989. In addition, the population census has been conducted nine times since 1911 by the National Statistical Office (Office of the Prime Minister). The population in Thailand is predominantly rural. The urban population is 30 percent of the total population. Most urbans live in the Bangkok Metropolitan Area with a registered population of 8 million (1994). There is an estimation of an additional 2 million people who commute to work in Bangkok daily and reside in neighboring provinces such as Samut Prakan, Nonthaburi, and Pathum Thani. The next largest centers constitute the regional capitals of Chiangmai, Hadyai, and Ubon Ratchathani, each having more than 250,000 in population.

Nutritional Problems

Three major undernourishment conditions have been identified as national public health problems since the Fourth National Economic and Social Development Plan (1977–1981). They are protein-energy malnutrition, iodine-deficiency disorder (IDD), and iron-deficiency anemia. Results of a survey in 1990 and 1991 that surveyed the whole country indicate that there are 27 percent of preschool children with malnutrition—25 percent, first degree; 2 percent, second degree; and none in the third degree.

IDD is regarded as a public health problem if goiter prevalence exceeds 10 percent in any area. It varies from 20 to 60 percent in the endemic areas in the north and northeastern provinces of the country. Iodate salt and iodate fish sauce, fortified salt, drinking water fortification, and iodized oil capsules are provided according to the severity of IDD problems. Iron-deficiency anemia is one of the most common nutritional problems in Thailand among schoolchildren and pregnant women, particularly in the northeastern and southern regions. Control measures include anemia survey, supply of ferrous supplementation tablets in health centers and schools, nutrition education, and hookworm control and treatment.

Overnutrition has started to be a problem in large cities where the Western-style diet is gaining popularity. Prevalence of obesity falls in the 35 to 54 age group. Community self-reliance has developed as the control strategy. Supporting strategies such as food composition and value analysis, multisectoral collaboration, monitoring and education, and food and nutrition manpower development are under way to diminish the nutritional problem.

Environmental Hazards

Environmental problems have become more and more serious in Thailand, especially in big cities such as Bangkok and Chiangmai. This may be due to the economic transitional period and effects of becoming an industrial community. Moreover, since the disparity of social class has been minimal, the power to buy materialistic values has become more widespread. At the same time, big cities have become increasingly congested with regard to traffic and population. Toxic pollution of rivers and streams due to overuse of pesticides and chemical fertilizers has been added to the environmental problems in rural areas.

The urban area environmental problems are linked with traffic jams and overpopulation. The consequences manifest in the form of air pollution, water pollution, noise, and waste disposal and drinking water problems. In addition, in the attempt to transform into a diversified agroindustrial society, the expansion of land cultivation has accelerated. The rapid decline of the country's forests is obvious and has brought about ecological problems demonstrated in two contrasting disasters: floods and mudslides.

PROVISION, UTILIZATION, AND IMPACT OF HEALTH SERVICES

The health service system in Thailand can be divided into three areas: the government sector, the nongovernmental organization sector, and the private sector.

Government Sector

Ministry of Public Health. The Ministry of Public Health has the responsibility for the organization, management, and administration of the public health services of the government, especially in the rural areas.

Other Governmental Agencies. Besides the Ministry of Public Health, which is responsible for direct health service delivery, many other ministries have

Table 5
Utilization of Health Services: Comparison Between Three Surveys, 1970, 1979, 1985

Type of Health Service	1970	1979	1985
Self treatment	51.4	42.3	28.6
Health Centers	4.4	16.8	14.7
Government Hospitals	11.1	10.0	32.5
Private Hospitals & Clinics	22.7	20.4	21.8
Traditional Healers	7.7	6.3	2.4
No treatment	2.7	4.2	--

Source: Ministry of Public Health 1991.

activities and responsibilities contributing to people's good health. In Thailand, the Ministry of Education, the Ministry of Interior, the Ministry of Public Health, the Ministry of Agriculture and Cooperatives, the Ministry of Commerce, and the Ministry of Industry are the six key ministries of importance for the achievement of health for all groups of the population. The Office of the Prime Minister is another key ministry governing different bodies that act as support units for overall development. At the same time, some other ministries or organizations carry out health-related activities or provide medical and health services such as the Ministry of University Affairs, the Ministry of Industry, the Ministry of Defence, and the Government Pharmaceutical Organization.

Nongovernmental Organizations Sector

Outside the sphere of the government sector, there are numerous nonprofit organizations with various charitable functions including health services. Some of these NGOs are totally charitable organizations aiming especially to render services to the public. Some are organizations with their own specific scope of work, both for its own benefit and for the public. NGOs must be registered with the Office of the National Cultural Committee in the Ministry of Education.

Private Sector

According to the most recent survey of utilization of health services (1985), 21.8 percent of the population used private and 32.5 percent government facilities when they became ill (Table 5). Self-treatment by buying drugs from the local drugstores accounted for 28.6 percent of the service used.

Most public health services for rural people are provided under the administration and supervision of the Ministry of Public Health, which has different units responsible for the following:

1. *Provincial health office.* Each of the nation's 72 provinces has a provincial chief medical officer (PCMO), who is nominally responsible for both administration and support of all medical and health facilities in the province including the provincial hospital and provincial health office. In practice, the day-to-day hospital operation of the provincial hospital is left to a hospital director, and the PCMO tends to focus on the supervisory aspects of technical and policy matters. The PCMO is responsible to the permanent secretary of the Ministry of Public Health, but he is also administratively responsible to the governor, the senior civil administrator of the province who reports to the Ministry of Interior.
2. *Regional and general hospital (provincial hospital).* Most provincial hospitals have 150 to 500 beds, but the regional referral hospitals (17) have 500 to 1,000 beds and provide training for a variety of medical and paramedical workers. Provincial hospitals are predominantly curative, but to a certain extent, promotive, preventive, and rehabilitative services are also offered. General hospitals are predominantly utilized by people in the immediate area of the provincial capital, whereas the bigger regional hospitals serve as a catchment area for the health center population in their respective regions.
3. *Community hospital (district hospital).* Almost 90 percent of the nation's districts have a district hospital (now called a *community hospital*). These hospitals normally have 10 to 60 beds; a few have 90 beds. A 10-bed hospital normally has two physicians. Thirty-bed, 60-bed, and 90-bed facilities can have three, four, and six physicians, respectively. Each community hospital provides curative, promotive, preventive, and rehabilitative health services and has official responsibility for overall supervision and technical support of health center activities and public health programs in the district where the hospital is located.
4. *District health office (DHO).* The DHO is basically an organization entity that includes technical and administrative staff. The DHO is directly responsible to the district officer, who reports to the Ministry of Interior. In practice, however, most of the DHO's technical and managerial support is coordinated by the provincial health office.
5. *Health center.* In each of the 6,754 *tambons*, there is at least one health center. Each health center is staffed by at least a technical nurse or midwife and a junior sanitarian. All of the major promotive and preventive health services are integrated into the tasks of these two health personnel. The midwife and sanitarian are responsible for immunization; prenatal, delivery, and postnatal services; nutrition; water supply; family planning; and sanitary activities. Health centers are also providing limited emergency services and treatment for minor illness beyond which they provide referral service to district and provincial hospitals. The health center also serves as a referral unit in the primary health care (PHC) delivery system. Likewise, it provides support to the village for the development and strengthening of its PHC program.
6. *Community health system station (CHSS).* The CHSSs are the smallest health facilities located in villages. The villages selected to have CHSSs are those that are perceived to be a national security risk, in remote areas of scattered population and/or in the areas of minority groups, such as the border villages and hill tribe villages.

Public and Private Health Insurance

The health care system in Thailand uses mainly public providers, funded by a combination of taxation and users' fees. A number of medical benefit and health insurance schemes have existed in Thailand for a long time, including the civil servant's Medical Benefit Scheme and the voluntary health card scheme, which covers the cost of care in government facilities. The 1990 Social Security Act (SSA) aims to extend considerably the use of social insurance funding for health services. The SSA covers all workers in companies of 20 or more employees, approximately 3 million people in total.

Health Service Provision and Payment System

The Thai model borrows from the idea of managed markets. At the beginning of each year, employees register with a hospital (which, as the main provider, is required to make primary care available to those registered with it). The hospital is then paid a capitation fee for each person registered. These fees covers all health services except identified expensive conditions for which a "special payment" schedule is used.

The option of registering with a different hospital at the beginning of each year was included in order to stimulate competition between providers to maintain a high quality of care. The capitation mechanism was designed to contain costs. The decision in choosing a hospital, which has to have a minimum of 100 beds, is made by the employer. As a consequence, employees have to travel long distances to obtain care, utilization rates are much lower than expected, and there is little incentive to provide a high quality of service. The scheme is financed by equal contributions from the insured persons (1.5 percent of salary), the employer, and the government. It is compulsory for all companies unless they can show that they provide a higher level of medical benefits through another scheme.

Health Card Program

A health card program has been in existence since the Sixth National Development Plan. The health card was designed to be used as a tool for increasing people's ability to become active in medical care. There are two types of health card coverage: (1) a maternal and immunization service and (2) a general medical care program.

Low-income health insurance is also provided by the Ministry of Health for the poor who cannot afford any health service. Through this system, they are provided medical care free of charge.

Approximately 44 percent of the Thai population are left out of the health insurance system. Health care expenses have reflected the inequality of the per capita resource consumption among different groups of the Thai population. Government officers and their families have the highest per capita expenditure

(U.S.$37), followed by those covered by the private health insurance group (U.S.$24).

Preventive Health Care

Preventive activities in the health care system include an expanded program on immunization, the Health Education and Public Relation Program, and a surveillance program. The national Expanded Program on Immunization (EPI) was launched by the Ministry of Public Health in 1977. This program now covers vaccination against tuberculosis, diphtheria, pertussis, poliomyelitis, tetanus, measles, and hepatitis. The impact of this program has shown the significant decline of vaccinated disease incidence when compared to previous incidence records. Vaccine coverage has also shown impressive results. In the future, the EPI program aims toward improving vaccination technique and the information system.

The Health Education and Public Relation Program has been integrated in all communicable disease prevention programs under the guidance of the Ministry of Public Health. Activities also cover a wide range of behavior change such as all forms of communication, community participation and mobilization, and skill development training. However, most activities deal with communication and materials distribution. A major program has been targeted to prevent the occurrence of diarrhea, tuberculosis (TB), malaria, dengue, hemorrhagic fever, parasitic diseases, hepatitis B, rabies, STDs, and acquired immunodeficiency syndrome (AIDS). The outcomes of this program on behavior change are very modest and show the inconsistency of preventive behavior change in the target population. Due to the AIDS epidemic, preventive program concentration nowadays is given to the AIDS & STD and TB prevention program. There is a policy to integrate AIDS & STD in all disease prevention programs delivered by the Ministry of Public Health as well as in all community activities that are delivered by other ministries. Other preventive health care delivered by the hospital services includes education activities to prevent the risk group from getting the disease, for example, diabetes mellitus and hypercholeresterolemia.

Relation Between Ambulatory and Hospital Health Care

Ambulatory care is provided in the hospital to a certain extent by nurse practitioners who are trained by the Faculties of Nursing. Ambulatory care has been carried out fully in only a very few university hospitals; other health centers or hospitals have applied only home visit activities.

Rehabilitation Services

Rehabilitation services under the supervision of the Ministry of Public Health are mostly provided in the mental health institutions in the form of occupational

Table 6
Distribution of Health Personnel, 1988–1990

Ration	1988	1989	1990
Health Personnel: Population			
Doctor: Population	1: 4,832	1: 4,361	1: 4,525
Dentist: Population	1:32,858	1:26,316	1:23,129
Pharmacist: Population	1:14,783	1:14,496	1:14,164
Nurse: Population	1: 1,065	1: 962	1: 998

Source: Health Statistics Division, Office of the Permanent Secretary for Ministry of Public Health (1988–1990).

therapy, recreational therapy, and so on. Four rehabilitation centers were established to provide services similar to halfway homes and day care. For the Bangkok Metropolitan Administration, rehabilitation service is provided for the drug-dependent person as an extension of drug detoxification service. Another type of rehabilitation service that is still limited is service for orthopedic or amputated patients. It is offered in some hospitals such as military hospitals and regional hospitals.

Self-Help Organizations

This type of service is not common in the health service system in Thailand. It has been developed by some nongovernmental organizations such as Samaritan or the Red Cross. Since the AIDS epidemic, the number of self-help organizations has increased in order to cope with the medical and psychological burdens to society. Community support groups are being developed by both governmental and nongovernmental organizations.

Accessibility and Equity of Services

According to Public Health Ministry statistics, there are about 15,000 doctors in the country, most of them employed by city and municipal councils and the ministry itself. Meanwhile, there are an estimated 2,500 doctors working in private hospitals.

The shortage of doctors in public hospitals (Table 6) is compounded by the failure of the University Affairs Bureau to produce enough medical graduates from its medical schools. The University Affairs Bureau has stated that due to budgetary constraints it would not be able to produce more than 880 medical students a year without compromising the quality of education. In Bangkok there is 1 doctor for every 1,000 people, while in the provinces, including urban areas, 1 doctor has to take care of 7,558 people. The doctor:patient ratio in Bangkok is closer to that of the industrialized countries of Asia: 1:650 in Japan and 1: 1,139 in South Korea. The ratio of rural Thailand falls in with most other developing countries because of the relative inaccessibility to proper health care in the provinces.

Beginning in 1995, the Public Health Ministry, jointly working with the University Affairs Bureau, will recruit more medical students and have them trained in medical schools and hospitals of the ministry as part of a program to boost the number of doctors. Moreover, the ministry has plans to improve the salaries and welfare benefits for doctors employed by government hospitals throughout the country by offering a minimum salary of U.S.$1,200 a month for new doctors.

THE INFRASTRUCTURE OF TRAINING AND RESEARCH IN PUBLIC HEALTH

The Committee for Medical Research was established under the National Research Council (NRC) in 1956. This committee is responsible for formulating policy, identifying research priorities, and promoting research activities through NRC grants.

Most universities and medical schools have their own policies and mechanisms for medical research administration. For the Ministry of Public Health (MOPH), research activities are carried out by various technical departments. In administering and setting research policy, there are three research subcommittees: the Research Project Review Subcommittee, the Ethical Review Subcommittee, and the Subcommittee on Research Capability Strengthening and Research Fund.

The Office of Technical Cooperation and Health Manpower Development was appointed to be the secretariat office in executing the research committee decision. Health systems research and science and technology research were initiated in the Seventh National Health Development Plan. The HSRI (Health System Research Institute) tailors the research to four areas: health policy and management, research and development on health service delivery, primary health care research, and health manpower development research. HSRI functions through two hierarchical bodies, the HSRI Governing Board and three HSRI sections (general administration, information center, and technical unit). The HSRI has three primary missions: to organize and support priority research, to promote the use of research studies, and to form an HSRI network. Science and technology research focuses on health promotion and technologies such as contraceptive technologies, pharmaceutical product distribution, local manufacture of local medical equipments and supplies, child growth and development, promotion of dental health, and prevention of iodine deficiency diseases. Traditional medicine development and pharmaceutical research especially on traditional herbal medicine are also promoted. Areas of research are directed toward the current public health problems in all areas: communicable disease, noncommunicable disease, environmental health, occupational health, and AIDS.

Public health personnel training is done through a formal process and provided by the universities and the MOPH public health colleges. Moreover, to cope with the shortage of health personnel as well as the changing patterns of public health problems, in-service and continuing education are also offered by the MOPH and other organizations both governmental and semigovernmental and local and international agencies. Different strategies are being developed and implemented to overcome the shortage of health personnel and increase people's participation. One major strategy developed in Thailand is the health training of community leaders to become village health volunteers and village health communicators.

Health Care Financing

Approximately 4.5 percent of the government budget is allocated to provide health care to the Thai society throughout the MOPH. Over 70 percent of the health budget is spent by the office of the permanent secretary in providing rural public health management all over the country. Approximately 8 to 10 percent of the budget is spent by the Medical Services Department and another 8 to 10 percent is spent in controlling communicable diseases under supervision of the Department of Communicable Diseases Control. An estimated 7 to 8 percent budget is spent by the Department of Health, while less than 1 percent is utilized by the Medical Sciences Department and Food and Drug Administrations.

The Ministry of Public Health annual budget is spent in different program areas.The largest allocation is the 57 percent spent on providing medical care, followed by that for health promotion activity (around 12 percent of the budget). Controlling communicable diseases takes 13 percent of the budget, while health manpower production and development activities spend 6 percent. Research and laboratory development receives approximately 5 percent. General administration and supplementary program activity spends 5 percent of the budget. When comparing the health budget allocations for the urban and rural public health programs, 1990 statistics indicated that medical care dollars were equally distributed to the urban and rural areas.

Additional health budget sources include the other ministries' government health budgets, foreign aid, private companies, and private insurance companies. In terms of health care expenditure, the national health care expenditure has increased gradually.

MAJOR CHALLENGES FOR THE HEALTH SERVICES

Surveillance and Monitoring

A surveillance program has long been established to monitor cases and deaths of major communicable and preventable diseases. Those diseases include: cholera, acute diarrhea, food poisoning, dysentery, enteric fever, hepatitis, conjunctivitis, influenza, rubella, chicken pox, pyrexia, meningococcal infection, measles, diphtheria, pertussis, tetanus, hemorrhagic fever, encephalitis, malaria, pneumonia, TB, leprosy, yaws, STD, rabies, leptospirosis, scrub typhus, occupational diseases, mumps, and other diseases (insecticide poisoning; lead poisoning; manganese, mercury, and arsenic poisoning).

In addition, due to AIDS, the Ministry of Health and the universities are attempting to develop a behavioral surveillance system to help monitor the risk behavior of the general population and to help design the appropriate behavior change. However, this behavior surveillance system is still in the development process, unlike the disease surveillance program.

Intervention and Evaluation

There are many interventions that Thailand has developed and implemented successfully. This chapter will select a few that are considered to have a nationwide impact. A major intervention in the Thailand public health system is the reorganizing of the health system by using the concept of primary health care. Over the last 15 years, with the technical and financial support of the World Health Organization (WHO), Thai PHC has recognized that training villagers to become potential change agents who play active roles in the community is the major intervention to achieve PHC service and the Health for All goal in Thailand.

Moreover, "Basic Minimum Needs," which was simultaneously developed as the strategy for the national rural development program and involved intersectoral action, has been an effective tool. The PHC Thai program also has other components that are uniquely designed to fit the society's values and culture. Those program components include self-management, self-financing, self-analysis, leadership development, and TCDV (technical cooperation among the developing villages). These innovative approaches have had a strong and positive impact on the progress and direction of national rural development and have extended health services to the rural population.

Another intervention that is considered to be a model and has attracted attention from the international community is the AIDS Control and Prevention Intervention. There are many intervention activities in the AIDS control program that have been implemented. The major intervention that has attracted global response is the level of political involvement, with the prime minister as chairman of the National AIDS Committee and the provincial governor as chairman of the Provincial AIDS Committee. This political involvement has resulted in expanding the AIDS education program to all ministries and reaching a larger number of the target population. The strategy used to get political involvement was bringing together media journalists leading nongovernmental organizations and the MOPH. As a result, the government decided to form a National AIDS Committee. A condom promotion intervention, a community participation intervention, a community mobilization intervention, and a clinical-based intervention have been designed and implemented. These interventions are still ongoing. Evaluation activities and indicators are being reported such as decrease of STD cases and increase of condom use. It is still premature to claim success in AIDS control and prevention. However, it can be concluded that the Thai AIDS prevention and control program has achieved a considerable amount of success in involving the Thai society in the prevention effort.

Specific Public Health Services for Defined Population

Mothers and interventions targeted to mothers and children include breast-feeding promotion, well child care and the EPI program, the Thai Model Mother Program, and the high-risk check card program. These interventions have been developed based on the realization of the insufficient number of maternal and child health (MCH) services in rural areas.

This target group has received attention for a long time since this group has a psychological and social nature that requires special interventions. Major campaigns and interventions focus on the issues of smoking cessation, condom promotion, drug addiction prevention, and so on. School health programs have long been established, and out-of-school youth programs have increased.

Intervention focused on the ''family'' has increased its importance. This may be due to changing disease patterns, the population structure, and socioeconomic growth of the society. However, health and social welfare services for the family are still limited. Public health personnel are now in the process of reorienting themselves toward the family approach.

This target group has just recently become the focus of attention due to the changes in the population structure. Policies to provide health care and social welfare facilities have been promoted. The elderly support group and medical service has been provided throughout the country. Despite these initiatives, there is a lot more work needed in the area of elderly and public health in Thailand.

Many public health campaigns have been carried out. These have applied traditional fear arousal or medical-oriented approaches more than behavior change and persuasive approaches. Recent behavior change campaigns such as stop-smoking campaigns and AIDS campaigns have tried to change their strategies from sending fear-arousal messages to promoting self-responsibility and community participation. Additional strategies such as law and legislation, fund-raising, and social mobilization are also included.

For environmental problems, there have been several campaigns. Preserving natural resources has long been promoted in Thailand under the leadership of the king and queen and their family. Nongovernmental agencies have campaigned on several issues and projects such as Magic Eyes, Think Earth. Recycling has just been started by private agencies. A few government offices under several ministries also have responsibility for protecting the environment; however, their job lies in enforcing the legislation rather than in introducing campaigns to protect the environment.

In view of demographic changes, Thailand has an increasing older population; this elderly group, later on, will be the group in society that stands to be left behind. They tend to have more health problems. Moreover, social changes such as urbanization and migration of the adults from the rural areas to cities will pose a threat to the well-being of the elderly. It is a challenge and a considerable burden on health services to cope with the aging population. Another challenge is the urban public health problem. Intervention will require not only medical knowledge but also technology and reorientation of social values toward Thai people's lifestyle.

REFERENCES

Division of Health Statistics, Bureau of Health Policy and Planning Office, Ministry of Public Health. (1992). *Public Health Statistics AD*. Bangkok, Thailand.

Faculty of Social Welfare. (1976). *Social Services in Thai Society: Way to Reality*. Bangkok: Thammasart University. (in Thai)

Health Department Association. (1995). *Public Health Calendar 1995*. Bangkok: Sahaprachanich.

Ministry of Public Health. (1991). *Thailand Health Profile, 1990*. Bangkok, Thailand.

National Environmental Committee. (1993). *Quality in Thailand 1987–1990*. Bangkok: Chomnum Sahakorn Karnkaset Printing Office.

National Statistical Office, Office of the Prime Minister. (1990). *Population and Housing Census: Whole Kingdom*. Bangkok: National Statistical Office.

Nopawan Chongwatana & Kuo Wongbasin. (1989). *Survey Report on Family Planning Behavior of Indo-China Refugee in Thailand in 1988*. Bangkok: Population Institute, Chulalongkorn University.

Office of the National Economic and Social Development Board. (1992). *Social Indicators*. Bangkok: Medsai Printing.

Survey Report. (1994). *Health Status and Policy Recommendations*. Bangkok. (in Thai)

Wiroj Tangcharoensathien. (1993). *Medical Expenditure for Inpatients Under the Civil Servant Medical Benefits Scheme*. Bangkok: Ministry of Public Health.

UNITED KINGDOM

Christopher Birt

ORIGINS OF BRITISH PUBLIC HEALTH

Although it is possible to identify earlier origins, British public health, as we now recognize it, began in the first half of the last century, when some of the large industrial cities first appointed medical officers of health. This was a response to the growing realization that the effects of rapid industrialization and urbanization over the previous century had resulted in major adverse effects on the health of the population. For several decades, these doctors, working in public health in Victorian Britain as employees of local government, sought to ensure that proper drainage systems were installed, that clean water was supplied to the population, and that a reasonable standard of food hygiene was maintained. From an early stage, these medical officers of health were guaranteed, through legal statute, very considerable security of employment, so that they could be able to speak openly on public health hazards, including when it became necessary to criticize their employing authorities (Frazer 1950). Toward the end of the last century, and early in this century, the developing local authority public health departments began to provide other services, particularly for mothers and small children, and also certain hospital services, for example, for those with venereal diseases (Evans, 1992), and for those with infectious diseases generally (Abel-Smith 1964).

After World War I, there was a major expansion in academic medicine in medical schools. By the 1930s, some doctors working in academic departments of medicine began to specialize in the study of the distribution of disease within society (i.e., epidemiology). From 1933 onward, starting in Oxford, some of these doctors began to separate from university departments of general medicine and to establish departments of epidemiology, at that stage often called departments of social and preventive medicine (Brockington 1966). During World War II, the government of the day set up a committee to review the training needs of doctors who would work in the health service to be set up after the war. This committee, the Goodenough Committee, reported that all doctors should be provided with training in epidemiology, and in social and preventive medicine, during their medical student studies, and that examination of these subjects should be a compulsory component of the final examinations for all medical students. Although it took more than a quarter of a century for these recommendations to be fully implemented (London University was the last to enforce them), they became universally applied from the late 1960s.

An emergency medical service was set up throughout the United Kingdom during World War II, and a similar administration was maintained to run the hospital service after the National Health Service (NHS) was established on July 5, 1948 (Forsyth 1966). Administrative doctors were employed to plan hospital services as according to need, and although they were very largely medical administrators, these doctors clearly carried out some public health functions. They were employed mainly in regional hospital boards, which were set up to administer the hospital sector within the National Health Service.

In the mid-1960s, the Wilson government set up a Royal Commission to study the future needs of medical education. The report, known as the *Todd Report*, was published in 1968 (Royal Commission on Medical Education 1968). Building on the recommendations of the Goodenough report, it recommended that epidemiological and public health skills should be made available to every health service district and, accordingly, that postgraduate training in this specialty should be developed for doctors wishing to specialize in this way. In the light of these recommendations, the three Royal Colleges of Physicians, of London, Edinburgh, and Glasgow, set up together a Faculty of Community Medicine (later to be renamed The Faculty of Public Health Medicine), and in 1973, three very differing groups of doctors (the local authority public health doctors, the academic epidemiologists, and the regional hospital board medical administrators) were invited to identify themselves as public health physicians by joining the Faculty.

Nonmedical Public Health Professionals

The Faculty of Public Health Medicine, established as the Faculty of Community Medicine in 1973, provided a specialist career structure for public health doctors. However, by this time, many nonmedical professional people were working in the field of public health, and more were to follow. For many years previously, the environmental health officer profession had developed within local authority public health departments, and these professional people carried out various routine public health activities on behalf of medical officers of health, many of these being concerned with control of communicable disease. Meanwhile, by 1970, information scientists, another group of public health department employees, were also growing in numbers. These people collected and collated data of an epidemiological nature, which medical officers of health required to enable them to make policy decisions. Over the same period, the rapidly developing academic departments of public health (or of social and preventive medicine) were employing increasing numbers of nonmedical epidemiologists, medical sociologists, and health economists.

Environmental health officers were able to establish a career structure for themselves after 1974, when local authorities ceased to employ medical officers of health. However, some of the other groups mentioned have had more difficulty establishing career structures, owing to the lack of availability of senior public health posts to nonmedical graduates (Watterson 1994). However, the Faculty of Public Health Medicine is currently considering the possibility of offering membership to nonmedical public health professionals (O'Brien 1995), thereby offering them assistance with career development in the future (Somervaille and Griffiths 1995).

NHS provider organizations also employ two other groups of professionals who work in public health. Health visitors are specially trained public health nurses, who are in particular concerned with the health of children and the elderly (Symond 1993), and health promotion officers are employed to coordinate the health education and health protection activities of health authorities and provider organizations.

Public Health Medicine in the NHS Since 1974

Since April 1, 1974, most nonacademic public health physicians have been employed by health authorities (whether or not they were previously employed by local authorities, regional health hospital boards, or even within academic departments). Area health authorities, which were the employers, although set up by a Conservative government, operated under a Labor government (elected in February 1974) until 1979. Following the victory of the Conservative Party in the election of 1979, area health authorities in England were replaced by a very much larger number of smaller district health authorities (Baggott 1994), causing disruption to the employment of many public health physicians, as they had to reapply for their jobs (in Scotland, Wales, and Northern Ireland there was very much less disruption at this time). Management of health authorities remained subject to a consensus procedure, which involved public health physicians in every district. However, following the establishment of district health authorities, the Conservative government subsequently enforced a system of general management, according to which each health authority had to appoint a chief executive to its board. There was nearly always a public health physician as a member of each board, and in a few cases, public health physicians were appointed as chief executives themselves.

Following 1989, the Conservative government enforced a much more radical reform of the National Health Service, introducing market forces and dividing the health service structure into ''purchasers'' (health authorities) and ''providers'' (hospitals and community services) (Baggott 1994).

Training arrangements for public health doctors are similar to those in any other United Kingdom medical specialty (Pearson, Carr, and Pouse 1993). Following qualification as a doctor, each medical graduate must work compulsorily in junior hospital posts for one year. In practice, most junior doctors work in such posts for rather longer. Subsequently, they apply for posts in the registrar grade, which provides general professional training (in this case, registrar posts in public health medicine).

During the two years normally spent in this grade, trainees are expected to pass Part 1 of the examination for membership in the Faculty of Public Health Medicine. They can then advance to a senior registrar post in public health medicine (higher specialist training), within which they will carry out work later to be written up and reported to the Faculty as part of the Part 2 examination for membership. When both parts of the membership examination have been passed, and following a period of sufficient time in training in the various aspects of public health medicine, accreditation is granted to each trainee. At this stage, a senior registrar is able to apply for consultant posts in the specialty, as these become available, usually following retirement of a previous post holder. However, continuing education is also a priority for public health physicians throughout their careers, as for other specialist doctors, and appropriate courses and other types of training are provided by various medical schools and other bodies (McEwen 1995).

MAJOR HEALTH PROBLEMS FACING THE UNITED KINGDOM

In the period 1991–1992, the British government published various health strategy documents for different parts of the United Kingdom. These were closely related to the World Health Organization's (WHO) Health for All program (Targets for Health for All 1985). They sought to address some of the major health problems in each country, and they set definite targets for improved health to be achieved over stated periods of time. The document for England was titled *The Health of the Nation*, and that for Scotland, *Scotland's Health: A Challenge to Us All*. Similar proposals were made by the relevant government departments for Wales and Northern Ireland.

Strategies to reduce morbidity and mortality from cardiovascular disease feature highly in each of these documents. Although the death rate from coronary heart disease appears to have peaked in the United Kingdom during the 1980s, with a subsequent fall particularly evident in younger men, the death rate from this condition, especially in Scotland and Northern Ireland, remains among the highest found anywhere in the world. The death rate from stroke has been falling fairly consistently over recent years. The government's health strategies include proposals to reduce tobacco smoking, to improve diet, to reduce the mean population blood pressure (as well as for more effective screening to identify those with existing hypertension), and to encourage more physical exercise.

Cancer also features highly in these documents. Lung cancer remains the commonest cancer in the United Kingdom, and it is nearly always fatal. The death rate among men is falling (following the marked reduction in the prevalence of smokers among the male population), but it is still rising among women. In Scotland, lung cancer now kills more women than does any other cancer, having overtaken breast cancer in this respect, and other parts of the United Kingdom are following this trend. Bowel cancer also has a high incidence. The government's strategies include various approaches designed to reduce cigarette smoking and also to provide more effective screening for both breast cancer and cervical cancer (both these types of screening are now provided systematically to the female population at risk throughout the United Kingdom).

Sexual health features prominently within the government's areas of concern, particularly on account of the hazards to public health posed by human immunodeficiency virus (HIV) infection and acquired immunodeficiency syndrome (AIDS). A major program for containment of this hazard continues to be implemented in the United Kingdom, including education for sexual health, provision of condoms, and provision of free needle exchange in many places for drug addicts who use intravenous injection of drugs.

Improved mental health appears within the strategy for England, with a target set for reduction in the suicide rate. In Scotland the emphasis is on dental health, with plans to provide fluoridated water supplies to the whole population, not hitherto carried out regularly in Scotland owing to particular legal difficulties in that country.

Reduction in the mortality and morbidity rates from accidents and injuries features in the government's strategies throughout the United Kingdom. Proposals were made for injury reduction in various sectors, including for road traffic accidents. Injury rates are falling, and it seems likely that the targets set by the government will be met.

One type of health problem received only a cursory reference within the government's strategy documents. This concerns the widening gap in health status between the more prosperous and the poorer parts of the United Kingdom population (Watkins 1994). *The Black Report*, published in 1981, provided well-documented evidence of the extent of the gap regarding expectation of life and health, as between the richer and poorer of the social classes (Townsend, Davidson, and Whitehead 1988). This evidence was reinforced in a further report entitled *The Health Divide*, published later in the 1980s (Townsend, Davidson, and Whitehead 1988). Further research has followed, and as the income gap between the richest and poorest parts of the British population has widened, so has the health gap (''The Unhealthy Poor'' 1994). However, it is not only the very poorest who are adversely affected. Health status deteriorates stepwise, class by class, as one reviews the position from the best-off social class to the poorest social class. Moreover, recent work in Southampton suggests that, notwithstanding these differences, countries with an egalitarian system for distribution of wealth enjoy better overall health status throughout the population than do those with inegalitarian systems of distribution (Davey Smith and Egger 1993).

PATTERN OF HEALTH SERVICE PROVISION

The UK population has enjoyed the benefits of a National Health Service since 1948, according to which most health service expenditure is paid for from general taxation. This health service is administered separately in each of the four UK countries, and accordingly, administrative arrangements differ considerably. However, since the most recent government reforms (Working for Patients 1989), implemented in 1990, health authorities (England and Wales), health boards (Scotland), and health and social services boards (Northern Ireland) have been responsible for identifying the health needs of the populations for which they are accountable and for purchasing appropriate health care from provider organizations (mainly National Health Service hospitals and community health services units). Purchasing organizations are accountable to a government health department in each country, and their performance is monitored by means of an annual review system. In England, owing to its large population, the government is establishing regional outposts of the Department of Health so that accountability reviews can take place at the regional level.

Most primary care is carried out by general practitioners. In Scotland and Northern Ireland, these doctors have always held contracts with health boards (Scotland) and with health and social services boards (Northern Ireland), and these bodies continue to purchase primary health care from general practitioners. In England, general practitioners have previously held contracts with family health service authorities, but plans are now being implemented to integrate these authorities with district health authorities, to provide all-purpose authorities for the purchase of health services. The general practice contract has changed quite markedly in recent years, however, and general practitioners now obtain approximately a third of their income from the health promotion activities that the government now wishes them to undertake.

Public Health in the 1990s

The vast majority of public health doctors are now employed by the health purchasing bodies in all parts of the United Kingdom. However, doctors working in the public health departments of these purchasing organizations find some difficulty in reconciling their public health professional role, which they feel bound to fulfill, with the expectations of their employer organizations regarding the work they should be doing. These public health doctors are aware of the public health tradition of which they are the current manifestation. They know that they are professionally obliged to maintain a watching brief over all aspects of the public health of their local populations, and they also know that if they are to maintain and improve health status, they need to work with a wide variety of organizations locally, in both the public and private sectors (Holland 1992). However, they are employed as part of purchasing organizations, and the managers of these organizations see their role as being the provision of epidemiological advice to purchasers regarding purchasing strategies mainly limited to the National Health Service itself (Bhopal 1993). This results in inevitable potential conflict, which in some places is resolved satisfactorily but, in other places, boils over from time to time. There has therefore been some recent professional uncertainty among some public health physicians and some poor morale (Milner 1994). Partly owing to these conflicts, there is debate concerning whether or not public health departments should remain within the National Health Service, or whether they should return to local government. This question will certainly be debated once again if the Labor Party returns to power after the next general election (*Health 2000* 1994).

Meanwhile, the environmental health departments of local authorities (and some other local authority departments) carry out many routine public health functions, and they are expected to obtain professional medical advice from the public health department of the NHS purchasing organization that corresponds geographically with each local authority environmental health department. However, the extent and quality of communication on public health matters, between NHS public health doctors and local authority environmental health officers, vary considerably across the country.

Another group of public health doctors continues to work in academic departments, mainly in medical schools. Although these departments generally maintain a standard of excellence in teaching and research, the medical staff working in them do perceive a number of problems. There is a feeling among them that they lack a proper career structure and training program, as while they are expected to undergo higher specialist training in public health (as for all public health doctors), and to pass the examination for membership in the Faculty of Public Health Medicine, both training arrangements and the examination itself tend to be slanted toward the needs of service-oriented doctors working in the NHS. Moreover, the government's recent changes to the health service have resulted in a number of difficulties being presented to those working in medical research in all specialties, including public health.

However, much research is being done, and a review of current public health research in academic departments throughout the United Kingdom was carried out for this chapter (Birt 1995). The findings provide an insight into the priorities for health research in the United Kingdom today, as perceived by public health doctors.

It is not surprising that a large amount of work is being carried out, throughout the country, in the field of general epidemiology—the measurement of health and disease (and of determinants of health). However, it is noteworthy that several academic departments are working to support their colleagues in NHS service public health departments in carrying out health needs assessments designed to be of assistance to health service purchasers. There is currently considerable epidemiological interest in rheumatoid arthritis and in systems for monitoring progress of this disease. Other departments are studying the health needs of the elderly, both mental and physical, the use they make of health services, and the need for long-term residential care for a number of elderly people. Various aspects of oncology, the effects on health of air pollution, and mental health are also common themes for general epidemiological studies. Some departments are studying epidemiology from a geographical point of view, such as a project in Nottingham for the mapping of rare diseases.

Just as cardiovascular disease continues to pose a major health problem in the United Kingdom, so cardiovascular epidemiology remains a consistently high priority for research in many academic departments. Currently, there is much interest in increasing our understanding of the effects of hyperlipedemic states, of the effects of *trans* fatty acids on the development of coronary heart disease, and on the manner in which cigarette smoking and fatty acid intake in the diet together contribute to the onset of this disease. The British Regional Heart Study, based at the Royal Free Hospital in London, has resulted in the publication of many papers that have increased our understanding of potential risk factors for heart disease. This same department has also been working on early influences in childhood for cardiovascular disease risk.

As already mentioned, it has been becoming increasingly clear that social deprivation provides a major determinant of poor health status, and there has been increasing interest in the development of more research in this field. Of particular note are the studies carried out by the academic department in Liverpool, by University College in London, and by the London School of Hygiene and Tropical Medicine.

Another major interest within several academic departments has been epidemiological methodology itself, and various groups have been working on ways of improving and clarifying the manner in which particular types of epidemiological studies can best be carried out and also on improving statistical analysis. Work carried out in the departments in Leicester and Liverpool is particularly noteworthy.

Considerable emphasis is evident in some departments on the study of the health of children, including in the Third World. Epidemiological study of the health of children in Peru, at the London School of Hygiene and Tropical Medicine, and on infant survival factors in Ethiopia, carried out in Leeds, should both be noted. However, within the United Kingdom, there is interest in the study of sexual abuse of children and in particular health problems of children, including common ones affecting all children such as accidents (childhood accident prevention is being studied at Queen's University, Belfast), as well as less common ones, including, for example, the needs of children with neurological disorders, studied at St. Mary's Hospital Medical School in London. A number of other departments are also studying particular aspects of the health of women (for example, at St. Bartholomew's Hospital Medical School in London).

Sexual health provides another common theme for research. Thus, sexual behavior in teenagers is being studied by various workers, partly in an attempt to understand better how to prevent the spread of HIV infection. The Nottingham department is studying teenage conception rates, and the Oxford department continues to demonstrate its long-standing interest in the study of fertility control. AIDS, needle exchange schemes, and condom distribution are, not surprisingly, providing subjects for much research, as is the assessment of hospital services for HIV and the cost of AIDS prevention. St. Mary's Hospital Medical School in London has been carrying out the largest study of sexual behavior in the United Kingdom ever. Meanwhile, perinatal mortality continues to be a subject of research interest, for example, in Leicester.

Medical sociology provides a most important subdivision of epidemiological research. The leading department is the Medical Research Council Medical Sociology Unit in Glasgow, where a major community study is based, carried out in the west of Scotland, of health and a number of relevant behaviorable variables. However, this unit is also carrying out many other types of work, including study of life events, socioeconomic status, and health; of family life and health; of influences on smoking behavior; of sexual behavior and knowledge; of the diet of adolescents; of the correlates of blood pressure and teenage behavior; and of many other issues, including ethnicity, religion, and health. Other sociological themes elsewhere include a study of the behavior of health professionals, carried out by Wessex Institute of Public Health; a study of participation in health, carried out by University College in London; and a study of smoking among medical students and nurses, carried out by the Royal Free's department.

Closely related to research in the field of medical sociology is the more obviously service-related field of health promotion research. Many departments have been involved in lifestyle studies (as an aid to improved planning and evaluation of health promotion projects), with the Nottingham department making a particular specialty of this. The Oxford department has been studying nutritional behavior, for example, with emphasis on school meals and on the benefits of vegetarianism. Other departments have been looking at nutrition in the elderly, at diet in those who have already suffered ischemic heart disease, and at dietary advice being offered to international travelers.

The health of ethnic minority groups in the United Kingdom is of particular interest to some academic departments. This is most evident within departments located in cities with substantial ethnic minorities, such as Leicester, Newcastle, and London. The London School of Hygiene and Tropical Medicine has been studying cardiovascular disease in ethnic minorities, and St. Mary's Hospital Medical School has been studying ethnicity and place of death.

Infectious diseases stimulated the earliest epidemiological studies, and they continue to be researched. Diseases commonly studied include tuberculosis, leprosy, meningitis, and hepatitis. The London School of Hygiene and Tropical

Medicine is carrying out a study of leishmaniasis in Latin America, while King's College Hospital Medical School in London is studying the manner in which general practitioners provide official notification of the infectious diseases they diagnose.

Access to health care facilities is another research interest. For example, the London School of Hygiene and Tropical Medicine has studied access to coronary artery bypass graft surgery in East Anglia and found five-fold differences, dependent upon where in East Anglia people happened to live. Primary care research is closely related to access to care, as primary care is, for most people, the gateway to other health services. The St. Mary's department has been particularly active in this field, studying the interface between primary and secondary care, and has been evaluating a new primary health care package called "Community Orientated Primary Care." This department has also been involved in the evaluation of the general practitioner fund-holding scheme in the United Kingdom, whereby general practitioners are provided with funds with which they can purchase secondary care for their patients. Academic departments have been researching counseling in general practice and the use of computers by general practitioners, while others have studied research and development for primary health care teams and have also been evaluating the value of general practitioner lifestyle checkups provided on a routine basis. Wider studies in other aspects of community health have included international comparisons in the developed world (the Sheffield department) and the evaluation of small-scale community health projects (the Liverpool department). Other work of note has included a study of informal care, community development approaches to health service provision, the particular health problems of people living on new housing estates, homelessness and ill health, housing and health, and good practice within locality commissioning of health services.

One of the most important components of research work carried out by academic departments of public health is health services research generally and, more specifically, the effectiveness of health services. Preeminent in this work is the Health Services Research Unit at Aberdeen, within which literally dozens of such studies are under way. The scope of these stretch from one to develop measures of patient outcome, to evaluation of services to manage asthma and diabetes, to use of patient data cards, to evaluation of stroke care, to evaluation of bone mineral screening, and to management of end-stage renal failure in Europe. Many other units are also carrying out major health services research studies, including evaluation of services and care for stroke patients (in Oxford), evaluation of legal abortion (in Nottingham), evaluation of services for severe head injury patients (also in Nottingham), evaluation of community nursing care (also in Nottingham), evaluation of child health surveillance (by the United Medical and Dental School in London), evaluation of primary prevention of cancer (in Liverpool), evaluation of rehabilitation services (Institute of Public Health in Wessex), and evaluation of screening of the elderly (Royal Free School of Medicine in London).

Another major research area, with close links to public health, is that of health economics. Research in this area is centered in particular in two specialist health economic centers, in Aberdeen and York, both of which are involved in various option appraisal exercises, in service evaluation and audit, in program budgeting research, and in modeling of health services. However, a number of other university departments also are involved in health economics research, such as the academic department of public health in Newcastle. Closely related to health economics research is research into a number of ethical issues, such as those being carried out at the University of Wales College of Medicine. Apart from a general analysis of various ethical issues, workers here have been reviewing the ethics of applying calculation of quality-adjusted life years (QALYs) to decisions on prioritization in health service purchasing, as well as to other areas of prioritization.

This brief review illustrates quite well that, in a somewhat difficult and rapidly changing environment, research in various aspects of public health is flourishing throughout the United Kingdom. This is being given further encouragement by the establishment of research and development directorates within central government health departments and also within large health authorities (Holland, Fitzsimons, and O'Brien 1994).

FUTURE CHALLENGES FOR PUBLIC HEALTH IN THE UNITED KINGDOM

Until recently, although many of those involved in public health in the United Kingdom have taken a lively interest in public health problems outside the United Kingdom, and especially in the Third World, and indeed have played a major part in international organizations such as WHO and its activities, health problems in the United Kingdom had always been seen as a matter of domestic concern, to be resolved by British people, using well-developed British systems, acting in a British political environment. The Maastricht Treaty (Treaty on European Union 1992) has changed all this, and for the first time, the institutions of the European Union now have a considerable opportunity to develop public health strategies and to implement programs. British public health practitioners are in many ways well positioned to take advantage of this new situation, as public health (including all the various disciplines that contribute to it) tends to be better developed in the United Kingdom than in many other European Union member states. However, if British public health practitioners are to play the part that they could in this new arena, bringing British public health knowledge and expertise to a wider European environment, a radical change of outlook will first have to take place within the various professions, and many complacent domestic attitudes will need to be challenged.

Although health administration is carried out separately in each of four nations within the United Kingdom, in recent years there has generally been increasing centralization of power and decision making in the United Kingdom. There is nowadays much discussion of devolution, to which the Labor Party is committed. Labor Party policy proposals envisage much greater autonomy for the four nations, and in England a system of regional government might be developed, with health as one of the main areas of responsibility for such regional government. Accordingly, a new challenge to public health in this situation would be the need to establish ways, within regions, to influence the planning and management of health services, so as to ensure that this takes place as according to established needs, and that evaluation of health services takes place as according to appropriate scientific criteria.

As already mentioned, public health in the United Kingdom currently functions as part of the National Health Service. This has some logic, but it results in public health physicians being required to give undue consideration to those health needs that should be met by health services themselves, at the cost of insufficient time being allocated for consideration of other health needs. There is current discussion, including within Labor Party circles (*Health 2000* 1994), regarding whether it may be more appropriate to make public health once again a local authority responsibility, as it was prior to 1974. If health services are to become a responsibility of regional government in the future, it may indeed become the case that these services themselves would in reality come under local authority control. However, whatever administrative changes the future may bring to management of health services, the challenge to public health physicians will be to respond appropriately to any changes, such that appropriate public health influence and advice can be fed into strategic decision making on health service planning at all levels.

Prior to the separation within the National Health Service of purchaser and provider organizations, public health doctors worked in much closer association with clinical colleagues in other specialties. Relationships are no longer so close, and there is now often a failure on the part of other doctors to understand the work of their public health colleagues (Voss 1992). Support and assistance from the whole medical profession is necessary if public health doctors are to work effectively. Here lies a challenge to arrange better systems of communication within the medical profession.

Current Issues in Health Services in the United Kingdom Today

There is general agreement that current systems for measuring effectiveness and efficiency of health services are, to say the least, rudimentary. Accordingly, a challenge to public health doctors is to collaborate with clinicians and health service managers in efforts to develop more accurate measures of effectiveness (health gain per unit resources invested) and in service efficiency (organization of a particular service of given effectiveness for minimum cost). As in most other economies in the developed world, this is because cost containment of health services generally has become a political necessity. As a contribution toward greater effectiveness, medical audit and clinical audit (Crombie 1993;

Hopkins 1994; Shaw 1990) are now becoming well-established practices in UK health services (much more so than in many other member states of the European Union). Moreover, other aspects of health service quality are receiving very considerable attention. However, further developments in the use of clinical audit and quality assurance are also essential.

New technology is bringing with it major changes in surgical practice, with the possibility to carry out many more surgical procedures by noninvasive means. This is resulting in it becoming possible to do much more surgery than hitherto on a day-case basis, and the alteration of practice from inpatient surgery to day-case surgery will continue to be a major challenge to health service organization in the future (Morgan 1992; Grainger and Griffiths 1994).

There is also a consensus that most future health service development will be in primary health care rather than in secondary care (Watkins 1994; Sheaff and Peel 1993; Shapiro 1994). More services than hitherto will be provided at the primary level, with particular emphasis on prevention and health promotion within primary care, and primary care practitioners will be increasingly more involved in the commissioning and purchasing of secondary care (Ham and Shapiro 1995; Winkler 1994). All of these developments pose major future challenges and problems to managers of health services.

In summary, it may be said that two main future challenges can in particular be identified: first, the development of more accurate and efficient means of carrying out health needs assessment in relation to population need for health services and, second, the development of better systems for measuring service effectiveness. These tools are essential if purchasing of health services is to be better targeted in the future.

REFERENCES

Abel-Smith, B. (1964). *The Hospitals 1800–1948*, London: Heinemann.

Baggott, R. (1994). *Health and Health Care in Britain*. London: St. Martin's Press.

Bhopal, R. S. (1993). Public health medicine and purchasing health care. *British Medical Journal*, 306 (6874), 381–382.

Birt, C. A. (1995). Personal communication.

Brockington, C. F. (1966). *A Short History of Public Health*. 2nd ed. Edinburgh: Churchill Livingstone.

Crombie, I. K. (1993). *The Audit Handbook: Improving Health Care Through Clinical Audit*. Chichester: John Wiley.

Davey Smith, G. & Egger, M. (1993). Socioeconomic differentials in wealth and health. *British Medical Journal*, 307 (6912), 1085–1086.

Evans, D. (1992). Tackling the hideous scourge—the creation of venereal disease treatment centers in early 20th century Britain. *Social History of Medicine*, 5 (3), 413–433.

Forsyth, G. (1966). *Doctors and State Medicine*. London: Pitman Medical.

Frazer, W. M. (1950). *A History of English Public Health 1834–1939*. London: Tindall & Cox.

Grainger, C. & Griffiths, R. (1994). Day surgery: How much is possible? *Public Health*, 108 (4), 257–266.

Ham, C. & Shapiro, J. (1995). The future of fundholding (editorial). *British Medical Journal*, 310 (6988), 1150–1151.

Health 2000. (1994). London: Labor Party.

Holland, W. W. (1992). The faculty of public health medicine. *Hospital Topics*, 70 (4), 7–10.

Holland, W .W., Fitzsimons, B. & O'Brien, M. (1994). Back to the future—public health research into the next century, *Journal of Public Health Medicine*, 16 (1), 4–10.

Hopkins, A. (Ed.). (1994). *Professional and Managerial Aspects of Clinical Audit*. London: Royal College of Physicians.

McEwen, J. (1995). *Continuing Professional Development for Public Health Medicine—Implementing the Next Stages*. Liverpool: Faculty of Public Health Medicine.

Milner, P. (1994). Unsettling times for public health. *Journal of Public Health Medicine*, 16 (1), 1–3.

Morgan, M. (1992). Surgeons' views of day surgery. *Journal of Public Health Medicine*, 14 (2), 192–198.

O'Brien, J. M. (1995). *Widening the Faculty's Membership*. Liverpool: Faculty of Public Health Medicine.

Pearson, V. A. H., Carr, R. J. & Pouse, A. (1993). Public health medicine training. *Medical Education*, 27 (2), 274–279.

Royal Commission on Medical Education. (1968). *Royal Commission on Medical Education 1965–1968*. London: HMSO.

Shapiro, J. (1994). *Shared Purchasing and Collaborative Commissioning Within the NHS*. Birmingham: NAHAT.

Shaw, C. D. (1990). Medical Audit: *A Hospital Handbook*. London: King's Fund Centre.

Sheaff, W. R. & Peel, V. J. (Eds.). (1993). *Best Practice in Health Care Commissioning*. Harlow: Longman.

Somervaille, L. & Griffiths, R. (1995). *The Training and Career Development Needs of Public Health Professionals*. Birmingham: Institute of Public and Environmental Health, University of Birmingham.

Symond, A. (1993). Health visiting and the new public health. *Health Visitor*, 66 (6), 204–206.

Targets for Health for All. (1985). *Targets in Support of the European Regional Strategy for Health for All*. Copenhagen: WHO.

Townsend, P., Davidson, N. & Whitehead, M. (1988). *Inequalities in Health. The Black Report and the Health Divide*. London: Penguin Books.

Treaty on European Union. (1992). *Maastricht Treaty*. 7 February 1992, HMSO, London.

The unhealthy poor. (1994). *Economist*, 331 (7866), 27–28.

Voss, S. (1992). Doctors' understanding of the specialty of public health medicine: A survey of general practitioners and junior hospital doctors. *Journal of Public Health Medicine*, 14 (4), 399–401.

Watkins, S. J. (1994). Public health 2020. *British Medical Journal*, 309 (6962), 1147–1149.

Watterson, A. (1994). Whither lay epidemiology in United Kingdom public health policy and practice—Some reflections on occupational and environmental health opportunities. *Journal of Public Health*, 16, 270–274.

Winkler, F. (1994). Commissioning and developing primary care. *Primary Care Management*, 4 (11), 5–7.

Working for Patients. (1989). *The Health Service: Caring for the 1990's.* London: HMSO.

UNITED STATES

Abdelmonem A. Afifi, Lester Breslow, and E. Richard Brown

POPULATION AND HEALTH

Population Development and Trends

In 1992, the population in the United States was 258.2 million and is expected to reach 300 million by the year 2010, and 392 million by 2050. As Figure 1 shows, the traditional pyramidal distribution of population was already breaking down by 1960. In 1993, the distribution was moving toward a rectangular form, with a bulge in the 30–39 age group due to the "baby boomers" born after World War II. By 2030, the rectangular distribution is expected to be clearly in evidence. Relative to the total population, the proportion of people under 40 will decrease, while the proportion of those 40 and older will increase. The greatest relative rate of increase is occurring in the 80 and over age group.

The U.S. population, historically one of the most diverse on earth, has become increasingly heterogeneous in the twentieth century. From 1920 to 1960, blacks comprised approximately 10 percent of the population. That percentage reached 12.4 percent in 1992 and is expected to climb to 15.7 percent by the year 2050. Hispanics represented 6.4 percent of the population in 1980, 9.5 percent in 1992, and are expected to reach 22.5 percent by 2050. Currently, however, the largest rate of increase is among Asian and Pacific Islanders who constituted only 1.65 percent of the population in 1980, rapidly increasing to 3.31 percent in 1992; they are expected to triple their numbers by 2050. Changing immigration patterns have dramatically affected ethnic composition. For example, the number of immigrants to the United States from Mexico and Central America (the largest group among all regions) has doubled from 1.65 million in the 1970s to 3.1 million in the 1980s; Asian immigrants, the second largest group, increased from

Figure 1
Population Structure in 1960, 1993, and 2030 (projected)

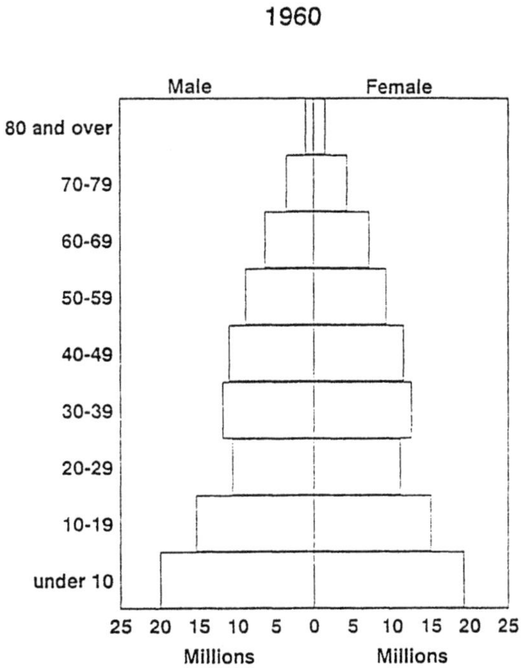

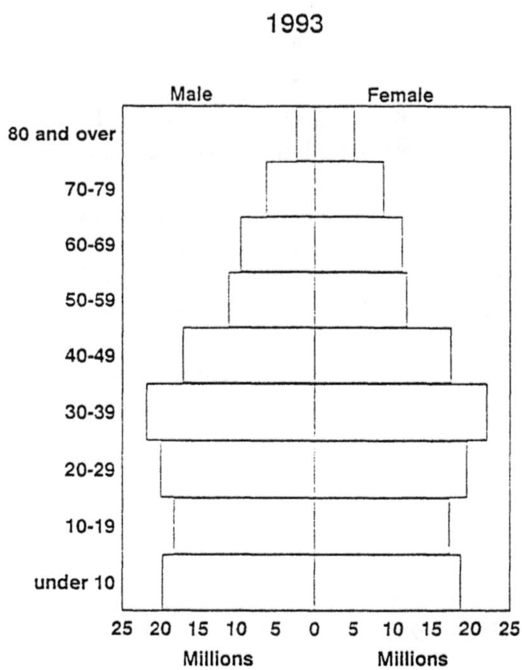

Figure 1 (Continued)

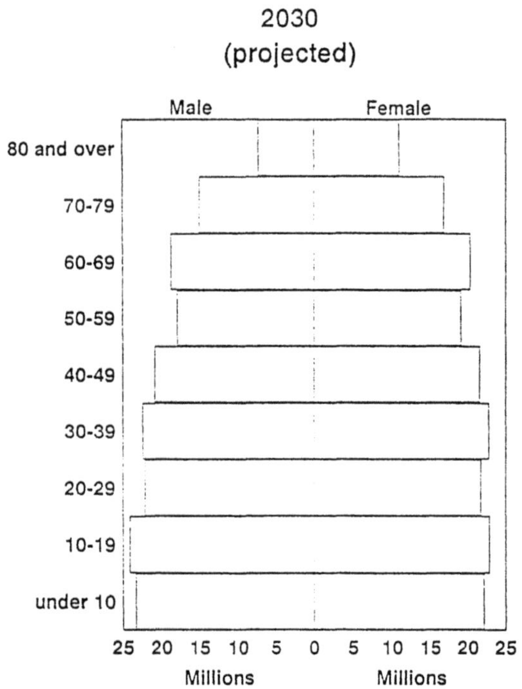

Source: U.S. Department of Commerce 1974, 1993.

1.63 million to 2.82 million; while European immigrants decreased from 0.8 million to 0.7 million during the same period (U.S. Department of Commerce 1994).

The U.S. population is also characterized by socioeconomic differences among the ethnic groups, as well as differences in infant mortality rates and life expectancy for various ethnic groups. In terms of income, 31 percent of blacks live below the poverty level. Hispanics are a close second (26.7 percent), with non-Hispanic whites having the lowest percentage (10.3 percent). In the first half of the 1980s, percentages below the poverty level increased for all ethnic groups. These percentages decreased steadily in the second half of the 1980s, but turned upward again at the beginning of the 1990s.

Between 1970 and 1991, the infant mortality rate in the United States decreased by 56 percent. A greater decline occurred among white and Hispanic infants (59 percent) than for black infants (46 percent). In 1991, this rate for black infants (17.6 percent) was 2.4 times that for white infants (7.3 percent). The average life expectancy for men and women in 1991 reached 75.5 years. From 1985 to 1991, the difference in this index between whites and blacks widened from 6 years to 7 years, while the gender difference narrowed from 7.4 to 6.9 years.

Infectious Diseases

Advances in public health have vastly reduced the occurrence of infectious disease, epidemics, and pandemics. Progress in medical science has made us less vulnerable to their devastation when they do occur. Nevertheless, the nation's current experience with the human immunodeficiency virus (HIV), as well as other infectious diseases such as Hanta virus and Lyme disease, is a sobering reminder that serious microbial threats to health remain. During the last decade, HIV infection has grown rapidly in the United States. Between 1987 and 1991, the age-adjusted death rate from HIV infection more than doubled, from 5.5 to 11.3 deaths per 100,000 population, placing HIV infection as the ninth leading cause of death, with clear differences in rates for blacks and whites. In 1991, acquired immunodeficiency syndrome (AIDS) ranked as the sixth leading cause of death for blacks but ranked tenth for whites. The age-adjusted death rate for black men (52.9 deaths per 100,000) was more than three times that for white men (16.7) and more than four times that for black women (12.0), while the rate for black women was more than nine times that for white women (1.3) (Table 1).

Vaccines are one of the most cost-effective means available for preventing disease. Although there are more than 20 diseases that can be prevented through the use of vaccines, there are many diseases for which no vaccine is available. These facts argue strongly for making vaccine development an important first consideration for controlling microbial threats to health.

Chronic Conditions

In 1980, the 10 leading causes of death in the United States were (1) diseases of the heart, (2) malignant neoplasms, (3) cerebrovascular diseases, (4) unintentional injuries, (5) chronic obstructive pulmonary diseases, (6) pneumonia and influenza, (7) diabetes mellitus, (8) chronic liver disease and cirrhosis, (9) atherosclerosis, and (10) suicide. By 1991, the first seven causes still headed the list, with the order of unintentional injuries and chronic obstructive pulmonary diseases being reversed; suicide jumped to eighth on the list, while HIV infection and homicide and legal intervention placed ninth and tenth, respectively (see Table 1).

Mental Health

Deinstitutionalization has been the "single most important issue" for those in the mental health sphere for the past three decades (Mechanic and Rochefort 1990). The most commonly cited statistic used to describe the course of dein-

Table 1
Leading Causes of Death in the United States (per 100,000 resident population)

Cause of Death (traditional)	Total (all races,sexes)	Male		Female	
		White	Black	White	Black
All Causes	513.7	634.4	1048.8	366.3	575.1
Heart Disease	148.2	196.1	272.7	100.7	165.5
Cerebrovascular Disease	26.8	26.9	54.9	22.8	41.0
Malignant Neoplasms	134.5	159.5	242.4	111.2	136.3
Malignant Neoplasms of Respiratory System	41.1	58.1	88.4	26.8	27.4
Chronic Obstructive Pulmonary Disease	20.1	27.4	25.9	16.1	11.3
HIV Infection	11.3	16.7	52.9	1.3	12.0
Motor Vehicle Crashes	17.0	24.2	26.2	10.4	8.7
Homicide	10.9	9.4	72.5	3.0	13.9
Suicide	11.4	19.9	12.5	4.8	1.9
Firearm Injuries	15.2	20.7	66.4	3.7	8.0

Source: National Center for Health Statistics 1994.

stitutionalization in the United States is the year-end count of resident patients in the state and county mental hospitals. In 1955, the number of inpatients was 559,000. During the next three decades, the total decreased by 81 percent. By 1990, the number of inpatients dropped to 110,000, with many of those deinstitutionalized remaining homeless. A major threat to mental health is homelessness. Estimates of the number of the homeless range widely, from 200,000 to 2 million, but there is broad agreement that the number has been growing. Also, it is believed that between a quarter and a half of the homeless have significant psychiatric symptoms.

Of all the age-related syndromes, perhaps the most age-associated one is dementia, described as a syndrome of generalized mental deterioration that causes functional impairment. Before the mid-1970s, dementia was considered a natural, indeed normal, consequence of aging. Alzheimer's disease was primarily considered a cause of presenile dementia, whereas so-called "senile dementia" (age 65+) was largely ignored by both the public and medical practitioners. It is now known that Alzheimer's disease affects adults of all ages but only rarely those under 60. The prevalence increases dramatically for each age group over age 65. Because of the high percentage of aging in most advanced societies, the past decade has seen increasing awareness that dementia is a problem of immense importance to public health.

Actual Causes of Death

McGinnis and Foege (1993) have attempted to identify and quantify the major external (nongenetic) factors that contribute to death in the United States. They call these the "actual" causes of death, as opposed to the disease-based "nominal" causes of death. The authors estimated that approximately half of all deaths that occurred in 1990 could be attributed to the following "actual causes" among Americans in 1990: (1) tobacco: 400,000 (19 percent); (2) diet/activity patterns: 300,000 (14 percent); (3) alcohol: 100,000 (5 percent); (4) microbial agents: 90,000 (4 percent); (5) toxic agents: 60,000 (3 percent); (6) firearms: 35,000 (2 percent); (7) sexual behavior: 30,000 (1 percent); (8) motor vehicles: 25,000 (1 percent); and (9) illicit use of drugs: 20,000 (1 percent). Tobacco contributes substantially to deaths from cancer, cardiovascular disease, lung disease, low birth weight and other problems of infancy, and burns. Dietary factors and activity patterns are associated with cardiovascular diseases, cancers, and diabetes mellitus. The related health, social, and economic consequences of alcohol extend far beyond the mortality tables. Many cirrhosis deaths, motor vehicle fatalities, home injuries, drownings, fire fatalities, job injuries, and cancer deaths can be attributed to alcohol. Once the leading killer in the United States, infections are still a prominent threat, especially to persons with other health impairments. The estimated deaths due to toxic agents may be quite uncertain because measurement techniques and the recognition of health effects are still evolving. The prominent, detrimental effect of firearms on overall death rates in the United States is unique in comparison with other countries. As indicated by the large number of deaths from sexually acquired HIV infection, unprotected intercourse now represents one of the most rapidly increasing causes of death in the country. Finally, it is estimated that some 3 million people in the United States have serious drug problems. Illicit use of drugs contributes to infant death, overdose, suicide, homicide, motor vehicle injuries, HIV infection, pneumonia, hepatitis, and endocarditis.

In addition, lack of access to a reliable source of primary care and poverty are also associated with an increased risk of death from a variety of "nominal" causes as well. People who are poor have higher mortality rates for heart disease, diabetes mellitus, high blood pressure, lung cancer, neural tube defects, injuries, and low birth weight, as well as lower survival rates from breast cancer and heart attacks. Efforts to improve health must take into account the special challenges among those who are poor or racially disadvantaged.

Between 1980 and 1991, the age-adjusted death rate for suicide remained stable, but rates varied among race-sex groups. In 1991, suicide rates were more than four times higher for white males than white females and nearly seven times higher for black males than black females (see Table 1). Between 1985 and 1991, the age-adjusted homicide rate increased 31 percent, reversing a downward trend in the first half of the 1980s. Homicides are more prevalent among black than white populations. In 1991, this rate was eight times higher for black males than for white males and nearly five times higher for black females than white females.

Prevention: Controlling Environmental and Nutritional Risk Factors

It is expected that the next decade will be filled with initiatives to improve environmental health. An emerging concept in the United States will be pollution prevention as opposed to remedial efforts alone. As the nation moves toward the twenty-first century, environmental challenges abound: hazardous and other waste dumps, radioactive waste from weapons production, toxic emissions, and groundwater contamination of unknown magnitude.

In order to protect U.S. citizens against the dangers posed by hazardous waste, the federal government created the Comprehensive Environmental Response, Compensation and Liability Act of 1980 (CERCLA). At the heart of CERCLA is the trust fund more popularly known as "Superfund," which was created to finance cleanup of hazardous waste sites. In the United States, approximately 50 percent of the population relies on groundwater for its potable water supply. Groundwater was overlooked in the flurry of the 1960s and 1970s environmental protection legislation. Today, the need for uncontaminated groundwater is rapidly moving to the front ranks of the nation's environmental protection concerns and priorities.

The Clean Air Act of 1970 made the Environmental Protection Agency the focal point of the federal effort to provide regulations. Since the passage of this law, there has been progress in improving air quality. For example, lead levels in urban air are down 87 percent from 1977. Sulfur dioxide levels have been reduced 37 percent; ozone and carbon monoxide have been reduced by 13 and 32 percent, respectively. Recycling has become an increasingly attractive option for handling waste as municipal dumps fill and as resistance mounts against landfills and incinerators. Today, only 10 percent of the country's solid waste is recycled. However, most experts agree that even well-run recycling programs might recover only 20 to 25 percent of reusable materials.

Thanks to an abundant food supply, fortification of some foods with critical trace nutrients, and better methods for determining and improving the nutrient content of foods, nutritional deficiency diseases, such as rickets, pellagra, and scurvy, are rare. But as the diseases of nutritional deficiency have diminished, they have been replaced by diseases related to dietary excess and imbalance—problems that now rank among the leading causes of illness and death in the United States. Four of the ten leading diseases causing death are associated with diet: coronary heart disease (CHD), some types of cancer, stroke, and non-insulin-dependent diabetes mellitus. Overweight is a risk factor for hypertension, and both are risk factors for CHD. Cirrhosis of the liver, unintentional injuries, suicide, and homicide have been related to excessive alcohol intake. While the nutritional deficiencies associated with alcohol abuse are still being defined, misuse of alcohol is one of the most preventable health problems in the United States. Recent trends suggest that both the intake of alcohol and its adverse health consequences are declining. There has also been a slow decline in deaths attributable entirely to alcohol-related causes since 1980. Awareness of the adverse health effects associated with a diet high in fat has increased from 8 percent in 1970 to 55 percent in 1989 among the American people. There has been a large shift from whole milk to low-fat and skim milk, and consumption of red meats and eggs has declined, while consumption of poultry, fish, fruits, and vegetables has increased. To help lead the way for the future, the federal government has developed a series of programs for monitoring and promoting nutritional improvement among the American people.

PRESSURES FOR CHANGE IN THE U.S. HEALTH CARE SYSTEM

In recent years, dissatisfaction with the health care system in the United States has become widespread. Nine out of ten Americans believe that the nation's health care system needs fundamental change or complete rebuilding (Blendon and Taylor 1989). Most chief executive officers of the nation's largest corporations have shared this view (Cantor et al. 1991).

Millions of Americans have no health insurance coverage, and millions more feel anxious about their coverage. The United States spends more on health care than any other country in the world—both absolutely and as a percentage of the gross domestic product (GDP)—and costs have been rising rapidly, as they have in other industrialized countries. Also, there is growing sentiment that the United States does not receive adequate value for what it spends on health care.

Incomplete Health Insurance Coverage

At least 39 million Americans have no coverage for medical expenses. The "uninsured" rate has grown from less than 14 percent in 1977 to 18 percent in 1992 (Kasper, Walden, and Wilensky n.d.; Brown et al. 1994). This estimate understates the extent to which lack of insurance affects American families; an estimated 64 million Americans—about one in four people—are uninsured for at least 1 month during each 28-month period.

Nearly nine out of every ten uninsured people are workers or in a family with at least one worker (Brown et al. 1994). Concern over insurance coverage is focused on widespread personal fears of loss of coverage, failure of insurance to pay for expensive medical bills, and workers staying with an employer because they are afraid that another job may not provide them with health insurance (Eckholm 1991).

Nevertheless, most people in the United States have some type of health insurance coverage. In 1992, 60 percent of the nonelderly population were covered by private health insurance obtained through their own or a family member's employment, down from 64 percent in 1989 (Brown et al. 1994). Medicaid, a welfare-based program established mainly for persons who are eligible for federal public assistance, covered 10 percent of the nonelderly population in 1992, including about half of the poverty population. Nearly the entire elderly population, 65 years of age or older, is covered by Medicare, a federal social insurance program that covers about half of the health care costs of the elderly. To pay for some of the expenses that Medicare does not cover, most of these elderly persons also have private insurance or Medicaid.

Compared to people with health insurance coverage, the uninsured have much less access to necessary medical care. Such reduced access may adversely affect health status, with especially serious consequences for pregnant women and their children and for persons with chronic illness (Lurie et al. 1986).

Although the uninsured get less care than the insured population, the costs of care they do receive are shifted to others. When the uninsured need urgent care, they usually go to hospitals and clinics. Individual and business taxpayers bear the financial burden of care provided by public hospitals to uninsured patients. However, these public facilities remain depressingly underfunded, understaffed, and ill equipped to meet this population's needs for medical care (Brown and Dallek 1990; Baker, Stevens, and Brook 1991).

Rising Health Care Costs

Health spending in the United States has climbed from 6 percent of the GDP in 1965 to 14 percent of GDP in 1993. The country spends 37 percent of national health expenditures on hospital care, 19 percent on physicians services, and about 1 percent on public health activities at all levels of government (Levit et al. 1991; unpublished data from U.S. Health Care Financing Administration).

Businesses and their employees have been hit very hard by these rising costs. Between 1965 and 1991, business health spending has grown from 2 percent of wages and salaries to 9.1 percent, and from 7.6 percent of pretax corporate profits to 61.8 percent (Cowan and McDonnell 1993).

Health care coverage for persons under age 65 in the United States is uncertain because individuals and families are not required to have coverage, nor are employers required to pay for it. At more than $5,000 a year for a family policy, health insurance is unaffordable to most families without a substantial contribution from an employer or the government. Most large employers do provide and help pay for health insurance for their employees, compelled by collective bargaining contracts with unions (which now represent only about one in seven American workers) or only by practices in their particular labor market.

Health care costs are high in the United States for many reasons. As insurance coverage expanded during the 1960s, hospitals competed for physicians and paying patients by investing in almost every new technology that came on the market. By 1975, the number of hospitals organized for short-term care peaked at 6,310, 53 percent of them private not-for-profit, 12 percent for-profit, and the remainder public. Cost containment pressures began to force down hospital capacity, although investment in technology was slower to respond to these pressures. By 1992, the number of hospitals had shrunk to slightly more than 5,600. The number of community hospital beds per 1,000 population followed a similar trend, increasing from 3.2 in 1940 to 4.5 in 1980 and then declining to 3.6 in 1991, as shorter lengths of stay (down to 7.4 days in 1991) reduced the need for hospital capacity (National Center for Health Statistics 1994, 192, 212, 215).

In response to a perceived shortage of physicians, the number of medical schools was increased from approximately 80 in 1963 to more than 120 by the late 1970s. By 1992, there were 236 physicians per 100,000 population in the United States. Nevertheless, the percentage of primary care physicians is among the lowest in the world, with less than 30 percent of practicing physicians in general or family practice or the specialties of internal medicine or pediatrics (National Center for Health Statistics 1994, 200, 202). The high proportion of specialists contributes substantially to the higher health care spending in the United States relative to other countries because specialists generate much higher expenditures per physician (Fuchs and Hahn 1990).

Demands for Change

Demands to control the growth in health care spending have dominated the health care reform debate, receiving strong support from business organizations and corporate leaders. Proposals to extend coverage to the uninsured receive support from most Americans, but this issue does not influence the debate about health care reform to the same extent as the issue of health care costs. This disparity in support reflects several factors, including the broad impact of health care costs on business, government, and families; the strength of individual corporations and of business organizations in American politics; and the relative weakness of both labor unions and the tradition of social solidarity principals in the United States, compared with a number of other industrialized countries.

Concerns are growing about the quality of health services provided and the value that society receives for its high expenditures. One frequent complaint is that the United States' pluralist health care financing generates excessive administrative costs, including profits. Private insurance companies spend an average of 14 cents of every dollar paid out in claims to administer their plans (Letsch et al. 1992). In comparison, the much larger, government-run Medicare program's administrative expenses are only 2 percent of paid claims, comparable to the Canadian national health insurance program. Overall, the United States spends about one fourth of its trillion-dollar health expenditures to administer private insurance plans, government programs, hospitals, doctors' offices, and other health services—a greater share of health resources devoted to "paper pushing" than other countries with national health programs.

As a result, public officials and some business health coalitions have pressed health plans and researchers for evidence that expensive medical procedures produce better outcomes than would be likely with less expensive techniques or no care at all. Proposals to extend coverage to all U.S. residents and to control the growth in health spending, advocated by President Bill Clinton and supported by many public and private sector leaders, also included specific requirements that would have compelled health plans and providers to measure and report indicators of health care quality and outcomes.

Market-Generated Changes in Health Care

Despite the failure of efforts to reform the U.S. health care system in 1994, pressures from employers and public programs, like Medicare and Medicaid, are transforming the health care system without extending coverage to the millions of uninsured Americans. Cost reduction procedures have fostered the growth of health maintenance organizations (HMOs), which constitute an alternative to traditional fee-for-service medical practice and payment systems that are unique to the United States. By 1993, HMOs enrolled 18.5 percent of the U.S. population, more than 47 million people, up from 15.9 percent in 1991. For-profit HMOs accounted for most of this growth. However, there is no evidence that managed care plans reduce the share of resources spent on administration and profit. On the average, HMOs with more than 50,000 enrollees spent more than 16 percent of their revenues on administration and profits, and those with fewer than 50,000 enrollees spent more than 18 percent of revenues on these nonmedical expenses (Marion Merrell Dow 1993).

Many large payers of health services are demanding discounts and price reductions from health plans and health care providers. Hospitals, physician groups, and other providers are forming "integrated delivery systems" (IDSs) to increase their vertical and horizontal control of regional medical marketplaces. Although advocates of this process argue that it will save money and produce better outcomes, at this time there is no evidence to support these claims. In fact, there is evidence that many of these IDSs add administrative costs and do little to improve outcomes (Shortell 1988).

The market-driven process of vertical and horizontal integration control raises a number of policy questions. The IDSs, together with large employers, employer coalitions, and state Medicaid programs, are restructuring the health care delivery system and the allocation of resources with little public accountability. The market has not provided effective accountability because buyers have inadequate information with which to judge differences in quality among health plans, and enrollees have little say over which plans are made available to them by their employer or their public program. At the present time, the U.S. system for delivering personal health services is undergoing rapid change, but in ways that do not address the fundamental problems of incomplete coverage, costs, and overall contributions to the population's health.

INFRASTRUCTURE OF TRAINING AND RESEARCH IN PUBLIC HEALTH

While schools of public health educate scientists and researchers, the most distinctive role of public health education lies in the preparation of public health professionals. The growing demand for professionals with formal education in public health has led to a substantial expansion in training programs during the latter half of this century. In 1958, there were 11 schools of public health in the United States with a total enrollment of fewer than 1,200 students. Today, the 27 graduate schools of public health have a combined enrollment of over 13,000 students, a tenfold increase over the past 35 years. In the fall of 1992, almost half (46 percent) of the students in accredited schools of public health were enrolled in Master of Public Health (MPH) programs, the leading professional degree in public health. Another 24 percent were enrolled in other master's programs, 23 percent were pursuing doctoral degrees, and 7 percent were nondegree students. Over the years, there has been a substantial increase in part-time students and students enrolled in nontraditional degree programs, as well as in the number of physicians graduating with public health degrees. While the areas of study emphasized in schools of public health have changed slowly, the content of courses in those areas has evolved more rapidly to reflect new epidemiologic and statistical methods, new discoveries in the laboratory, new findings about health-related behaviors, and new ways of thinking about social and policy problems.

Both public and private universities offer education in public health schools and programs. All universities rely on the following sources of funding:

- Federal funds in the form of training and research contracts and grants;
- Institutional funds including state budgets for public universities, endowment income for private universities, as well as tuition fees in most cases; and
- Other funds, such as private gifts and foundation-sponsored contracts and grants.

Expenditures at the schools have increased almost fivefold ($122 million to $618 million) from 1975 to 1992. Today, public health educators firmly believe that there is no substitute for the fundamental role of the federal government in public health education. The private sector's focus on bottom-line profits and the volatile budgets of many states leave the federal government as the only stable source of funding.

MAJOR CHALLENGES FOR THE HEALTH SERVICES

Although the federal Public Health Service and state and local health departments are well-established agencies, they confront serious challenges. Changes in the nature of the nation's health problems over the past half century, the difficulty of redirecting programs in governmental departments, and the trend in the United States to downplay the role of public agencies in dealing with major social problems confront health providers, educators, and a public in need of quality health care. These changes precipitated a crisis in public health documented in a report by the Institute of Medicine of the National Academy of Science (IOM 1988; see also Afifi and Breslow 1994).

Traditionally, health departments provided protection against epidemic communicable diseases and the health hazards of pregnancy and childhood. As these conditions came under increasing control (with the exception of AIDS), a whole new set of problems, mainly the noncommunicable diseases, replaced them. Health departments are now redirecting their efforts to deal with them.

Surveillance

Monitoring the health of the population and the factors responsible for it is a fundamental public health responsibility that is carried out reasonably well at the federal level. The federal Public Health Service operates excellent systems for collecting and reporting mortality and communicable disease data and surveys the population's health and related factors, such as tobacco consumption. However, states and localities have lagged in systematic observation of trends in noncommunicable health conditions and their causes.

Behavior and Health

Health-related behavior evolves in the physical and social circumstances in which people live. Public health officials, however, with few exceptions, have left these matters in the hands of social activists. Governmental health leaders have generally avoided tackling social forces that must be overcome, principally the tobacco and gun industries and segments of the food industry. Some elements of society place priority on achieving profit, for example, by selling guns that facilitate violence, which must be countered by emphasizing social responsibility for health. More subtle influences lead to nutritional imbalance, such as in widespread obesity. Public health agencies should take the lead and vigorously seek allies among media, political, and other socially influential groups in developing an effective strategy for achieving patterns of behavior that favor health.

The Environment

Preventing the spread of microbial infections through water and food has been a central feature of public health from its beginning. That task continues, as evidenced by the recent outbreaks of water- and meat-borne disease. But environmental control measures must now be extended to provide protection against a host of toxic chemicals and physical agents that pervade workplaces, homes, and the atmosphere. While basic sanitary engineering and inspections of water and food services sufficed in the past, more extensive efforts to evaluate and intervene are needed to curtail the hazards of modern industrial life.

Availability of Personal Health Services

When public health agencies implemented widespread immunization programs to benefit the U.S. population, public health departments provided direct services to the economically disadvantaged as well as oversight of health services to prevent the spread of communicable disease. More recently, however, the public health role has been limited to caring for those who cannot afford private sector care. Separate public agencies, apart from health departments, have often been established to organize, deliver, and/or pay for personal health services for the poor. Three factors, however, have made ensuring personal health services of adequate quality to the population a major, present challenge to public health: (1) development of many effective medical procedures to safeguard health; (2) wide variation in access to, and quality of, personal health services; and (3) growing acceptance of the idea that access to quality medical services is a social right.

Special Population Groups

Public health has long focused its efforts on vulnerable groups of people. Children and adolescents, who are victims of family disruption and poverty, and the elderly poor currently stand in particular need of quality health care. Ethnic minorities and the homeless suffer from social and economic discrimination and need special attention in public health. Ensuring that these groups receive preventive services as well as adequate health education has become a public health challenge.

Resources

In the allocation of health resources, public health agencies' emphasis on preventive services has long taken second place to curative health agencies. Public health officials must find ways to obtain a proper allocation of the resources for health. Also, they face the task of allocating resources that are available to them to support activities that deal with major problems now affecting people's present and future health, reducing commitments to outmoded services, and enhancing services that are more pertinent to present problems.

REFERENCES

Afifi, A. A. & Breslow, L. (1994). The maturing paradigm of public health. *Annual Review of Public Health*, 15, 223–235.

Baker, D. W., Stevens, C. D. & Brook, R. H. (1991). Patients who leave a public hospital without being seen by a physician: Causes and consequences. *Journal of the American Medical Association*, 266(8), 1085–1090.

Blendon, R. J. & Taylor, H. (1989). Views on health care: Public opinion in three nations. *Health Affairs*, 8, 149–157.

Brown, E. R. & Dallek, G. (1990). State approaches to financing health care for the poor. *Annual Review of Public Health*, 11, 377–400.

Brown, E. R., Valdez, R. B., Wyn, R., Hongjian, Y. & Cumberland, W. (1994). *Policy Report: Health Insurance Coverage of Californians, 1989–1992*. Los Angeles: UCLA Center for Health Policy Research.

Cantor, C., Barrand, N. L., Desonia, R. A., et al. (1991). Business leaders' views on American health care. *Health Affairs*, 10(1), 98–105.

Cowan, C. A. & McDonnell, P. A. (1993). Business, households, and government: Health care costs, 1991. *Health Care Financing Review*, 14(3), 227–248.

Eckholm, E. (1991). Health benefits found to deter job switching. *New York Times*, 26 September, A1, A12.

Fuchs, V. R. & Hahn, J. S. (1990). How does Canada do it? A comparison of expenditures for physicians' services in the United States and Canada. *New England Journal of Medicine*, 323, 884–890.

Institute of Medicine (IOM), Committee Study of the Future of Public Health. (1988). *The Future of Public Health*. Washington, D.C.: National Academy Press.

Kasper, J. A., Walden, D. C. & Wilensky, G. R. (n.d.). *''Who Are the Uninsured?'' National Health Care Expenditures Study*. Data Preview 1. Hyattsville, MD: National Center for Health Services Research.

Letsch, S. W., Lazenby, H. C., Levit, K. R. & Cowan, C. A. (1992). National health expenditures, *Health Care Financing Review*, 14(2), 1–30.

Levit, K. R., Lazenby, H. C., Letsch, S. W. & Cowan, C. A. (1991). National health care spending, 1989. *Health Affairs*, 10(1), 117–130.

Lurie, N., Ward, N. B., Shapiro, M. F., et al. (1986). Termination of Medi-Cal benefits: A follow-up study one year later. *New England Journal of Medicine*, 314. 1266–1268.

Marion Merrell Dow. (1993). *Managed Care Digest*, Updated. Kansas City, MO: Marion Merrell Dow.

McGinnis, J. M. & Foege, W. H. (1993). Actual causes of death in the United States. *Journal of the American Medical Association*, 270, 2207–2212.

Mechanic, D. & Rochefort, D. A. (1990). Deinstitutionalization: An appraisal of reform. *Annual Review of Sociology*, 16, 301–327.

National Center for Health Statistics. (1994). *Health United States 1993*. Washington, D.C.: U.S. Department of Health and Human Services.

Nelson, C. & Short, K. (1990). *Health Insurance Coverage, 1986–88*. Washington, D.C.: U.S. Bureau of the Census.

Schieber, G. J., Poullier, J. P. & Greenwald, L. M. (1993). Health spending, delivery, and outcomes in OECD countries. *Health Affairs*, 12, 120–129.

Shortell, S. (1988). The evolution of hospital systems: Unfulfilled promises and self-fulfilling prophecies. *Medical Care Review*, 45, 177–197.

U.S. Department of Agriculture and U.S. Department of Health and Human Services. (1992). *International Conference on Nutrition Paper*. Submitted by the United States of America. Washington, D.C.: Government Printing Office.

U.S. Department of Commerce. (1974, 1993). *Current Population Reports: Population Estimates and Projections*. Washington, D.C.: Department of Commerce, Bureau of the Census.

U.S. Department of Commerce. (1994). *Statistical Abstract of United States 1994*. Washington, D.C.: Department of Commerce, Bureau of the Census.

PART III

Addresses of Public Health Organizations

AFRICA

ALGERIA

École Nationale de Santé Publique, El Marsa, Boumerdes 35320

BENIN

Institut Régional de Santé Publique, BP 918, Cotonou

CONGO

Centre Inter-États d'Enseignement Supérieur de Santé Publique d'Afrique Centrale (CIESPAC), BP 14513, Brazzaville

Departement de Santé Publique Institut Supérieur de Sciences de la Santé (INSSSA), Université Marien Ngouabi, BP 2672, Brazzaville

EGYPT

Department of Community Medicine, Public Health and Preventive Medicine, Faculty of Medicine, Al-Azhar University, Madinet Nasr, Cairo

Department of Health, Preventive Medicine and Industrial Hygiene, University of Mansûra, Mansûra

Department of Public Health, Faculty of Medicine, University of Alexandria, Alexandria

Department of Public Health and Industrial Medicine, University of Zagazig, Zagazig

Department of Public Health, Preventive Medicine and Industrial Hygiene, University of Cairo, Kasr-el-Eini, Cairo

Department of Public Health, Preventive Medicine and Industrial Hygiene, University of Tanta, Tanta

Departments of Community, Environmental and Occupational Medicine, Faculty of Medicine, Ain Shams University, P.O. Box 38, Abbassia, Cairo

High Institute of Public Health, University of Alexandria, 165 El-Horreya Avenue, Alexandria

ETHIOPIA

Department of Community Health, Faculty of Medicine, Addis Ababa University, P.O. Box 1176, Addis Ababa

IVORY COAST

Institut Régional de Santé Publique, BP V47, Abidjan

KENYA

Department of Community Health, Faculty of Medicine, University of Nairobi, P.O. Box 19676, Nairobi

LAGOS

Department of Community Health, College of Medicine, University of Lagos, Private Mail Bag 12003, Lagos

LEBANON

School of Public Health, American University of Beirut, P.O. Box 11-0-236, Bliss Street, Beirut

MOZAMBIQUE

Institute of Public Health, Ministry of Health, P.O. Box 264, Maputo

NIGERIA

Department of Community Health, College of Health Sciences, Usmani Danfodiyo University, Sultan Abubakar Road, P.O. Box 02254, Sokoto, Sokoto State

Department of Community Health, College of Medicine, University of Nigeria, Teaching Hospital, PMB 01129, Enugu

Department of Community Health, Institute of Health, Ahmadu Bello University, Zaria, Kaduna State

Department of Community Health, University of Benin, PMB 1154, Benin City

Department of Preventive and Social Medicine, College of Medicine, University of Ibadan, PMB 5116, Ibadan, Oyo

SENEGAL

Institut de Santé et Développement, BP 6259, 20, Allée des Jambaar, Dakar, Étoile

SOUTH AFRICA

Council for Scientific and Industrial Research, P.O. Box 395, Pretoria 0001

Department of Community Health, Faculty of Medicine, Medical University of Southern Africa, P.O. Box 219, Medunsa 0204

Department of Community Health, University of Cape Town, Medical School, Private Bag, Rondenbosch 7700

Department of Community Health, University of Natal, Medical School, P.O. Box 17039, Congella

Department of Community Health, University of Pretoria, P.O. Box 667, Pretoria 0001

Department of Community Health, University of Stellenbosch, Medical School, P.O. Box 19063, Tygerberg

Department of Community Health, University of the Free State, P.O. Box 339, Bloemfontein 9300

Department of Community Health, University of the Transkei, Medical School, Private Bag X1 Unitra, Umtata

Department of Community Health, University of the Witwatersrand, Medical School, 7, York Road, Parktown 2193, Johannesburg

Transvaal School of Public Health, Private Bag X385, Pretoria 0001

Western Cape School of Public Health, c/o University of the Western Cape, P.O. Box X 17, Modderdam Road, Belville 77535

SUDAN

Department of Community Medicine, Faculty of Medicine, University of Khartoum, Khartoum

TANZANIA

Institute of Public Health, College of Health Sciences, University of Dar es Salaam, United Nations Road, Upangu, P.O. Box 65015, Dar es Salaam

UGANDA

Institute of Public Health, Makerere University Medical School, P.O. Box 7072, Mulago-Kira Road, Kampala

ZAIRE

École de Santé Publique, Université de Kinshasa, BP 11.850, Kinshasa 1

ZIMBABWE

Department of Community Medicine, University of Zimbabwe, Medical School, Box A178, Avondale

ASIA

BANGLADESH

National Institute of Preventive and Social Medicine, Mohakhali, Dhaka 1212, Bangladesh, Telephone: 880-2-881236; Fax: WHO Dhaka, 880-2-863-247

BURMA

Postgraduate School of Public Health, 56 U Wisara Road, Rangoon

CHINA

Beijing Medical University, School of Public Health, Beijing 100083, People's Republic of China, Telephone: 86-1-201-7601; Fax: 86-1-201-5681

China Medical University, Institute of Preventive Medicine, 150 N. Nanjing Road, Shenyang 110001, People's Republic of China, Telephone: 86-24-386-3731, ext. 2431; Fax: 86-24-387-5539

Hunan Medical University, Faculty of Public Health, Post Box 422, Changsha, Hunan 410078, People's Republic of China, Telephone: 86-731-448-111; Fax: 86-731-444-329

Shanghai Medical University, School of Public Health, 138 Yi Xue Yuanh Road, Shanghai 200032, People's Republic of China, Telephone: 86-21-431-1900; Fax: 86-21-433-0543

Sun Yat-Sen University of Medical Sciences, School of Public Health, Zhongshan Road 2, Guangszhou 510089, People's Republic of China, Telephone: 86-20-778-5223; Fax: 86-20-776-5679

West China University of Medical Sciences, School of Public Health, Chengdu Sichuan 610041, China, Telephone: 86-28-558-1130, ext. 3201; Fax: 86-28-558-3252

Xi'an Medical University, School of Public Health, 16 Scarlet Bird Avenue, Xi'an, Shaanxi 710061, China, Telephone: 86-29-526-5564; Fax: 86-29-525-0501

INDIA

Andhra Pradesh

Department of Postgraduate Public Health, Osmania Medical College, Osmania University, Hyderabad 500001

Department of Social and Preventive Medicine, Andhra Medical College, Andhra University, Visakhapatnam

Bihar

Department of Social and Preventive Medicine, Patna Medical College, Patna University, Patna

Delhi

Center for Community Medicine, All-India Institute for Medical Sciences, Ansari Nagar, New Delhi 110 029

Center for Social Medicine and Community Health, School of Social Sciences, Jawaharlal Nehru University, Block III, NAA Campus, New Delhi 110 067

Department of Social and Preventive Medicine, Lady Hardinge Medical College, University of Delhi, New Delhi 110 001

International Institute of Health and Family Welfare, New Mehrauli Road, Munirka, New Delhi 110 067

Gùjarat

Department of Community Medicine, Government Medical College, South Gùjarat University, Outside Majura Gate, Surat 395001

Department of Community Medicine, Medical College, Maharaja Sayajirao University of Baroda, Baroda 390001

Department of Preventive and Social Medicine, B.J. Medical College, Gùjarat University, Ahmedabad 380016

Department of Preventive and Social Medicine, Smt. N.H.L. Municipal Medical College, Gùjarat University, Ellisbridge Ahmedabad 380006

Kerala

Department of Social and Preventive Medicine, Trivandrum Medical College, University of Kerala, Trivandrum 11

Maharashtra

Department of Preventive and Social Medicine, Armed Forces Medicine College, University of Pune, Pune 411001

Department of Preventive and Social Medicine, Dr. Vaishampayan Memorial College, Shivaji University, Sholapur 413003

Department of Preventive and Social Medicine, Government Medical College, University of Nagpur, Nagpur

Department of Preventive and Social Medicine, Grand Medical College, University of Bombay, Byculla, Bombay 400008

Department of Preventive and Social Medicine, Medical College, Marathwada University, Aurangabad 431001

Department of Preventive and Social Medicine, Seth G.S. Medical College and K.E.M. Hospital, University of Bombay, Acharya Donde Marg. Parel, Bombay 400012

Department of Preventive and Social Medicine, Topiwala National Medical College and B.Y.L. Nair Charitable Hospital, University of Bombay, Dr. A. L. Nair Road, Byculla, Bombay 400008

Orissa

Department of Preventive and Social Medicine, M.K.C.G. Medical College, Berhampur University, Berhampur 760004

Punjab

Department of Community Medicine, Government Medical College, Guru Nanak Dev University, Amritsar

Rajasthan

Department of Community Medicine, R.N.T. Medical College, University of Rajasthan, Udaipur 313001

Department of Preventive and Social Medicine, Sadar Patel Medical College, University of Rajasthan, Bikaner

Department of Preventive and Social Medicine, Swai Mensingh Medical College, University of Rajasthan, Jaipur

Tamil Nadu and Pondicherry

Department of Community Medicine, Christian Medical College, University of Madras, Bagayam, Vellore 632002

Department of Community Medicine, Jawaharlal Institute of Postgraduate Medical Education and Research, University of Madras, Pondicherry 605006

Uttar Pradesh

Department of Preventive and Social Medicine, Ganesh Shanker Vidhyarthi Memorial Medical College, Kanpur University, Kanpur

Department of Preventive and Social Medicine, Jawaharlal Nehru Medical College, Aligarh Muslim University, Aligarh 202001

Department of Preventive and Social Medicine, M.L.N. Medical College, University of Allahabad, Allahabad

Upgraded Department of Preventive and Social Medicine, K.G. Medical College, University of Lucknow, Lucknow 226003

West Bengal

All-India Institute of Hygiene and Public Health, 110 Chittaranjan Avenue, Calcutta 700073

INDONESIA

Airlangga University, Program Study of Public Health, Faculty of Medicine, UI Darmahusada 47, Surabaya 60131 Indonesia, Telephone: 62-31-40251, ext. 34; Fax; 62-31-402-2472

University of Indonesia, Faculty of Public Health, Kampus UI, Depok, Jawa Barat, Indonesia, Telephone: 62-21-727-0037; Fax: 62-21-727-0153

JAPAN

The Institute of Public Health, Shirokanedai, Minato-ku, Tokyo 108, Japan, Telephone: 81-3-3441-7111; Fax: 81-3-3446-4314

University of the Ryukus, School of Health Sciences, Faculty of Medicine, 207 Uchara Nishihara Nakagami, Okinawa 903-01, Japan, Telephone: 81-98-895-3331; Fax: 81-98-895-2841

University of Tokyo, School of International Health, Faculty of Medicine, Hongo, Bunkyo-Ku, Tokyo 113, Japan, Telephone: 81-3-3812-2111, ext. 3696; Fax: 81-3-5684-3198

University of Tokyo Hongo, School of Health Sciences and Nursing, Faculty of Medicine, Bunkyo-ku, Tokyo 113, Japan, Telephone: 81-3-3812-2111, ext. 3509; Fax: 81-3-3815-0258

KOREA

Department of Health Administration, College of Health Science, Yonsei University, 234 Maeji-Ri, Hungob-Myon, Wonju, Kangwon-Do 222-701

Department of Health Care Management, College of Health Science, Inje University, 607 Obang-Dong, Kmhae, Kyongnam 621-749

Department of Health Education, College of Education, Ewha Womans University, 11-1 Daehyun-Dong, Seodaemun-Ku, Seoul 120-750

Department of Health Science, Dongduck Women's University, 23-1 Wolgok-Dong, Sungbuk-Ku, Seoul 136-714

Department of Health Science, Kosin University, 149-1 Dongsan-Dong, Youngdo-Ku, Pusan 606-701

Department of Health Science, Kyungsan University, 75 Chomchom-Dong, Kyongsan, Kyongbuk 712-240

Department of Public Health, College of Natural Science, Keimyung University, 1000 Shindang-Dong, Dalseo-Gu, Taegu 704-701

Department of Public Health Administration, College of Social Science, Wonkwang University, 344-2 Shinyong-Dong, Iri, Chonbuk 570-749

Graduate School of Health Science and Management, Yonsei University, C.P.O. Box 8044, Seoul 120-752

Graduate School of Public Health, Chungnam National University, 6 Munhwa-Dong, Jung-Ku, Taejeon 301-130

Graduate School of Public Health, Inje University, 607 Obang-Dong, Kimhae, Kyongnam 621-749

Graduate School of Public Health, Kosin University, 34 Amnan-Dong, Suh-Ku, Pusan 602-702

Graduate School of Public Health, Kyungpook National University, 101 Dong-In-Dong, Chung-Gu, Taegu 700-422

Graduate School of Public Health, Kyungsan University, 75 Chomchon-Dong, Kyongsan, Kyongbuk 712-240

Graduate School of Public Health, Seoul National University, 28 Yeunkun-Dong, Cnongro-Ku, Seoul 110-799

School of Public Health, Inje University, 18-3 Obang-dong, Kimhae, Kyongsangnam-do 621-749 Korea, Telephone: 82-525-347-121 or 82-514-631-341; Fax: 82-525-340-712

Seoul National University, School of Public Health, 28 Yunkeun-Dong, Chongno-Ku, Seoul 110-450, Korea, Telephone: 82-2-740-8851; Fax: 82-2-745-9104

LAO

University of Health Sciences, School of Public Health, Vientiane, Lao PRD; Fax: 856-21-214055

MALAYSIA

University of Malaya, Department of Social Obstetrics and Gynecology, Faculty of Medicine, 59100 Kuala Lumpur, Malaysia, Telephone: 60-3-750-2342; Fax: 60-3-755-7740

MONGOLIA

University of Mongolia, Medical Education Services, National Medical, Jamyangunee Str. 4, P.O. 48, Box 111, Ulaanbaatar, Mongolia, Telephone: 976-1-323-032; Fax: 976-1-727-313

NEPAL

Tribhuvan University, Department of Community Medicine, Institute of Medicine, P.O. 2844, Maharajgunj, Kathmandu, Nepal, Telephone: 977-1-414-792; Fax: 977-1-228-349

PHILIPPINES

University of Philippines, College of Public Health, P.O. Box EA-460, Ermita, Manila, Philippines, Telephone: 63-2-502-1703; Fax: 63-2-521-1394

SINGAPORE

National University of Singapore, Department of Community Occupational and Family Medicine, Faculty of Medicine, National University Hospital, Lower Kent Ridge Road, Singapore 0511, Republic of Singapore, Telephone: 65-772-4299; Fax: 65-779-1489

TAIWAN

National Taiwan University, College of Public Health, No. 1, Jen Al Road, 1st Section, Taipei, Taiwan, Republic of China, Telephone: 886-2-391-4424; Fax: 886-2-391-1308

THAILAND

Mahidol University, Faculty of Environment and Resource Studies, Nakorn Pathom 73170, Thailand, Telephone: 66-2-441-9335; Fax: 66-2-441-9510

Mahidol University, Faculty of Public Health, 420/1 Rajvithi Road, Bangkok 10400, Thailand, Telephone: 66-2-245-5521; Fax: 66-2-246-7765

Sukhothai Thammathirat Open University, Bang Pood, Pakkred, Nonthaburi 11200, Thailand, Telephone: 66-2-573-5805; Fax: 66-2-573-5817

VIETNAM

Hanoi Medical University, School of Public Health, 138A Giang Vo Street, Hanoi, Vietnam, Telephone: 84-4-25303; Fax: 84-4-25247

AUSTRALIA

University of Sydney, Department of Public Health, Sydney, New South Wales 2006, Australia, Telephone: 61-2-692-4367; Fax: 61-2-692-4179

EUROPE

Association of Schools of Public Health in the European Region, (ASPHER), Hôpital Nationale de St. Maurice, 14 Rue du Val D'Osne, F-94229 H Saint Maurice, Prof. Jacques Bury, Executive Director

AUSTRIA

School of Public Health, Department of Social Medicine, University of Innsbruck, Sonnenburgstr. 16, 6020 Innsbruck

BELGIUM

Department of Public Health, University Hospital, de Pintelaan 185, 9000 Gent

Dienst voor Hygiëne en Sociale Geneeskunde, Rijksuniversiteit te Gent, Akademisch Ziekenhuis, de Pintelaan 135, Gent

Ecole de Santé Publique, 3, avenue de l'Hôpital, Bât B 23, 4000 Liège

Ecole de Santé Publique, Université Catholique de Louvain, Chapelle aux Champs 30-34, 1200 Bruxelles

Ecole de Santé Publique, Université Libre de Bruxelles, Campus Erasme—CP/591, Route de Lennik 808, 1070 Bruxelles

European Public Health Alliance, 1 Place du Luxembourg, 1040 Brussels

Institute de Médecine Tropicale Prince Léopold, Nationalestraat 155, 2000 Antwerpen

School voor Maatschappelijke Gezondheitszorg, Katholieke Universiteit Leuven, Vital Decosterstraat 102, 3000 Leuven

School voor Maatschappelijke Gezondheitszorg, Vrije Universiteit Brussel, Laarbeeklaan 103, 1090 Brussel

School voor Maatschappelijke Gezondheitszorg (School of Public Health), Kapucijnenvoer, 35, 3000 Leuven

BULGARIA

Medical Academy, Ulica D. Nesterov 15, Sofia 1431

BYELORUSSIA

Belorusskij Institut UsoverěnstvovanijaVracej, Ul. Petrusja Brovki 2, 220714 Minsk

CROATIA

Škola narodnog zdravlja "Andrija Štampar" ("Andrija Štampar" School of Public Health), Medical Faculty, University of Zagreb, Rockefellerova 4, 41,000 Zagreb

CZECH REPUBLIC

Department of Public Health, Institute of Public Health and Preventive Medicine, 2nd Medical Faculty, Charles University, Vúvalu 84, 15018 Praha–Motol

Institute of Public Health, Karlovo nam. 40, 12800 Praha 2

Institute of Social Health and Public Health, Medical Faculty of University of Masaryk, Joštova 10, 66243 Brno

National Institute of Public Health, IPVZ, Ruská 85, 10000 Praha 10

Postgraduate Medical School, Ruská 85, 10005 Praha 10

University of Palacky, Theoretical Institutes, Hnevotínská 3, 77600 Olomouc

DENMARK

Department of Social Medicine, University of Copenhagen, Panum Institute, 3, Blegdamsvej, 2200 Copenhagen

World Health Organization (WHO), Regional Office for Europe, Scherfigsvej 8, 2100 Copenhagen

FINLAND

Department of Community Health and General Practice, University of Kuopio, P.O. Box 1627, 70211 Kuopio

Department of General Practice and Primary Health Care of the University of Helsinki, Lääkärinkatu 8 F, 00250 Helsinki

FRANCE

Départment d'Epidemiologie, Economie de la Santé et Santé Communautaire, Université Toulouse III, Faculté de Médicine, 37, Allées Jules Guesde, 31073 Toulouse Cedex

Ecole de Santé Publique, Faculté de Médicine, Université de Nancy I, 9 avenue de la Forêt de Haye, BP 184, 54505 Vandoeuvre les Nancy Cedex

Ecole Nationale de la Santé Publique, Avenue du Professeur Léon Bernard, 35043 Rennes Cedex

U.E.R. de Médecine en Santé tropicale, Université d'Aix-Marseille, 27 boulevard Jean Moulin, 13005 Marseille

GEORGIA

Tbilisskij Gosudarstvennyj Institut Usoveršenstvovanija Vracej, Prospekt Cavcavadze 33, 380030 Tbilisi

GERMANY

Abteilung Epidemiologie und Sozialmedizin, Medizinische Hochschule Hannover (Department of Epidemiology and Social Medicine, Hannover Medical School), Konstanty-Gutschow-Str. 8, 30625 Hannover

Akademie für das öffentliche Gesundheitswesen, Bayerisches Staatsministerium für Arbeit und Sozialordnung, Familie, Frauen und Gesundheit, Winzererstr. 9, 80797 München

Akademie für öffentliches Gesundheitswesen, Auf'm Hennekamp 70, 40225 Düsseldorf

Department of Medical Informatics, Biometry and Epidemiology, Marchionistr. 15, 83177 München

Fakultät für Gesundheitswissenschaften/School of Public Health, University of Bielefeld, P.O. Box 10 01 31, 33501 Bielefeld

Institut für Gesundheitswissenschaften, Technische Universität Berlin, Gesundheitswissenschaften/Public Health, -HH 7-, Steinplatz 1, 10623 Berlin

Institut für Medizin-Soziologie, Universitäts-Krankenhaus Eppendorf, Martinistr. 52, 20251 Hamburg

Institut für Tropenhygiene und öffentliches Gesundheitswesen am Südasien-Institut, Universität Heidelberg, Im Neuenheimer Feld 324, 69120 Heidelberg

Medical School, Heinrich-Heine-University, Institute of Medical Sociology, Moorenstr. 5, 40225 Düsseldorf

Technische Universität Dresden, Medizinische Fakultät, Carl Gustav Carus, Public Health, Fiedlerstr. 27, 01307 Dresden

Zentrum für Angewandte Gesundheitswissenschaften, Universität Lüneburg und Fachhochschule Nordostniedersachsen, Am Schifferwall 1, 21335 Lüneburg

GREECE

National School of Public Health, 196, Alexandras Avenue, 11521 Athens

HUNGARY

Department of Public Health, University Medical School of Pècs, Szigeti U 12, 7643 Pècs

Department of Social Medicine, University Medical School of Debrecen, P.O. Box 2, 4012 Debrecen

Orvostovábbképzö Intézet (Postgraduate Medical University, Institute of Public Health Medicine), Szabolcs u. 35, 1389 Budapest III

IRELAND

Department of Community Medicine and Epidemiology, Faculty of Medicine, University College, Earlsfort Terrace, Dublin 2

European Healthcare Management Association (EHMA), Vergemount Hall, Clonskeagh, Dublin 6

ISRAEL

School of Public Health and Community Medicine, The Joseph and Belle Braun Hebrew University—Hadassah, P.O. Box 12 21 72, Jerusalem 91120

ITALY

Cattedra di Medicina di Comunità, Dipartimento di Pediatria, 35100 Milano

Dipartimento di Igiene e Medicina di Comunità, Via Santena 5, 10126 Torino

Dipartimento di Medicina Preventiva, Viale Forlanini 2, 27100 Pavia

Dipartimento di Sanità Publica, Via R. Orazio 8—Tor Vergata, 00173 Roma

Dipartimento di Sanità Publica, Via S. Zeno 35, 56100 Pisa

Dipartimento di Sanità Publica, Via T. Cannizzaro 278, 98100 Messina

Dipartimento di Sanità Publica, Viale Morgagni 48, 50134 Firenze

Istituto di Igiene e Medicina Preventiva, Via Istria 65, 34100 Trieste

Istituto di Igiene e Medicina Preventiva, Via L. Armanni 5, 80100 Napoli

Istituto di Igiene e Medicina Preventiva, Via Pansini 5, 80131 Napoli

Istituto di Ricerche Farmacologiche Mario Negri, Consorzio Mario Negri Sud, Via Nazionale 1, 66030 Santa Maria Imbaro

KAZAKHSTAN

Alma-Atinskij Institut Usoveršenstvovanija Vracej, Ul. Capaeva 34, Alma-Ata

LUXEMBOURG

European Commission, Directorate of Health and Safety GD V/F/1 "Public Health," L-2920 Luxembourg

THE NETHERLANDS

Department of Public Health, Leidse Hogeschool, Faculty of Health Sciences, Endegeesterwatering 2, 2333 CG Leiden

European Public Health Association (EUPHA), University of Amsterdam, Institute of Medicine, Meibergdreef 15, 1105 AZ Amsterdam

Faculty of Health Sciences, University of Limburg, P.O. Box 616, 6200 MD Maastricht

Hogeschool von Amsterdam, Tafelberg 51, 1105 BD Amsterdam

Instituut voor Sociale Geneeskunde, Vrije Universiteit, Van den Boechorststraat 7, Amsterdam-Buitenveldert

Instituut voor Social-Medische Wetenschap der Rijksuniversiteit, Bloemsingel 1, 9713 BZ Groningen

Koninklijk Instituut voor de Tropen (Royal Tropical Institute), 63 Mauritskade, 1092 AD Amsterdam

Nederlands Instituut voor Preventieve Gezondheidszorg, TNO, Wassenaarseweg 56, 2353 AL Leiden

Netherlands School of Public Health, Admiraal Helfrichlaan 1, 3527 KV Utrecht

Stichting Sociale Gesondheidszorg, Leidseweg 83, 3531 BG Utrecht

Vahgroep Sociale Geneeskunde, Katholieke Universiteit, Verlengde Groenenstraat 75, 6525 EJ Nijmegen

NORWAY

Videreutdanning i Folkehelsevitenskap (Tromsø School of Public Health), University of Tromsø, Institute of Community Medicine, 9037 Tromsø

POLAND

Centrum Medyczne Kształcenia Podyplomowego, Studium Medycyny Spolecznej (Medical Centre of Postgraduate Education, Faculty of Social Medicine), Ul. Kleczewska 61/63, 01-823 Warsaw

School of Public Health, Collegium Medicum of the Jagiellonian University, Ul. Grzegórzecka 20, 31-531 Kraków

School of the Public Health, Nofer Institute of Occupational Medicine, P.O. Box 199, 8 Teresy Str., 90-950 Lodz

PORTUGAL

Escola Nacional de Saúde Pública, Av. Padre Cruz, 1699 Lisboa Codex

ROMANIA

Institute of Hygiene, Public Health, Health Services and Management, 1-3 Dr. Leonte Str., 76256 Bucharest

RUSSIA

Central'nyj Ordena Lenina Institut Usoveršenstvovanija Vracej, Barrikadnaja 2, 123242 Moscow

International Academy of Science, International Institute of Restorative Medicine, P.O. Box 44, 125284 Moscow

Irkutskij Institut Usoveršenstvovanija Vracej, Deputatskaja Ul. 45/2, Irkutsk 664023

Kazanskij Gosudarstvennyi Institut Usoveršenstvovanija Vracej, Ul. Komleva 11, 420012 Kazan 12

Leningradskij Institut Usoveršenstvovanija Vracej, Ul. Saltykova-Ššedrina 41 St. Petersburg

Novokuzneckij Institut Usoveršenstvovanija Vracej, Ul. Krupskoj 3, Penza 440039

Uralskij Institut Usoveršenstvovanija Vracej, Prospekt Pobedy 287, Celjabinsk 454026

SERBIA

Institut za strucno usavršavanje i specializaciju zdravstvenih radnika (Postgraduate Medical Institute), Nušiceva 25/1, Belgrade

Institute of Public Health of Serbia, 5, Dr. Subotica Street, 11000 Belgrade

SLOVAKIA

School of Public Health, Postgraduate Medical School, Limbovà 12, 833 03 Bratislava

SPAIN

Area de Medicina Preventiva y Salud Pública, Universidad de Oviedo, Av. Julian Claveria, Oviedo (Asturias)

Centro Universitario de Salud Pública, General Oraá, No 39, 28006 Madrid

Escola Nacional de Sanidad, Facultad de Medicina, Universidad Complutense de Madrid, Ciudad Universitaria, Pabellon 1, Madrid 3

Escuela Andaluza de Salud Pública, Campus Universitario de Cartuja, Apdo. 2070, Granada 18080

Instituto de Ciencias de la Salud de Cantabria, Escuela de Salud Pública, C/ Antonio Lopez, 30, 8° Izda, 39009 Santander

Instituto Valenciano de Estudios en Salud Pública, Juan de Garay, 21, 46017 Valencia

SWEDEN

Faculty of Health Sciences, Center for Public Health, Master of Public Health Program, 581 85 Linköping

Karolinska Institute, Department of Environmental Hygiene, P.O. Box 60400, 104 01 Stockholm

Nordiska Hälsovårdshögskolan (Nordic School of Public Health), Medicinaregatan, S-413 46 Göteborg

SWITZERLAND

Department of Social and Preventive Medicine, University of Bern, Finkenhubelweg 11, 3012 Bern

Human Resources Division, OMS/WHO, Avenue Appia, 1211 Geneva 27

Swiss Tropical Institute, Department of Public Health and Epidemiology, Socinstr. 57, 4002 Basel

Unité de Santé communautaire, Faculté de Médecine, Université de Genève, 24 rue Michel Servet, 1211 Geneva 4

TURKEY

Department of Public Health, Cerrahpasa School of Medicine, Istanbul University, Istanbul

Department of Public Health, Faculty of Medicine, Akdeniz University, Ankara

Department of Public Health, Faculty of Medicine, Cumhuriyet University, Sivas

Department of Public Health, Faculty of Medicine, Dicle University, Diyarbakir

Department of Public Health, Faculty of Medicine, Dokuz Eylül University, Izmir

Department of Public Health, Faculty of Medicine, Ege University, Izmir

Department of Public Health, Faculty of Medicine, Gazi University, Ankara

Department of Public Health, Faculty of Medicine, I19 Mayis University, Samsun

Department of Public Health, Faculty of Medicine, Istanbul University, Istanbul

Halk Sagligi Ana Bilim Dali (Department of Public Health), Faculty of Medicine, Anadolu University, Eskisehir

Halk Sagligi Ana Bilim Dali (Department of Public Health), Faculty of Medicine, Çukurova University, Adana

Halk Sagligi Ana Bilim Dali (Department of Public Health), Faculty of Medicine, Hacettepe University, Ankara

Halk Sagligi Anabilim Dali (Department of Public Health), Faculty of Medicine, Uludag University School of Medicine, 16059 Görükle Bursa

Hifzissihha Okulu (School of Public Health), Cemal Gürsel Caddesi 18, Yenisehir, Ankara

UKRAINE

Kievskij Institut Usoveršenstvovanija Vracej, Ul. Dorogozickaja 9, 252112 Kiev 112

Ukrainskij Institut Usoveršenstvovanija Vracej, Ul. Artema 8, Har'Kov 310002

Zaporozskij Institut Usoveršenstvovanija Vracej, Ul. Vintera 20, Zaporoz'e 330010

UNITED KINGDOM

Department of Community Medicine, University of Edinburgh, Usher Institute, Warrender Park Road, Edinburgh EH9 1DW

Department of Community Medicine, University of Glasgow, Ruchill Hopsital, Bilsland Drive, Glasgow G20 9NB

Department of Community Medicine and General Practice, School of Medicine, University of Leeds, 32 Hyde Terrace, Leeds LS2 9LN

Department of Epidemiology and Public Health Medicine, University of Bristol, Canynge Hall, Whiteladies Road, Clifton, Bristol BS8 2PR

Department of International Community Health, Liverpool School of Tropical Medicine, Pembroke Place, Liverpool L3 5QA

Department of Public Health, University of Liverpool, P.O. Box 147, Liverpool L69 3BX

Department of Public Health Sciences, University of Edinburgh, Medical School Buildings, Teviot Place, Edinburgh EH8 9AG

Institute of Public Health and Environmental Health, University of Birmingham, The Medical School, B15 2TT Birmingham

London School of Hygiene & Tropical Medicine, University of London, Keppel Street, London WC1E 7HT

Nottingham School of Public Health, Queen's Medical Center, Nottingham NG7 2UH

The Royal Institute of Public Health and Hygiene, 28 Portland Place, London W1N 4DE

Welsh Combined Centres for Public Health, University of Wales, College of Medicine, Cardiff

World Federation for Medical Education (WFME), The University of Edinburgh, Centre for Medical Education, 11 Hill Square, Edinburgh EH8 9DR

UZBEKISTAN

Taškentskij Institut Usoveršenstvovanija Vracej, Ul. Generala Petrova 51, 700007 Taškent

LATIN AMERICA AND THE CARIBBEAN

Asociación Latinoamericana y del Caribe de Educación en Salud Pública (ALAESP), Dr. Arnaldo Augusto Franco de Siqueira, Secretaria Ejecutiva, ALAESP, Director da Faculdade de Saúde Pública, Universidade de São Paulo, Av. Dr. Arnaldo 455–2° andar, 01246-00 São Paulo

ARGENTINA

Centro de Estudios Estrategicos en Recursos Humanos para la Salud (CERSA), Obispo Trejo 661, 5000 Córdoba

Universidad de Buenos Aires, Escuela de Salud Pública, Facultad de Medicina, Marcelo T. de Alvear 2202, C.P. 1122 Buenos Aires

Universidad Nacional de Córdoba, Escuela de Salud Pública, Pabellon Argentina, Ciudad Universitaria, Estafeta 32, 5000 Córdoba

Universidad Nacional del Litoral, Escuela Superior de Sanidad "Dr. Ramón Carrillo," Salvador Caputto 3353, 3000 Santa Fé

BOLIVIA

Comisión de Desarrollo Social, República de Bolivia, H. Senado Nacional, Casilla 9997, La Paz

Maestría en Salud Pública, Avda. Capitán Ravelo No. 2199, La Paz

BRAZIL

Escola de Saúde Pública, Av. Ipiranga, 6311, 90610-001 Porto Alegre, RS

Escola Nacional de Saúde Pública, Rua Leopoldo Bulhões 1480, Manguinhos, Rio de Janeiro

Universidade de São Paulo, Departamento de Medicina Preventiva, Faculdade de Medicina, Av. Dr. Arnaldo 455–2° andar, 01246-00 São Paulo, SP

Universidade de São Paulo, Departamento de Medicina Social, Faculdade de Medicina de Riberão Preto, Av. Bandeirantes 3900, 14049-900 Riberão Preto, SP

Universidade de São Paulo, Faculdade de Saúde Pública, Av. Dr. Arnaldo 715, São Paulo 01255

Universidade Federal da Bahia, Departamento de Medicina Preventiva, Rua Padre Feijó–20–4° andar, 40110-170 Salvador, BA

CHILE

División de Desarrollo Social, CEPAL, Casilla 179, D-Santiago

Escuela de Salud Pública, Avenida Independencia 939, Casilla 6537, Correo 7, Santiago

COLOMBIA

Universidad de Antioquía, Facultad Nacional de Salud Pública, Calle 62, N° 52-19, Apartado Aéreo 51922, Medellin

Universidad del Valle, Departamento de Medicina Social, Facultad de Salud, San Fernando, Apartado Aéreo 2188, Cali

Universidad Nacional de Colombia, Departamento de Medicina Preventiva y Social, Facultad de Medicina, Edificio Facultad de Medicina, Ciudad Universitaria, Santafé de Bogotá D.C.

CUBA

Facultad de Salud Pública, Apartado Aéreo 9082, Zona 9, La Habana

Instituto de Desarrollo de la Salud, Apartado de Correo 9082, Zona Postal 9, La Habana

ECUADOR

Universidad Central de Quito, Escuela de Salud Pública, Leyton 1248, Quito

JAMAICA

University of the West Indies, Department of Social and Preventive Medicine, Mona, Kingston 7

MEXICO

Departamento de Salud Pública, 6° piso Edificio "B," Facultad de Medicina, Universidad Nacional Autónoma de Mexico, Cuidad Universitaria, Apartado Postal 70-443, 04510 Mexico, D.F.

Departamento de Salud Pública, Instituto de Ciencias de la Salud, Ernesto Ortíz Medina No. 1, Esq. Av. Xalapa, Apdo. Postal 57, Yalapa, Veracruz 91020

Escuela de Salud Pública de México, Instituto Nacional de Salud Pública, Avenida Universidad 655, Colonia Santa María Ahuacatitlán, C.P. 62508, Cuernavaca, Morelos

Facultad de Salud Pública de la Universidad Autónoma de Nuevo León, C.P. 64460, Eduardo Aguirre Pequeño y Yuriria Col. Mitras Centro, Monterrey, Nuevo León

Instituto Nacional de Salud Pública, Av. Universidad No. 655, Col. Sta. María Ahuacatitlán, C.P. 62508, Cuernavaca, Morelos

Maestría en Medicina Social, Departamento de Atención a la Salud, Universidad Autónoma Metropolitana, Unidad Xochimilco, Calzada del Hueso No. 1100, Vial Quietud, Coyacán, 04960 Mexico, D.F.

PANAMA

Escuela de Salud Pública, Facultad de Medicina, Cuidad Universitaria Octoavio, Mendez Pereira, Estafeta Universitaria, Panamá

PERU

Escuela de Salud Pública, 3558 Avenida Brasil, Lima 17

VENEZUELA

Escuela de Salud Pública, Complejo Hospitalario "José I. Baldó," El Algodonal, Apartado de Correos 62231, Antimano, Caracas

NORTH AMERICA

CANADA

Dalhousie University, Department of Community Health and Epidemiology, 5848 University Ave., Halifax, Nova Scotia, B3H 4H7

McGill University, Department of Epidemiology and Biostatistics, 1020 Pine Avenue West, Montreal, Quebec, H3A 1A2

McMaster University Medical Center, Department of Epidemiology and Biostatistics, 1200 Main St. West, Hamilton, Ontario, L9H 2S4

Memorial University of Newfoundland, Division of Community Medicine, Faculty of Medicine, St. John's, Newfoundland, A1B 3V6

Queen's University, Department of Community Health and Epidemiology, Abramsky Hall, Kingston, Ontario, K7L 3N6

Université de Laval de Québec, Departement de médecine sociale et preventive, Faculté de Medecine, Pavillon de l'EST, Sainte-Foy, Quebec, G1K 7P4

Université de Montréal, Department d'administration de la santé, Faculté de Médecine, C.P. 6128 Succursale Centre-ville, Montreal, Quebec, H3C 3J7

University of Alberta, Department of Public Health Sciences, Faculty of Medicine, 13-103 Clinical Sciences Building, Edmonton, Alberta, T6G 2G3

University of British Columbia, Department of Health Care and Epidemiology, Faculty of Medicine, 5804 Fairview Avenue, Vancover, British Columbia, V6T 1Z3

University of Calgary, Department of Community Health Sciences, Faculty of Medicine, Health Sciences Center, 3330 Hospital Drive. NW, Calgary, Alberta, T2N 4N1

University of Guelph, Department of Population Medicine, Ontario Veterinary College, Guelph, Ontario, NIG 2W1

University of Manitoba, Department of Community Health Sciences, Faculty of Medicine, 750 Bannantyne Avenue, Winnipeg, Manitoba, R3E OW3

University of Montreal, Department of Social and Preventive Medicine, Faculty of Medicine, 2375 Cote Ste. Catherine, Montreal, Quebec, H3C 3J7

University of Ottawa, Department of Epidemiology and Community Medicine, 451 Smyth Road, Ottawa, Ontario, K1H 8M5

University of Prince Edward Island, Department of Health Management, Atlanta Veterinary College, Charlottetown, Prince Edward Island, CIA 4P3

University of Saskatchewan, Department of Community Health and Epidemiology, College of Medicine, Saskatoon, Saskatchewan, S7N 0W0

University of Toronto, Graduate Department of Community Health, Faculty of Medicine, McMurrich Building, 12 Queens Park Crescent West, Toronto, Ontario, M5S 1A8

The University of Waterloo, Department of Health Studies and Gerontology, Faculty of Applied Health Sciences, Waterloo, Ontario, N2L 3G1

The University of Western Ontario, Department of Epidemiology and Biostatistics, Clinical Sciences Building, London, Ontario, N6A 5C1

UNITED STATES OF AMERICA

Association of Schools of Public Health (ASPH), 1660 L Street, NW, Suite 204, Washington, DC 20076

Boston University, School of Public Health, School of Medicine, 80 East Concord Street, Boston, MA 02118-2394

Columbia University, School of Public Health, 167 West 168th Street, New York, NY 10032

Emory University School of Public Health, 1599 Clifton Road NE, Atlanta, GA 30329

Harvard University School of Public Health, 677 Huntington Avenue, Boston, MA 02115

Health Resources and Services Administration, 5600 Fishers Lane, Rockville, MD 20857

International Health Institute of Medicine, National Academy of Sciences, 2101 Constitution Avenue, NW, Washington, DC 20418

The Johns Hopkins University School of Hygiene & Public Health, 615 North Wolfe Street, Baltimore, MD 21205-2179

Loma Linda University School of Public Health, Hill Street, Loma Linda, CA 92350

Saint Louis University School of Public Health, O'Donnell Hall, 4th Floor, 3663 Lindell Blvd. St. Louis, MO 63108

San Diego State University Graduate School of Public Health, San Diego, CA 92182-0405

State University of New York (SUNY), University at Albany School of Public Health, Two University Place, Albany, NY 12203-3399

Tulane University Medical Center School of Public Health & Tropical Medicine, 1430 Tulane Avenue, New Orleans, LA 70112

University of Alabama at Birmingham School of Public Health, 720 South 20th Street, University Station, Birmingham, AL 35294-0008

University of California at Berkeley School of Public Health, 19 Earl Warren Hall, Berkeley, CA 94720

University of California at Los Angeles School of Public Health, Center for the Health Sciences, Los Angeles, CA 90024-1772

University of California at Los Angeles School of Public Health, International Epidemiology Association (IEA), Los Angeles, CA 90024-1772

University of Hawaii School of Public Health, 1960 East-West Road, Honolulu, HI 96822

University of Illinois at Chicago School of Public Health, Health Sciences Center, M/C 922, Post Office Box 6998, Chicago, IL 60680

University of Massachusetts School of Public Health, 108 Arnold House, Amherst, MA 01003-0037

University of Michigan School of Public Health, 109 South Observatory Street, Ann Arbor, MI 48109-2029

University of Minnesota School of Public Health, Box 197, 1360 Mayo Memorial Building, 420 Delaware Street, SE, Minneapolis, MN 55455-0381

University of North Carolina at Chapel Hill School of Public Health, CB-7400, Rosenau Hall, Chapel Hill, NC 27599-7400

University of Oklahoma College of Public Health, Health Sciences Center, 801 N.E. 13th Street, Oklahoma City, OK 73104-5072

University of Pittsburgh Graduate School of Public Health, 111 Parran Hall, 130 De Soto Street, Pittsburgh, PA 15261

University of Puerto Rico School of Public Health, Medical Sciences Campus, G.P.O. Box 5067, San Juan, Puerto Rico 00936

University of South Carolina School of Public Health, Sumter and Greene, Columbia, SC 29208

University of South Florida College of Public Health, 13201 Bruce B. Downs Boulevard, Tampa, FL 33612-3805

University of Texas School of Public Health, Health Science Center at Houston, Post Office Box 20186, Houston, TX 77225

University of Washington School of Public Health & Community Medicine, Mail Drop SC-30, Seattle, WA 98195

Western Consortium for Public Health, 2001 Addison Street, Suite 200, Berkeley, CA 94704-1103

Yale University Department of Epidemiology & Public Health, School of Medicine, Post Office Box 3333, 60 College Street, New Haven, CT 06510

Graduate Programs in Community Health Education

California State University—Long Beach MPH and US' Programs in Community Health Education, Health Science Department, College of Health & Human Services, 1250 Bellflower Boulevard, Long Beach, CA 90840

California State University—Northridge MPH Program in Community Health Education, Department of Health Science, Schools of Communication & Professional Studies, 18111 Nordhoff Street, Northridge, CA 91330

East Stroudsburg University MPH Program in Community Health Education, Health Department, East Stroudsburg, PA 18201

Hunter College MPH Program in Community Health Education, School of Health Sciences, 425 East 25th Street, New York, NY 10010

New York University MPH Program in Community Health Education, Department of Health Education, School of Education, Health, Nursing and Arts Professions, 35 W. 4th Street, Suite 1200, New York, NY 1,0003

San Jose State University MPH Program in Community Health Education, Department of Health Science, School of Applied Sciences and Arts, San Jose, CA 95192

Temple University MPH Program in Community Health Education, Department of Health Education, College of Health, Physical Education, Recreation & Dance, 304 Seltzer Hall, Philadelphia, PA 19122

University of Illinois at Urbana-Champaign MSPG Program in Community Health Education, Department of Community Health, 1206 South Fourth Street, Champaign, IL 61820

University of Northern Colorado MPH Program in Community Health Education, Department of Community Health & Nutrition, College of Health & Human Sciences, Greeley, CO 80639

University of Wisconsin at LaCrosse MPH Program in Community Health Education, Health Education Department, 203 Mitchell Hall, LaCrosse, WI 54601

Graduate Programs in Community Health and Preventive Medicine

Florida International University Graduate Program in Public Health, Department of Public Health, North Miami Campus, 3000 N.E. 145th Street, North Miami, FL 33181-3600

George Washington University MPH Program, School of Medicine & Health Sciences, 2150 Pennsylvania Avenue, NW, Washington, DC 20037

Medical College of Wisconsin MPH Program, Department of Preventive Medicine, 8701 Watertown Plank Road, Milwaukee, WI 53226

Ohio State University Graduate Program in Preventive Medicine & Community Health, Department of Preventive Medicine, College of Medicine, Starling Loving Hall, 320 W. 10th Avenue, Columbus, OH 43210-1228

Tufts University School of Medicine Combined MD/MPH Program, Department of Community Health, 136 Harrison Avenue, Boston, MA 02111

Uniformed Services University of the Health Sciences MPH and MTM & H Graduate Programs, Department of Preventive Medicine & Biometrics, School of Medicine, 4301 Jones Bridge Road, Bethesda, MD 20814-4799

University of Colorado MSPH-Program, Department of Preventive Medicine & Biometrics, School of Medicine, Health Science Center, 4200 E. Ninth Avenue, Box C-245, Denver, CO 80262

University of Connecticut Master of Public Health Program, Department of Community Medicine & Health Care, School of Medicine, Farmington, CT 06032-1910

University of Medicine & Dentistry of New Jersey—Robert Wood Johnson Medical School, Rutgers, The State University of New Jersey Graduate Program in Public Health, Department of Environmental & Community Medicine, 681 Frelinghuysen Rd., Piscataway, NJ 08854

University of Miami MPH Programs, Department of Epidemiology & Public Health, School of Medicine, Post Office Box 016069, Miami, FL 33101

University of Rochester, MPH Program, School of Medicine & Dentistry, 601 Elmwood Avenue, Rochester, NY 14642

University of Southern Mississippi MPH Program, Center for Community Health, College of Health & Human Sciences, Southern Station, Box 5122, Hattiesburg, MS 39406-5122

University of Tennessee at Knoxville MPH Program, Department of Health, Leisure & Safety, College of Education, 1914 Andy Holt Avenue, Knoxville, TN 37996-2700

University of Utah MPH and MSPH Programs, Department of Family & Preventive Medicine, Medical Center, 50 North Medical Drive, Salt Lake City, UT 84132

SELECTED BIBLIOGRAPHY

Afifi, A. A. & Breslow, L. (1994). The maturing paradigm of public health. *Annual Review of Public Health* 15, 223–235.

American Public Health Association. (1991). *Guide to Implementing Model Standards.* Washington, D.C.: APHA.

Arnold, M. (1991). *Health Care in the Federal Republic of Germany.* Köln: Deutscher Ärzte-Verlag.

Baggott, R. (1994). *Health and Health Care in Britain.* London: St Martin's Press.

Barnard, K. & Köhler, L. (1994). Creating a learning environment in a school of public health. *European Series on Training and Research in Public Health*, 2, 20–28.

Blendon, R. J. & Taylor, H. (1989). Views on health care: Public opinion in three nations. *Health Affairs*, 8, 149–157.

Brockington, C. F. (1966). *A Short History of Public Health.* 2nd ed. Edinburgh: Churchill Livingstone.

Brown, E. R. & Dallek, G. (1990). State approaches to financing health care for the poor. *Annual Review of Public Health*, 11, 377–400.

Crombie, I. K. (1993). *The Audit Handbook: Improving Health Care Through Clinical Audit.* Chichester: John Wiley.

Deutsche Forschungsgemeinschaft (DFG). (1995). *Gesundheitssystemforschung in Deutschland.* Memorandum. (Ed.: F. W. Schwartz). Weinheim: VCH.

Epp, J. (1986). *Achieving Health for All: A Framework for Health Promotion.* Ottawa: Health and Welfare Canada.

Evans, R. G., Barer, M. L. & Marmor, T. R. (Eds.). (1994). *Why Are Some People Healthy and Others Not? The Determinants of Populations.* New York: Aldine de Gruyter.

Fineberg, H. V., Green, G. M., Ware, J. H. & Anderson, B. L. (1994). Changing public health training needs: Professional education and the paradigm of public health. *Annual Review of Public Health*, 15, 237–257.

Forsyth, G. (1966). *Doctors and State Medicine*. London: Pitman Medical.

Frazer, W. M. (1950). *A History of English Public Health 1834–1939*. London: Tindall & Cox.

Frenk, J. (1993). The new public health. *Annual Review of Public Health*, 14, 469–490.

Hancock, T. (1985). Beyond health care: From public health policy to healthy public policy. In: Beyond Health Care: Proceedings of a Conference on Healthy Public Policy. *Canadian Journal of Public Health*, 76 (Supp. 1), 9–11.

Holland, W. W., Detels, R. & Knox, G. (Eds.). (1984). *Oxford Textbook of Public Health*. Oxford: Oxford University Press.

Holland, W. W., Fitzsimons, B. & O'Brien, M. (1994). Back to the future—public health research into the next century. *Journal of Public Health Medicine*, 16 (1), 1, 4–10.

Hurrelmann, K. (1989). *Human Development and Health*. New York: Springer Verlag.

Hurrelmann, K. & Laaser, U. (Eds.). (1993). *Gesundheitswissenschaften. Handbuch für Lehre, Forschung und Praxis*. Weinheim: Beltz.

Hurrelmann, K. & Lösel, F. (Eds.). (1990). *Health Hazards in Adolescence*. Berlin: De Gruyter.

Köhler, L. (1991). Public health renaissance and the role of schools of public health. *European Journal of Public Health*, 1, 2–9.

Laaser, U. (1994). The contribution of the schools of public health to public health in Europe. *German Journal of Public Health*, 2, 109–118.

Lasser, U., de Leeuw, E. & Stock, C. (Eds.). (1995). *Scientific Foundations of a Public Health Policy in Europe*. Weinheim: Juventa.

Milner, P. (1994). Unsettling times for public health. *Journal of Public Health Medicine*, 16 (1), 1–3.

Pearson, V. A. H., Carr, R. J. & Pouse, A. (1993). Public health medicine training. *Medical Education* 27 (2), 274–279.

Peckham, M. (1991). Research and development for the National Health Service. *Lancet*, 338, 367–371.

Pederson, A., O'Neill, M. & Rootman, I. (1994). *Health Promotion in Canada: Provincial, National and International Perspectives*. Toronto: W. B. Saunders.

Rachlis, M. & Kushner, C. (1994). *Strong Medicine: How to Save Canada's Health Care System*. Toronto: HarperCollins Publishers.

Schieber, G. J., Poullier, J. P. & Greenwald, L. M. (1993). Health spending, delivery, and outcomes in OECD countries. *Health Affairs*, 12, 120–129.

Schwartz, F. W. & Badura, B. (Eds.). (1991). *Public Health*. Berlin: Springer Verlag.

Shortell, S. (1988). The evolution of hospital systems: Unfulfilled promises and self-fulfilling prophecies. *Medical Care Review*, 45, 177–197.

Townsend, P., Davidson, N. & Whitehead, M. (1988). *Inequalities in Health. The Black Report and the Health Divide*. London: Penguin Books.

U.S. Department of Health and Human Services. (1980). *Promoting Health/Preventing Disease: Objectives for the Nation*. Washington, D.C.

U.S. Department of Health and Human Services. (1990). *Healthy People 2000. National Health Promotion and Disease Prevention Objectives*. Publication no. PHS 91–50212. Washington, D.C.

U.S. Department of Health, Education and Welfare. (1979). *Healthy People: Surgeon General's Report on Health Promotion and Disease Prevention*. Publication no. PHS 79–55071. Washington, D.C.

Watkins, S. J. (1994). Public health 2020. *British Medical Journal*, 309 (1962), 1147–1149.

WHO/EURO. (1994). *Training and Research in Public Health. Copenhagen:* WHO.

Winett, R. A., King, H. C. & Altman, G. D. (1989). *Health Psychology and Public Health.* New York: Pergamon.

World Bank. (1993). *Investing in Health. World Development Report.* Washington, D.C.: World Bank.

World Health Organization. (1980). *Classification of Impairments, Disabilities and Handicaps.* Geneva: WHO.

INDEX

ABOUT THE EDITORS AND CONTRIBUTORS

EDITORS

Klaus Hurrelmann is professor of sociology and public health at the University of Bielefeld and director of the Research Center on Prevention and Intervention in Childhood and Adolescence in Germany. He is presently dean of the Bielefeld School of Public Health.

Ulrich Laaser is professor of epidemiology and social medicine at the University of Bielefeld and director of the Institute of Population Research and Social Policy. He was the president of the Association of Schools of Public Health in the European Region (ASPHER) from 1993 to 1995.

CONTRIBUTORS

ABDELMONEM A. AFIFI is professor at the School of Public Health, Center for Health Sciences, University of California, Los Angeles, California, USA.

MARTIN ALILIO is research fellow at the National Institute for Medical Research, Dar es Salaam, Tanzania.

JANE C. BALTAZAR is professor at the College of Public Health, University of the Philippines, Manila, Philippines.

CHRISTOPHER BIRT is research fellow at the Health Services Management Centre, Birmingham University, Park House, Birmingham, United Kingdom.

LESTER BRESLOW is professor at the School of Public Health, Center for Health Sciences, University of California, Los Angeles, California, USA.

E. RICHARD BROWN is professor at the School of Public Health, Center for Health Sciences, University of California, Los Angeles, California, USA.

JACQUES BURY, M.D., is director at the World Health Organisation, Office of Europe, Copenhagen, Denmark.

G. DENNIS CALVERT is professor at the Medical Research Unit, University of Wollongong, Wollongong, New South Wales, Australia.

JOSÉ CARVALHO DE NORONHA is professor at the Universidade UERJ, Instituto de Medicina Social (IMS), Rio de Janeiro, Brazil.

FRANCO CAVALLO is professor at the Department of Hygiene and Community Medicine, University of Torino, Torino, Italy.

DAVID CHINITZ is research fellow at the School of Public Health, Hebrew University Hadassah, Jerusalem, Israel.

ROGER DETELS is professor at the Department of Epidemiology, School of Public Health, University of California, Los Angeles, California, USA.

D. PHILIPPE DUPRAT is professor at the Management Department, Ecole National de la Santé Publique (ENSP), Rennes, France.

LEON EPSTEIN is research fellow at the School of Public Health, Hebrew University Hadassah, Jerusalem, Israel.

GRACĪELA FREYERMUTH ENCĪSO is professor at the Centro de Investigaciones en Antropología Social, San Christóbal de las Casas, Chiapas, Mexico.

KEYOU GE is professor at the Chinese Academy of Preventive Medicine, Institute of Nutrition and Food Hygiene, Beijing, China.

ATSUAKI GUNJI is professor at the Department of Health Administration, Faculty of Medicine, University of Tokyo, Tokyo, Japan.

PALTI HAVA is research fellow at the School of Public Health, Hebrew University Hadassah, Jerusalem, Israel.

AXEL HOFFMANN-MARKWALD is research fellow at the Department of Medical Sociology, Albert-Ludwig Universität, Medizinische Fakultät, Freiburg, Germany.

WALTER W. HOLLAND is professor at the United Medical and Dental Schools, Department of Public Health Medicine, St. Thomas's Campus, London, United Kingdom.

CAREL B. IJSSELMUIDEN is professor at the School of Public Health, Medical University of Southern Africa (MEDUNSA), Pretoria, South Africa.

PETER KILIMA is research fellow at the National Institute for Medical Research, Dar es Salaam, Tanzania.

JONG-GYU KIM is research fellow at the Graduate School of Public Health, Seoul National University, Seoul, Korea.

YONG-WOOK LEE is research fellow at the Graduate School of Public Health, Seoul National University, Seoul, Korea.

EDUARDO LEVCOVITZ is research fellow at the Universidade UERJ, Instituto de Medicina Social (IMS), Rio de Janeiro, Brazil.

WAH-YUN LOW is research fellow at the Faculty of Medicine, University Malaya, Kuala Lumpur, Malaysia.

CYRIL PERVILHAC is research fellow at the National Institute for Medical Research, Dar es Salaam, Tanzania.

JAIME PAGE PLIEGO is research fellow at the Centro de Investigaciones en Antropología Social, San Cristóbal de las Casas, Chiapas, Mexico.

MONIKA PRZETAKIEWICZ-KOZIEJ is research fellow at the Institute of Oncology, Maria Sklodowska-Curie Memorial Cancer Center, Warsaw, Poland.

GIOVANNI RENGA is professor at the Department of Hygiene and Community Medicine, University of Torino, Torino, Italy.

EITAN F. SABATELLO is research fellow at the School of Public Health, Hebrew University Hadassah, Jerusalem, Israel.

ROBERT A. SPASOFF is professor at the Université d'Ottawa, Faculté de Medicine, Epidemiologie et Medicine Sociale, Ottawa, Ontario, Canada.

ULRICH STÖßEL is research fellow at the Department of Medical Sociology, Albert-Ludwig-Universität, Medizinische Fakultät, Freiburg, Germany.

SOMJIT SUPANNATAS is research fellow at the Faculty of Public Health, Mahidol University, Rajathvee, Bangkok, Thailand.

HEIZO TANAKA is professor at the Department of Epidemiology, Medical Research Institute, Tokyo Medical and Dental University, Tokyo, Japan.

VALERY E. TCHERNJAVSKY is professor at the Public Health Institute "MedSocEconInform," Ministry of Health of Russia, Moscow, Russia.

TEODORA V. TIGLAO is professor at the College of Public Health, University of the Philippines, Manila, Philippines.

JÜRGEN VON TROSCHKE is professor at the Department of Medical Sociology, Albert-Ludwig-Universität, Medizinische Fakultät, Freiburg, Germany.

XUDONG YANG is professor at the Chinese Academy of Preventive Medicine, Institute of Nutrition and Food Hygiene, Beijing, China.

KHAIRUDDIN YUSOF is professor at the Faculty of Medicine, University Malaya, Kuala Lumpur, Malaysia.

WITOLD ZATOÑSKI is professor at the Institute of Oncology, Maria Sklodowska-Curie Memorial Cancer Center, Warsaw, Poland.

SITI NORAZAH ZULKIFLI is research fellow at the Faculty of Medicine, University Malaya, Kuala Lumpur, Malaysia.

www.ingramcontent.com/pod-product-compliance
Ingram Content Group UK Ltd.
Pitfield, Milton Keynes, MK11 3LW, UK
UKHW020226290926
15470UKWH00001B/397

9 780313 295003